Reflexes, Movement, Learning & Behaviour

Endorsements

I am delighted with this new book from Sally Goddard, an authority and tireless advocate of the fundamental role of the early reflexes in learning. Her clear and concise explanations help demystify many of the behaviors and difficulties children exhibit during their development. Readers in search for ways to maximize the child abilities and facilitate school readiness will greatly benefit from Sally's insights and extensive experience.

This is a 'must read' book for parents, educators, and childcare professional interested in a 'bottom up' approach to learning and who view the child's wellbeing as key for optimizing their performance.

Paul Madaule
Founder of The Listening Centre, Toronto
Author of *When Listening Comes Alive*
(1993, updated e-book version 2015)

Provides a readable yet comprehensive overview of primitive and neonatal reflexes and postural control. These are holistically integrated into descriptions of human senses, neural structures and systems, along with their relevance for learning delays, disorders, and psychological conditions. Her expositions and recommendations draw on empirical-scientific analysis, many years of therapeutic experience, and a phenomenological-symptomology, offering readers from wide ranging backgrounds her unique theoretical and therapeutic insights into reflexes and learning.

Associate Professor Sebastian Suggate
University of York

If you view a learner as just a brain carried around by a body, it is rather like servicing a car engine without checking the brakes and tyres. That might be fine, but often you will waste fuel and occasionally you will crash. Sally is one of the leading experts in understanding how the body and mind work together, how to spot where there is a problem and then what to do about it. These issues are not simple, but they are important for thousands of children. Reflexes, Movement, Learning and Behaviour will give you a comprehensive resource to work with.

David Morgan
Creator of *The Easyread System* and *All Aboard Phonics*.

At a time when parents and professionals emphasise and analyse school readiness and learning yet children are the most sedentary in history, Sally Goddard Blythe has put the horse back before the cart. Physical literacy and movement have always been the poor cousin to proper cerebral learning, until now. This book provides an excellent comprehensive overview of this emerging area.

Dr Aric Sigman
Child health education lecturer, author of *Getting Physical*
Winner of *The Times* Educational Supplement's Information Book Award.

Every ounce of Sally Goddard Blythe's passion and commitment to her career-long quest to analyse and unblock neuro-motor immaturity is captured in this book. It is essential reading for anyone wanting the fullest picture of this important field.

Mike Boulton
Emeritus Professor of Child Psychology at the University of Chester.

Published by Hawthorn Press, Hawthorn House,
1 Lansdown Lane, Stroud, Gloucestershire, GL5 1BJ, UK
Tel: (01453) 757040
E-mail: info@hawthornpress.com
Website: www.hawthornpress.com

Cover design by Bruce Winslade
Typesetting by Winslade Graphics, Stroud, Gloucestershire, GL5 2AJ
Printed by Short Run Press Ltd, Exeter

Printed on paper sourced from sustained managed forests and elemental chlorine free.

British Library Cataloguing in Publication Data applied for.

ISBN 978-1-912480-78-4

Reflexes, Movement, Learning & Behaviour

Analysing & unblocking neuro-motor immaturity

Sally Goddard Blythe

Hawthorn Press

Dedicated to my grandchildren

Henry, William, Chloë, Harry, Jemima, Isabella and Evie

'The good teacher does not bid you enter the house of his wisdom, but rather leads you to the threshold of your own mind.'

***Kahlil Gibran**, The Prophet*

Contents

Appendices

Foreword

About two decades ago, I remember reading in a newspaper clipping complaints from teachers about how children entering school were unable to use a pair of scissors or draw properly, thereby showing inadequate physical readiness for school learning. The observation was fascinating, sparking in me the notion that movement was more linked to cognition and learning than I had previously encountered in my psychology degree. Around that time, during data collection in a school for my PhD in New Zealand, a teacher proceeded to zealously recount the work of a woman who had made a 'discovery' about movement reflexes. If I remember correctly, amongst descriptions of the importance of crossing the midline during crawling, such reflexes could fail to be inhibited in development resulting in later learning difficulties. Interesting. I proceeded to observe children in one class conducting various movement exercises, I believe with the purpose of, although my memory may be tricking me, integrating primary and postural reflexes. Although I am not 100 percent certain, I believe that this was my first encounter with the work of Sally Goddard-Blythe, about 15 years ago and 12,000 miles away.

At the time, I remember feeling a little sceptical, even smiling to myself inwardly in the shadow of the teacher's conviction – unfortunately with a touch of the usual condescension prone to the scientifically-trained, who have not yet learned that the questions in life are far more important than the answers. I thought that although the idea was certainly interesting, it seemed like a bit too much of a stretch to implicate reflexes in later learning, especially since we had covered primary and neonatal reflexes in developmental psychology courses and surely, were it true, the importance of these for learning would have been mentioned by the lecturer. As it happens, I have often looked back on this conversation, along with anecdotal reports of increasingly poor motor skills in children – and my doctoral findings that children who attend school earlier have no advantage later on in reading – as a significant turning point in my thinking. A seed was planted and I began, about ten years ago, to study motor processes in child development and learning. I quickly realised that this was a path seldom trodden, that much knowledge was spread across diverse disciplines encompassing medicine, psychology, sport science, occupational therapy and special education. No one seemed to have developed the necessary oversight across these disciplines, drawing together what threads existed, and combining this with practical knowledge to be able to work effectively with these ideas. Or so I thought.

> Nothing is in the mind that wasn't previously in the senses... except for the mind itself.
>
> *G. W. Leibniz*

There has been longstanding interest in how physical development imprisons, shapes, and liberates the mind. It is said that the Ancient Greeks saw the importance in cultivating both the mind and the body as a high form of education, art and culture. However, recent times have seen a carving up of the human being into two supposedly separate domains, the physical and the mental. Thus, many educators and therapists, philosophers and scientists, often avoid examining the physical body and sensorimotor system as a potential cause of learning difficulties.

Arguably, the roots for this great separation are to be found in science and philosophy, with its dichotomy of 'two worlds', an inner subjective 'rational' and an outer observable 'empirical' world. In this inner subjective and rational world, abstract thought dominates and in the outer empirically observable world, many have felt comfortable trusting only what can be seen with the physical senses giving rise to great philosophical debates (e.g. Cartesian dualism, parallelism, monism, fatalism). Separating human experience so clearly and firmly into body and mind is philosophically problematic, with detrimental consequences educationally and therapeutically. However, instead of relying solely on philosophical arguments and speculation, careful observation and study of both physical and mental sides of human existence is called for, as Goddard Blythe illustrates in this book.

Perhaps one reason why physical development is often overlooked is that much of human sensorimotor development occurs early and unconsciously, starting in utero and takes enormous strides in early childhood. Without doubt, most adults can no longer recall what an effort it was to learn to crawl, build block towers, ride a bicycle, write, or even type, despite the latter occurring in adolescence for most of us. Further, I have yet to meet an adult who remembers grappling with and inhibiting innate reflexes in childhood. The result is that adults forget just how much of the mental world is shaped and governed by the development of our physical apparatus, which requires fine tuning and integration of the senses and mastery of the fine and gross motor systems.

In the context of education there is a great danger that overlooking physical development results in educational approaches that can overly stimulate abstract thinking before the sensorimotor foundations of thought have properly developed. With this in mind, there is reason to question how appropriate it is to introduce young children into the abstract modes of thought inherent in reading, writing, arithmetic and reasoning too early. Each of these processes rests on sensorimotor foundations; reading on visual and auditory processing and learning abstract letter-sound associations; writing on great sensorimotor control; arithmetic on internalised spatial relations, and reasoning on intuitive physics derived from the external world. Thus, many approaches, such as the Steiner-Waldorf approach which inspired our book *Reclaim Early Childhood* (2019), focus instead on gently nurturing the senses, allowing these to unfold and integrate gently with mental development. Accordingly, the current book is without doubt significant for those working in early childhood settings.

How then do we best treat children exhibiting learning difficulties? There is good reason to suggest that children should be given time and allowed to practise in order to develop motor control, process sensory input, and as argued in this book, regulate and inhibit physical reflexes. Disruption of the regulatory systems is known to play a role in dyslexia and attention-deficit hyperactivity disorder, for instance. Such regulatory systems are also, in part, central to motor control. Difficulties processing sensory input are common to developmental (e.g. autism) and psychological (e.g. conduct, anxiety) disorders. The author goes further, drawing detailed links between arousal and adrenal systems and various disturbances – ideas and therapeutical notions that many practitioners now trained by Goddard Blythe and her colleagues swear by, yet many scientists have yet to study seriously.

Although not focusing specifically on reflexes, in recent decades research on integrative paradigms on links between sensorimotor and cognitive processes has exploded. The terms embodied or grounded cognition are no longer peripheral phenomena but are developing into comprehensive models supplementing or challenging 'centrist' cognitive psychological models. Such centrist models maintain that cognition is independent of the senses, much like a computer with the printer being the limbs, the camera the eyes, and the thinking done in the CPU. In reality, the brain cannot be studied separately from the senses, sensorimotor systems, and the broader environment (e.g. through gravity, stimuli). Areas of the brain that were previously thought to be involved in movement only (e.g. cerebellum, primary motor cortex) have now been shown to be involved in language and thought. Researchers in these fields, such as myself, will certainly receive much food for thought after reading this book!

Importantly, the senses themselves are becoming better understood and in a more nuanced way than previously, a phenomenon which is also integrated into Goddard Blythe's framework. Although vision research still dominates the other senses, it is generally acknowledged that there are between seven and nine senses in total, each of which needs to be integrated during development. Depending on how you categorise the senses, these include vision, hearing, smelling, tasting, touching, balancing, and proprioception (body movement and position in space). Understanding the different senses in interplay with reflexes, as the author describes, provides insight into how reflexes can shield or expose the organism to excessive external input.

As Goddard Blythe points out comprehensively in this book, fine motor skills require a complicated integration of senses, built on the regulation of innate reflexes, to prosper. In my own work with my colleagues, we have found in many empirical studies that children's fine motor skills are linked to their language, reading, writing, mathematic, and cognitive development. Thus, fine motor skills are not only important enablers of learning, they also indicate that the body has attained a sufficient degree of maturity and mastery over itself, thereby providing a foundation of learning and development. This is also a key tenet of Goddard Blythe's thesis.

However, what is particularly unique about the current book, is the broad and detailed integration of numerous findings and insights into a broad therapeutical approach. Goddard Blythe provides a detailed overview of the primary reflexes, including tests for the existence and integration of these. She integrates this work into descriptions of relevant neural structures and systems, providing informative and clearly articulated depictions of neural anatomy. Further, she delineates relevant sensory and motor systems and relates reflexes to a number of common learning delays, disorders, and psychological conditions. Her expositions and recommendations are founded on a mixture of empirical-scientific analysis, many years of therapeutical experience, and a phenomenological-symptomology, providing readers from a wide range of backgrounds with unique theoretical and therapeutic insight.

Sebastian P. Suggate PhD

University of York and University of Regensburg
October 2022

Acknowledgements

Catharina Johannesson Alvegård, who first developed this work in Sweden.

Dr Kjeld Johansen for his tireless work on understanding the role of audition and auditory processing in the presentation of dyslexia, and in developing the method now known as Johansen Individualised Auditory Stimulation Therapy (JIAST).

Professor Birger Kaada at the University of Stavanger, whose work on the Fear Paralysis Response provided a vital link, and **Ernest Keeling**, who first introduced the Institute for Neuro-Physiological Psychology (INPP) to the fear paralysis response.

To students who over the years have practised and developed this work further.

To all international principals of INPP who have gone on to provide training to others through the INPP international network of trainers, tirelessly translating materials and continuing to provide an international standard of training in the INPP method.

To teachers who have implemented the INPP developmental movement programme in schools and provided reports and data on the incidence of neuromotor immaturity in children in mainstream schools and on the efficacy of the programme.

To many, many other people whose work behind the scenes, discussion, argument and ideas have contributed to the development of the INPP method.

To my children, **James, Thomas and Gabriella**, who allowed me to grow up a second time with them.

Most of all, to my beloved late husband Peter, who introduced me to all the knowledge contained in this book, encouraged me to follow what I saw in the face of scepticism and criticism and who always believed that behind every failure or emotional disorder there is a reason.

> *It is our sincere hope that as a result of what has been accomplished, many children and adults who have previously been unresponsive to educational and medical remediation will now have the opportunity to emerge from the shadows in which they have been surviving.*
>
> ***Peter Blythe*** *and* ***David McGlown****, 1979*

Introduction

Despite years of educational theory and knowledge of child development, modern education tends to view children's educational progress through the wrong end of the telescope, measuring success by performance rather than ability, and outcomes instead of processes.

Learning takes place best when new information meets a child where they are in terms of their current understanding or ability, and the ground on which the seeds of learning are scattered is fertile and prepared. Physical development is crucial in this preparation process, since experience and opportunity for maturation provide the foundations for later learning success.

This interrelationship between environment and well-being was described in a different context by the pathologist Rudolf Virchow (1949) when he said that malaria could not be blamed solely on the malaria-carrying mosquito, since the mosquito could proliferate because the swamp was there. In other words, the terrain is everything.

Terrain was described from another perspective by Ray Barsch in a series of books he wrote on motor perceptual efficiency in the 1960s, in which he described the young child as being a 'terranaut', or explorer of space on terra firma (see 1968). It was his belief that one of the first skills a child needs to learn is to become master or mistress of their own body in space – to achieve competence and confidence in standing and moving in a gravity-based environment. This physical competence provides the apparatus with which to explore the unknown, become cognisant with the known, feel secure in the physical self and integrate sensory experience with new experience.

Today, such theories fit into new terms such as 'physical literacy' and 'embodied cognition', but labels have a tendency to limit the scope of processes.

Physical development is a lifelong process which goes through its most prodigious period of education in the first years of life, but which continues to influence every aspect of experience, emotions and understanding for the remainder of one's life.

Parents are usually the first to recognise when a child has a problem; they will sense that 'there is something different about my child'. Early signs may include being difficult to settle, prone to tantrums, either slightly late in achieving or simply omitting some developmental milestones such as crawling, learning to walk and/or learning to talk. These early signs may be so subtle or marginal that they are overlooked and the child seems to catch up at a later stage or parents are told not to worry, that the child 'will simply grow out of it'. Other children may be referred for further investigations or therapy such as speech and language therapy (SALT) or occupational therapy (OT), or it may be suggested the parents need help in improving their child management skills.

Although it is certainly true that many children do grow out of early problems and there are many individual variations in the recognised parameters of development, there also exists a group of children who to all outward appearances are developing normally but who are immature in other aspects of their development. If these immaturities persist, they will be at risk of experiencing a range of learning and behaviour difficulties at various stages in their lives.

Research in the area of neural plasticity has shown us that the wiring of the central nervous system is open to change, particularly in its phases of most rapid growth or maturation, and that this rewiring has a profound impact upon a child's ability to interact effectively with both their social and physical environment. Galaburda (2001) suggests that problems can arise from two levels in the brain: higher- and lower-order processing. Although it is generally accepted that during the process of maturation higher centres in the brain should take increasing control and direction over lower centres, the persistence of lower-level involvement in certain functions will also influence functioning, learning and behaviour.

Most education and many remedial techniques aim to teach higher centres in the brain. A neurodevelopmental approach identifies the lowest level of dysfunction and targets therapy at that area – starting from the point where the child is and building connections upwards from there. This was described by one of my students in his exams as being a 'bottom-up' as opposed to a 'top-down' approach to tackling specific learning difficulties.

All learning takes place in the brain; the body acts as receptor for information and then becomes the vehicle through which knowledge is expressed. In this respect, movement lies at the heart of learning. Learning, language and behaviour are all linked in some way to the function of the motor system and control of movement. Before children learn to talk, they communicate through gesture, alteration in posture, rhythm of movement, and pitch, volume and tone of voice. These are the non-verbal aspects of language which both precede spoken language and also contribute up to 90 per cent of effective communication in supporting verbal language.

Speech as a skill is dependent upon the motor system for the combination of movements involved in coordinating the larynx, the pharynx, the tongue and the muscles at the front of the mouth. Reading depends largely on oculo-motor skill involving precise eye movements, and writing involves hand–eye coordination with the support of the postural system. Most academic learning depends on basic skills becoming automatic at the physical level. If a child fails to develop automatic control over balance and motor skills, many other aspects of learning can be affected negatively, even though the child has average or above average intelligence.

Control of the body also lays the foundation for self-control. Immaturity in the functioning of the nervous system is often accompanied by signs of emotional immaturity such as poor impulse control, difficulty in reading the body language of others (social cues), and unsatisfactory peer relationships. One parent described his child as being 'ten years old on the outside and three years old on the inside'. No amount of behaviour modification made a difference to his son's emotional behaviour until the underlying problem of neuromotor immaturity had been addressed.

Making the child fit the system…

When children first enter formal school (in the UK at rising five years of age), it is generally assumed that they will be able to sit still, pay attention, hold a writing implement and get their eyes to make the movements necessary to follow along a line of print. Many children do acquire these skills without difficulty; others take longer because they enter the school system at a definite disadvantage in terms of their neurological development and therefore lack the necessary physical abilities to succeed. In the higher grades these children run the risk of experiencing what are labelled specific learning difficulties, not because they lack intelligence, but because the basic systems fundamental to learning were not fully in place at the time they started school. Attention, balance and coordination are the primary A, B and C upon which all later academic learning depends.

The concept of maturational readiness for learning is not new. As early as 1947, it was noted that reading readiness seemed to coincide with the shedding of the first milk teeth and that individual variation in the timing of the eruption of the second tooth might be indicative of other aspects of neurological maturity related to reading readiness (Ames 1967). In 1999, Bax and Whitmore investigated whether it would be of value to include a short test battery of neurodevelopmental tests in school entrant medical examinations (cited in Whitmore et al. 1999). They found that there were significant links between neurological maturity and performance on cognitive psychological tests. Despite an increasing body of evidence to support the value of neurodevelopmental milestones at the time of school entry, these tests have still not been integrated into standard school pre-assessment. Chronological age alone still remains the criterion on which we allow a child to enter school.

Such a blanket approach to starting a child's formal education can adversely affect at least two groups: those children whose birthdays fall in the summer and who are therefore up to twelve months younger than some of their peers, and those children who are delayed in certain aspects of development related to the automatic control of balance and coordination and who therefore lack the ability to focus and sustain attention. The former can benefit from delaying the time of school entry by several months and thus allowing the child to enter as one of the older children in the next year's group. Those who have not yet achieved certain developmental milestones would benefit from an extended period of a more informal curriculum that included activities to foster physical and sensory development.

In what was then Czechoslovakia, two simple tests were used to assess school readiness: Could the child draw a circle in both a clockwise and anticlockwise direction? (This basic movement is involved in forming letters when writing.) And could the child touch one ear with the opposite hand and repeat this on the other side? (This shows whether a child is able to cross the midline of the body – a skill needed for the acts of reading and writing.)

Independent research has found similar connections between control of automatic balance and later learning abilities, and a number of tests such as the 'wobble test' (Nicolson and Fawcett 1994) and the 'one leg stand' (Schrager 2001) have been incorporated into more extensive test batteries to identify children who have, or are at risk of having, dyslexia and other specific learning disabilities. Although these tests provide indications of what is wrong, they do not tell us why one child has gained a degree of control over balance and coordination and another child has not.

It is the purpose of this book to provide not only the why, but also to suggest how to identify the child at risk and overcome the obstacles that keep children from succeeding in school and in life. ■

Chapter 1

Primitive Reflexes: Their Influence on Life and Learning

What are primitive reflexes?

Before birth, the developing foetus is largely protected from external sensory stimuli. They feel the motion and sounds of the mother's body, the chemical changes that take place in her body in response to what she eats and drinks, to stress and to pleasure. From about the 24th week after conception, the foetus responds to some external sounds, but even these are experienced within a narrower range of frequencies than in the outside world. All of this changes at birth. In addition to light, sound, temperature, touch and smell, for the first time, the newborn encounters the full force of gravity and must develop postural control and muscle tone to counteract it.

In the first days and weeks of life, the neonate does not understand these new sensations. If they are too strong or sudden, the baby will react to them, but they do not have conscious control over their own reaction, nor do they understand the feelings that those reactions engender. This is the stuff on which later emotional development will be built. The baby's first tasks are to learn to breathe, to feed, to seek fulfilment of their own needs and to learn to use their body to help themself. Mastery of their own body in space is the very first stepping stone to independence.

The infant is supported in the first months of life with a set of primitive reflexes designed to ensure immediate response to this new environment and to changing needs. Primitive reflexes are automatic, stereotyped movements, directed from the brainstem and executed without cortical involvement. In addition to aiding survival in the first few weeks of life, they also provide rudimentary mechanisms for training many later voluntary skills, but their active presence is time sensitive and, having seen the infant through the first weeks and months of life, they should be inhibited by higher centres in the developing brain as neural pathways are formed. This occurs through a dual process of maturation (hardwired into the developing nervous system at birth) and experience (the environmental software) through which the nervous system learns to adapt.

The primitive reflexes, however, should have only a limited lifespan and, having helped the baby to survive the first hazardous months of life, they should be inhibited or controlled by higher centres of the brain. This allows the development of the more sophisticated neural structures involved in the control of voluntary action and response.

If the primitive reflexes remain active after six months of age, they are said to be 'aberrant'; they are evidence of a structural weakness or immaturity within the central nervous system. As primitive reflexes are inhibited in the first six months of life, some become integrated into more mature patterns of response while others are replaced by more mature postural reflexes or reactions.

Primitive reflexes are not eliminated but become redundant and are put to sleep in the brainstem only to be reawakened if there is damage to, or insufficiency in functioning of, higher brain centres or systems. This can occur in later life as a result of degenerative and demyelination diseases such as Alzheimer's disease, multiple sclerosis, or brain damage following a stroke or head injury. If damage has occurred at or around the time of birth, such as in cerebral palsy (CP), primitive reflexes remain active and provide diagnostic signs of CP. These examples, where there is a pathological reason for the retention of primitive reflexes, are well recognised in the medical profession.

Less recognised is the fact that primitive reflexes can persist beyond infancy in the absence of identified pathology. In these cases, the reflex is not necessarily retained at full strength under all testing conditions and may vary according to the position from which it is assessed. One or more reflexes may remain in this lesser form, providing evidence of immaturity in the functioning of the central nervous system, interfering with specific functions and affecting performance of higher skills that are either dependent on or involve postural and motor systems.

Primitive reflex activity that is evident beyond the first six months of life can also impact on the development of the succeeding postural reflexes. Postural reflexes, sometimes described as 'postural reactions', develop from birth and take up to three-and-a-half years of age to be fully developed. They provide a basis for subconscious control of posture, balance and coordination in a gravity-based environment, enabling a child to maintain control of posture and change their position without the need for conscious thought.

When a cluster of primitive reflexes and/or underdeveloped postural reactions exist beyond three-and-a-half years of age, these reflexes are described as 'aberrant'; they are indicative of immaturity in the functioning of the central nervous system. Currently, school-aged children as well as adults who fit this profile constitute a 'grey area' on the periphery of a number of professional domains. This may be because the presenting signs and symptoms are not quite 'bad enough' to receive a medical diagnosis, but these individuals will not have acquired all of the tools they need to cope with the demands of the environment. A discrepancy will arise between innate ability and achievement, not only educational attainment but also aspects of emotional regulation. One parent described his child as 'having an infant attitude still active within a ten-year-old's body.' This was despite the child having been assessed as having above average intelligence. Often, the higher the level of intelligence, the greater the frustration, hence the emergence of secondary behavioural problems in childhood and emotional issues in adult life.

Neonatal reflexes

Although reflex actions are complex, most reflexes can be simplified into four basic steps:

- A stimulus is received by nerve endings involving one of the senses: balance, proprioception (interoreceptor systems), taste, sense, sight, smell, hearing or touch (exteroreceptor systems).
- Energy created by the stimulus is conducted through the nerves to the central nervous system.
- Impulses generated by the stimulus are transmitted to the nerves that stimulate muscle action.
- Finally, the muscles, and sometimes certain glands, respond with an action.

Any variation in or absence of response at key stages in development may be a sign of immaturity in the pathways involved. This may be described as a sign of 'neuromotor immaturity' (NMI).

Depending on the degree of aberrant reflex activity, this poor organisation of nerve fibres can affect one or all areas of functioning: not only gross muscle and fine muscle coordination, but also sensory perception, cognition and avenues of expression.

Emergence and inhibition

Primitive reflexes emerge in utero, are present at birth of a baby born at full term (40 weeks' gestation) and should be inhibited by six months of age – or 12 months at the latest. Some primitive reflexes may not be fully developed at the time of birth in infants who are born prematurely, depending on the gestational age of the neonate.

In normal development, inhibition of a reflex frequently correlates with the acquisition of a new skill, and hence knowledge of reflex chronology and normal child development may be combined to predict which later skills may be impaired as a direct result of retained primitive reflexes. In much the same way that the parent used the analogy of an infant remaining active in a schoolboy's body, it may be said that an individual's aberrant reflexes can give us clues as to what is hindering later skills.

Detection of primitive reflexes can help to isolate some of the underlying mechanical causes of a child's problem so that remedial training can be targeted more effectively. If the reflex profile is only marginally abnormal, teaching strategies alone will usually be sufficient. Children with a moderate degree of reflex immaturity may benefit from a combination of specialised teaching and some motor training designed to improve balance and coordination. If, however, a cluster of aberrant reflexes are present they provide evidence of NMI. In such cases, long-term improvement is only likely to be sustained after they child has undergone a reflex stimulation/inhibition programme designed specifically to treat their aberrant reflex profile (Figure 1.1).

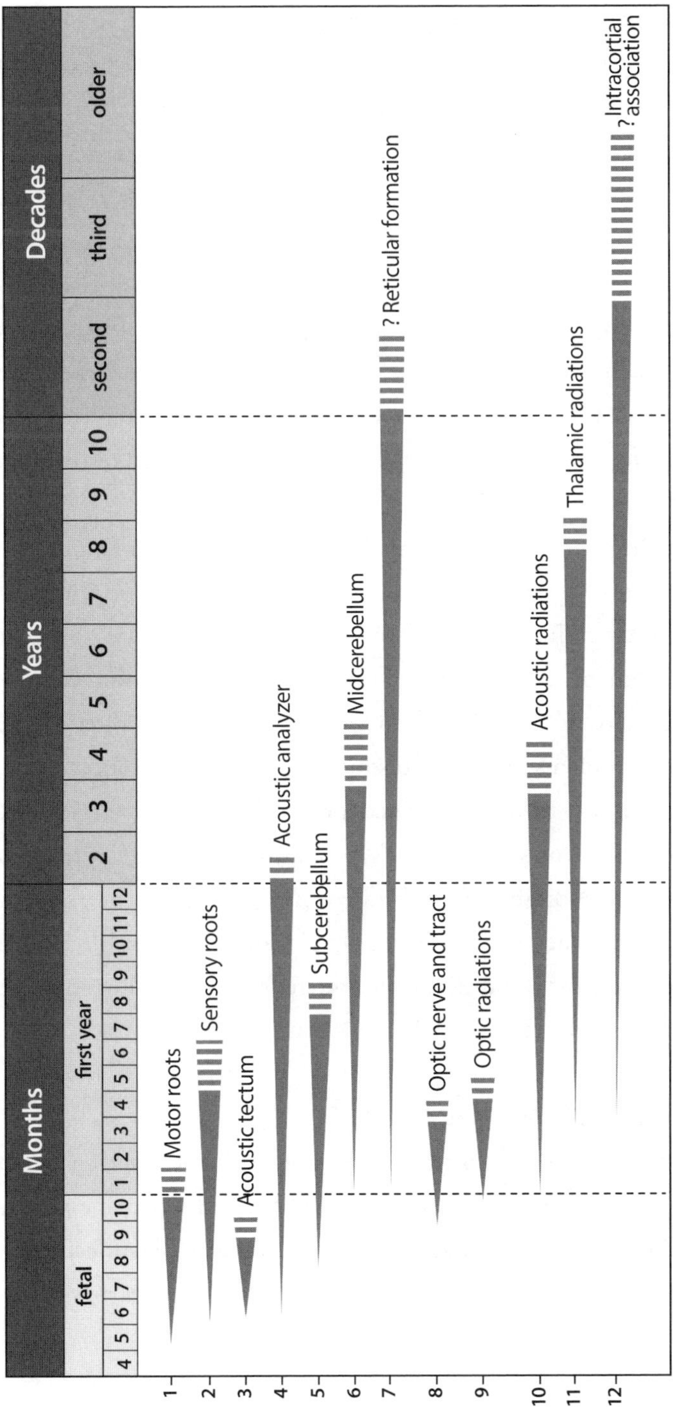

Figure 1.1: Periods of intensive myelination in different neural systems from before birth to beyond the third decade of life.

Reflex stimulation and inhibition programmes

A reflex stimulation/inhibition programme consists of specific physical, stereotyped movements practised for approximately five to ten minutes per day over a period of nine to twelve months. The movements are based upon a detailed knowledge of reflex chronology and normal child development. Thelan (1979) observed that all human babies make a series of stereotyped movements during their first year of life. The Institute for Neuro-Physiological Psychology (INPP) maintains that specific movement patterns made instinctively in the first months of life contain within them a natural inhibitor/integrator of the reflexes, and that these movements can be harnessed and replicated a second time if stages of movement development were either omitted or disorganised in the first year of life.

Through the application of stylised sequential movements, practised daily, it is possible to give the brain a second chance to register the reflex inhibitory movement patterns that should have been accomplished at the appropriate stage in development – an example of the body training the nervous system. As aberrant reflex activity is modified, many of the presenting physical, academic and emotional problems of the child start to go into remission.

Here, it is useful to mention anecdotally that as children's reflex profile improves over the course of a year's programme, parents often forget the reasons why they brought their child for assessment in the first place and are surprised when they are reminded several months later of the presenting symptoms, gross motor coordination and reflex and oculo-motor profile at the time of assessment (Figure 1.2).

What do primitive reflexes do?

Each reflex has a vital part to play in setting the stage for later functioning. In order to understand what goes wrong when reflexes become aberrant, it is important to realise the role that individual reflexes perform at the time their presence is normal. To do this, we need to return to the earliest weeks of an embryo's life – just five weeks after conception.[1]

At five-and-a-half to seven weeks, the embryo starts to show signs of response

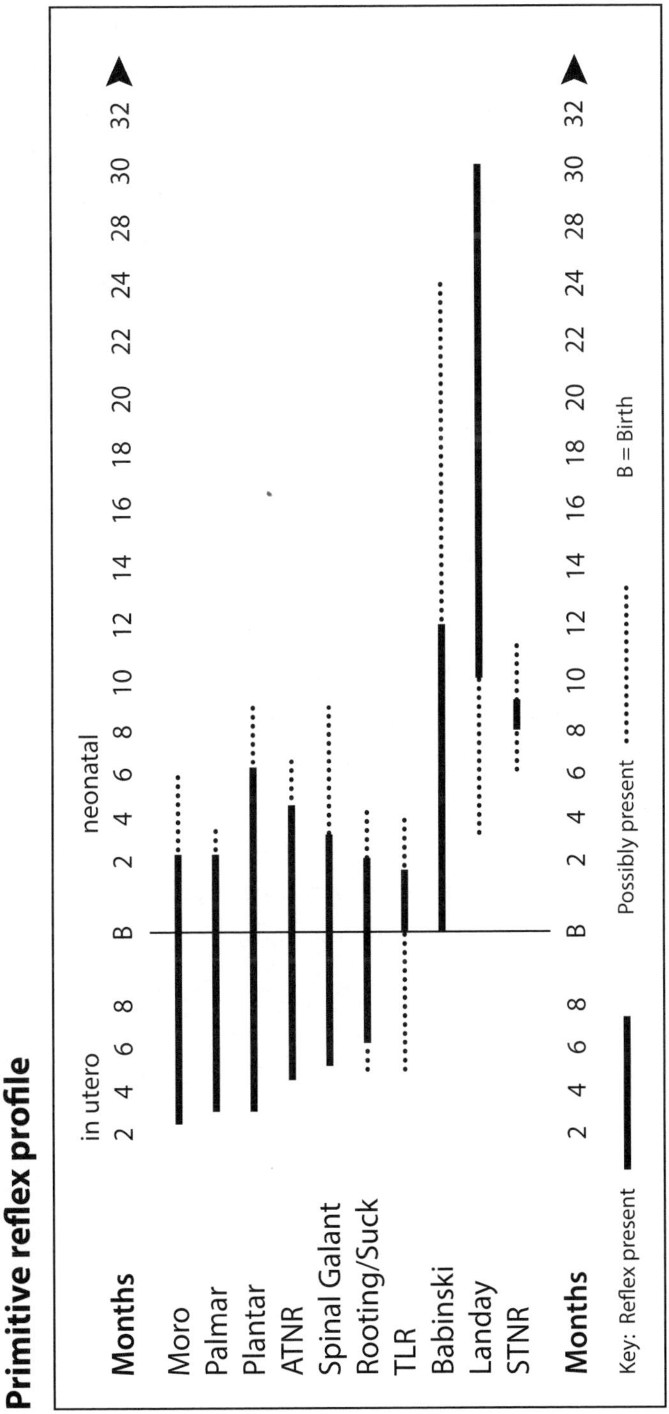

Figure 1.2. Primitive reflex profile – periods of activity in normal development.

to external stimuli. Gentle touch to the upper lip will cause the embryo to withdraw immediately from the stimulus – in an amoebic-like response. Only a few days later, this area of sensitivity will be spread to include the palms of the hands and the soles of the feet, until eventually the entire body surface is responsive to touch. At this stage, however, the response is always one of withdrawal from the source of contact and is a total body reaction. As tactile responses develop, withdrawal upon contact gradually diminishes.

Moro reflex

Emerges:	9 weeks in utero
Developed:	32 weeks in utero
Birth:	fully present
Inhibited:	2–4 months of life

As withdrawal responses are maturing, at circa nine weeks in utero, the first of the primitive reflexes – the Moro reflex – emerges. The earliest signs of the Moro reflex appear at 9–12 weeks post-conception (p.c.); it continues to develop up to 32 weeks p.c. so that the reflex will be fully present at birth in an infant born at full term (Figure 1.3).

The Moro reflex is a composite series of rapid movements made in response to sudden stimuli. It consists of a sudden symmetrical movement of the arms upward and outwards (abduction) from the body, with opening of the hands,

Figure 1.3: Moro reflex

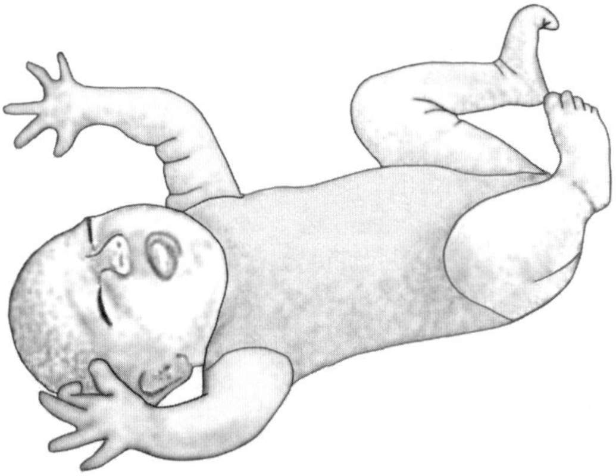

momentary freezing and then a gradual return of the arms across the body (adduction) into a clasping posture. The abduction is accompanied by a sudden intake of breath. Adduction facilitates the release of that breath (Figure 1.3).

In 1918, Moro emphasised his belief that this is essentially a 'grasping' reflex, analogous to the one seen in young apes, who instinctively cling to their mothers. He called it *Umklammerungsreflex*, which means 'clasping reflex'.

The Moro reflex is an involuntary reaction to a sudden unexpected stimulus. The baby cannot yet analyse incoming sensation to assess whether or not it indicates a threat. The brainstem releases the Moro reflex as if an emergency switch is tripped automatically; it acts as the earliest form of fight or flight response. It may be elicited occasionally in later life in situations of extreme danger. Essentially, however, it should be inhibited in its crude form between two and four months of age, to be replaced by an adult startle reflex or Strauss reflex.

Its role as a survival mechanism in the first months of life is to alert, to arouse and to summon assistance. It is also thought to play a part in supporting the development of the baby's breathing mechanism in utero, coinciding with the earliest 'practice' breathing-like movements observed in the womb. It can act as a secondary mechanism to facilitate the first breath of life at birth if breathing has not started naturally as a result of the normal physiological changes that occur at birth (compression of the lungs during passage down the birth canal, mild hypoxia and altered sensory stimulation) and it helps to open the airway if there is a threat of suffocation.

If the Moro reflex fails to be inhibited between two and four months of life, the child may continue to have an exaggerated startle reaction, which can result in hypersensitivity in one or several sensory channels, giving rise to overreaction to certain stimuli. Sudden noise, light, movement, change of temperature or alteration of position or balance – any of these may elicit the reflex at unexpected moments, increasing reactivity, and the experience of uncomfortable or distressing feelings and sensations, and leading to hypervigilance.

As a fight or flight reaction, activation of the Moro reflex releases hormones associated with fight or flight into the system – the stress hormones. These same hormones increase arousal and influence thresholds of sensitivity and reactivity so that both the trigger and the response are built into the system. Such a child may present a paradox: acutely sensitive, perceptive and imaginative, on the one hand, but immature and overreactive, on the other. They may learn to cope in one of two ways: by being the fearful child who 'withdraws' from situations, has difficulty in socialising and can neither accept nor demonstrate physical affection easily. On the other hand, they may become the overactive, aggressive child who is highly excitable, cannot read body language and needs to dominate situations. Either child will tend to be manipulative as they attempt to find strategies that give them some measure of control over their own reactions, physical sensations and emotional fallout.

Adrenaline and cortisol are two of the body's chief defences against allergy and infection. If heightened levels of arousal and reactivity are a recurring theme, these hormones may be diverted from their primary function, depleting stores that should normally be available to support immune response and a regulated response to potential allergens, thereby reducing natural resistance to infections and increasing inflammatory responses.

A child with a residual Moro reflex may be the child who has a history of recurrent infections in the pre-school and first school years, and repeated need for antibiotics, and who is sensitive to certain foods or food additives, which in turn can affect behaviour and concentration.

Overreactive inflammatory responses can be linked to imbalance in the biodiversity and neurotransmitters present in the gut. Neurotransmitters are chemical substances responsible for sending messages from one neuron to the next, and all neurotransmitters used as chemical messengers by the nervous system are present in the gut. Michael Gershon, in *The Second Brain*, describes how nerves talk with a chemical language and the gut is an independent site of neural integration and processing. 'The enteric nervous system is thus not a slave of the brain but a contrarian, independent spirit in the nervous organisation of the body.' From this alone, it can be seen that rarely is there a single cause of presenting symptoms linked to immaturity in the functioning of the central nervous system; rather, dysregulation in one system can have a spreading and profound influence on the functioning of the whole. A retained Moro reflex is not necessarily the primary cause of any of the above. Rather, it can act or react to existing dysfunction or dysregulation in other systems.

A child who is hypersensitive or stimulus bound in one or several sensory channels and whose system is prone to overarousal pays attention to too many things at the expense of being able to focus on salient stimuli. This scattering of response and attention is energy inefficient and in biochemical terms is rather like turning on every light in the house to read a book in one room. It can result in a child who metabolises blood sugar more rapidly than other children, which will contribute to swings in mood (meltdowns). Svea Gold describes this in *If Kids Just Came With Instruction Sheets*:

> When the child's cortex gets this overload, it sends messages to the adrenal gland and the pituitary. Now the glands have no perception of danger of their own. They can't tell us if it is a real emergency or not. All they can know is that they got a signal to squirt out their chemicals. It's the same as if there were a tiger out there somewhere, and the body had to get ready to fight. So each time, when they get the signal, the adrenals squirt out adrenaline and cortisol. Pretty soon the adrenals get exhausted. As the adrenals get exhausted, allergies start to show up along with psychosomatic illnesses, headaches and migraines, colitis, ulcers and high blood pressure. This is the basis for psychosomatic medicine. (Gold 1998)

Extreme effects of low blood sugar are well known in patients who have insulin-dependent diabetes and for whom it is crucial to maintain a balance between glucose-producing nutrition and insulin. In the case of diabetes, if the balance goes wrong and insulin levels in the body become too high then blood sugar can rapidly drop to dangerous levels – a hypoglycaemic episode. In extreme cases, this can result in coma and death, but at the point that blood glucose levels start to fall below the normal margin, concentration declines and anxiety, agitation and aggression all increase as cortical control recedes. This is because glucose is vital to the functioning of the cortex. Regulation of blood sugar levels can be erratic in some children and the resulting behavioural symptoms that can be seen are similar to those described above.

There can be many reasons for poor regulation of blood glucose (a diet high in sugars and refined carbohydrates can contribute). Again, the Moro reflex is not the cause, but if the threshold to elicited the reflex is too low it may be one factor, or, conversely, it may be a temporary symptom of dysregulation in blood sugar levels.

The child who still has a Moro reflex will tend to experience the world as being too full of bright, loud and abrasive sensory stimuli. The eyes will tend to be drawn towards changes in light and to movement on the periphery of the visual field. They may have difficulty filtering auditory stimuli, occluding background noise or protecting themself from loud sounds. They are, in effect, 'stimulus bound' in much the same way, but to a lesser degree, as an infant is naturally stimulus bound in the first months of life.

One example of this can be seen in the first two to four months of life. At the time when the Moro reflex is active, it is normal for an infant's visual attention to be drawn to the outside edges of shape and form and to sudden movement or change of light on the periphery of vision. However, if this continues, the child will have difficulty ignoring peripheral visual stimuli and maintaining visual attention on the centre. This can contribute to visual distractibility in the older child.

Arnheim (1969) describes how this affects information processing: 'Too many impressions which arrive from several sensory sources and which fall simultaneously on a mind which has not yet experienced them separately, will fuse for that mind into a single undivided object.'

What, then, are the symptoms that a parent or a teacher might recognise as suggestive of a strongly residual or retained Moro reflex? (Please note that the following lists do not comprise inevitable consequences of a retained Moro reflex.)

Triggers to the Moro reflex:

- sudden, unexpected occurrence of any kind
- stimulation of the labyrinth by change in head position (vestibular)
- noise (auditory)
- sudden movement or change of light in the visual field (visual)
- pain, temperature change, or being handled too roughly (tactile)

Physical response to the Moro reflex:

- instantaneous arousal
- rapid inhalation, momentary 'freeze' or 'startle', followed by expiration, often accompanied by a cry
- activation of fight or flight response, which automatically alerts the sympathetic nervous system and results in:
  - release of adrenaline and cortisol into the system (the stress hormones)
  - increase in the rate of breathing, particularly in the apices (upper lobes) of the lungs (hyperventilation)
  - increase in heart rate
  - rise in blood pressure
  - reddening of the skin
- possible outburst, e.g. anger or tears

Possible long-term response:

- poorly developed CO_2 reflex

The CO_2 (carbon dioxide) reflex causes spontaneous inhalation in the upper and lower part of the lungs. When CO_2 levels become too high in the blood, chemical changes take place in the medulla, which will then open the arteries to increase blood supply to the brain and at the same time stimulate deep breathing.

A feature of extreme anxiety can be repeated episodes of excessive shallow breathing in response to anxiety or fear. Symptoms are manifold, ranging from sensations of breathlessness, dizziness, parasthesis and chest pains to generalised weakness, syncope (fainting) and several others. This tendency may be exacerbated by a poorly developed CO_2 reflex, setting up a chain reaction so that the Moro reflex is linked to an inadequate CO_2 reflex, increasing the tendency to hyperventilate, which in turn induces physiological sensations associated with fear and/or extreme anxiety. These processes can become mutually reinforcing.

Possible long-term effects of retained Moro reflex:

- vestibular-related problems such as motion sickness, poor balance and coordination, particularly seen during ball games
- physical timidity
- oculo-motor and visual-perceptual problems, e.g. stimulus-bound effect (cannot ignore irrelevant visual material within a given visual field, so the eyes tend to be drawn to the perimeter of a shape, much to the detriment of perception of internal features)
- difficulty processing information in environments presenting multisensory stimuli
- poor pupillary reaction to light, photosensitivity, difficulty with black print on white paper, and easy tiring under fluorescent lighting[2]
- possible auditory confusion resulting from hypersensitivity to specific sounds, including poor auditory discrimination and have difficulty shutting out background noise
- poor regulation of stamina
- dislike of change or poor adaptability to surprises
- poorly developed CO_2 reflex

Whereas other residual reflexes tend to have an impact on specific skills, the Moro has an overall effect on the emotional profile of the child.

Possible secondary psychological symptoms:

- free-floating anxiety or 'angst' (continuous anxiety seemingly unrelated to reality)
- overreactivity
- irritability
- frustration leading to mood swings and labile emotions
- tense muscle tone (body armouring)
- difficulty accepting criticism, since the child finds it so difficult to change

- cycle of hyperactivity followed by excessive fatigue
- difficulty making decisions
- weak ego, low self-esteem
- insecurity/dependency
- need to control or manipulate events

The Moro reflex is the only one of the primitive reflexes to be connected in some way to each one of the senses. As the earliest primitive reflex to emerge, it forms a cornerstone for the establishment of reaction patterns in later life. It is needed to support survival in the first months of life, but its effects can be profound if it fails to be inhibited at the correct time and transformed into an adult startle response.

The adult startle response consists of a shrugging movement of the shoulders, followed by a turn of the head to locate the source of the disturbance (orientation to stimulus) and a cortical decision as to whether to react to the stimulus as a threat or to ignore it and carry on with whatever one was doing. This is different from the Moro reflex response, in which the individual reacts first and only a few seconds later becomes able to identify the nature of the stimulus. By this time not only the reflex reaction but the physiological responses of fight and flight have already entered the system, so that although the child may subsequently recognise that the stimulus was nothing to be scared of, everything physically and emotionally feels as if it had been real. This can lead to a conflict between 'what I feel' and 'what I know' as well as a build-up of tension and overarousal. 'If there is a conflict between feelings and logic and the feelings are too strong, then feelings will always win.'[3]
Benett (1988) describes how:

> In early neonate life, the brain and spinal cord are not fully connected and there is no perception (that is to say, the neonate receives impulse stimuli via the eyes and the ears etc. but has no ability to interpret their meaning, and is therefore unable to make sense out of what is experienced). As the neonate develops in the early months after birth, the brain has to learn to differentiate between threat stimuli and harmless stimuli. Where the Moro reflex does not become inhibited, there is a presence of two similar reactions: one of the 'shock' reflex, the other, the 'surprise' reflex (Moro and adult Startle

> or Strauss reflexes), and the brain has difficulty in discriminating between sudden harmless stimuli and true threats. (Benett 1988)

Both Blythe and Bennet viewed this distinction as playing a key role in the possible later development of extreme anxiety states and panic disorder. Bennet observed that in adults the continued presence of the Moro reflex could be masked by the development of protective muscle tension that could make it difficult for the clinician to elicit the reflex even though it was still present. He went on to outline a profile of possible traits that he observed were often present with this type of body 'armouring' whereby muscle tension was habitually used as a way of concealing and containing emotions:

- low self-esteem
- difficulty making and/or maintaining friendships
- history of multiple ultimately unsuccessful romantic relationships
- history of frequent medical investigations and/or treatments (often for minor problems)

Blythe had previously described this tendency in a paper on a somatogenic basis for neuroses, in which he observed that, although these individuals were often viewed as hypochondriacs because no medical reason could be found for their symptoms, they did indeed feel physically unwell because they were hypersensitive. Bennet's profile went on to list the following traits:

- often prone to excessive fear, worry and anxiety and will often have physical manifestations of this (shallow breathing, tachycardia, muscle pains, etc.)
- can be emotionally rigid or even prudish
- easily shocked by stressors and tend to be trouble or accident prone
- frequently hypersensitive to sound or antipathetic to a noisy environment
- may have an air of tension/readiness
- tendency to nightmares or insomnia revisiting events of the day or reviewing events to come

- often feel mildly threatened if someone moves too close to them, i.e. invades their personal zone
- tendency to feelings of panic in unexpected situations

The above profile observed in adults found to have an active Moro reflex can be masked for years by the process of conscious compensation and emerge in the form of minor, disparate physical (somatic) symptoms.

Palmar reflex

Emerges:	11 weeks in utero
Birth:	Fully present
Inhibited:	2–3 months of life
Transformed:	Gradual development from involuntary grasp to release and refined finger control. Replaced by the pincer grip at 36 weeks of age.

The palmar reflex forms a part of the group of reflexes that develop in utero and whose common characteristic is to grasp (Figure 1.4). A light touch or pressure to the palm of the hand will result in closure of the fingers with the thumb underneath. By 18 weeks after conception the response will have extended to include a gripping reflex in response to a pull against the finger tendons. Both of these responses should strengthen during uterine life, to be fully developed at birth.

They should be strongly active for the first 12 weeks of life and transformed by four to six months of age, so that the child can learn to hold an object between their thumb and index finger in a pincer grip.

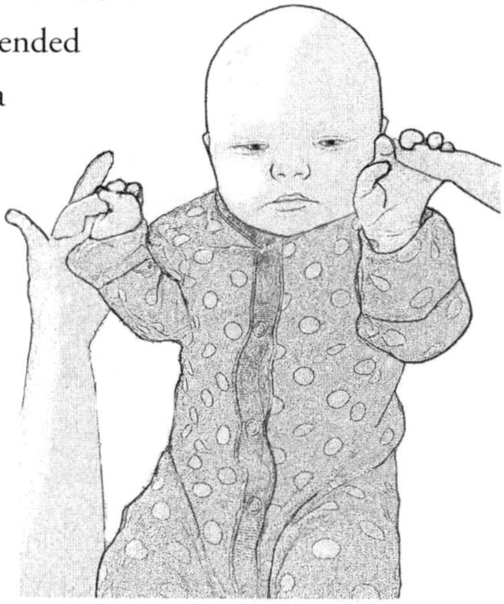

Figure 1.4: Palmar reflex

The ability to release an object follows some weeks later, to be practised many times before the child can acquire good manual dexterity. This is the stage when an infant may be sitting in a high chair or buggy and, having dropped a favourite toy, whimpers for an adult to retrieve it. Soon after the object has been returned, the infant drops it again. Adults quickly tire of this game, but for the infant this is the first time they have been able to 'let go' voluntarily – the more they do it, the better they become – and they do not tire of repetition.

Both the palmar and the plantar reflexes are thought to be a continuation of an earlier stage in human evolution, when it was still necessary for the neonate to cling to their mother for safety. There is also a direct link between the palmar reflex and feeding in the early months of life. The palmar reflex can be elicited by sucking movements, and the action of sucking may elicit simultaneous kneading movements of the hands (Babkin response). The mouth and the hands are the major fields of exploration and expression during the neonate period. Continued reflex activity in the palm of the hand can have a lasting adverse effect upon fine muscle coordination, speech and articulation if the reflexes fail to be inhibited and therefore uncoupled.

The effects of this neurological loop that connects stimulation of the palms with movements of the mouth can often be seen when the child first learns to write or to draw. Until these skills come easily, the child will lick his lips, or twist his mouth in some other way. Teachers will often admonish, 'You're not writing with your tongue!' Developmental optometrists call this 'overflow' and consider the child to have made visual progress when this overflow disappears.

If the palmar reflex remains, the child cannot proceed through the subsequent stages of voluntary release and thumb and finger opposition.

Gesell (1939) describes how this process unfolds:

> Voluntary grasping, such as reaching, indicates a proximo-distal course of development. Early grasping consists of crude palming movements in which the three ulnar fingers predominate, whereas the thumb is practically inactive. This type of grasp is later succeeded by a refined fingertip prehension, characterised principally by thumb opposition, forefinger dominance, readiness for manipulation and the adaption of a finger pressure to the weight of the object.

This can only occur as the palmar reflex becomes inhibited. When older children are assessed, if the palmar reflex is present, difficulty may be evident on tests for dysdiadochokinesis in the fingers (ability to carry out rapid sequential movements). This ability is a precursor to being able to hold, direct and control a writing instrument using a pincer grip. These children can learn to write, but often adopt an immature writing grip that impedes the wrist and finger movements needed to develop neat, legible and fluent handwriting.

Long-term effects of a retained palmar reflex:

- poor manual dexterity (the palmar reflex will interfere with independent thumb and finger movements)
- lack of pincer grip, which will affect pencil grip when writing
- a history of speech difficulties – if there is a continuing relationship between hand and mouth movement via the Babkin reflex (the Babkin reflex can result in hand and mouth movements remaining coupled beyond the stage when independent control of the fingers and muscles at the front of the mouth should have developed, which can then affect oral articulation)[4]
- palm of the hand may remain hypersensitive to tactile stimulation
- movements made with the mouth when trying to write or draw

A retained or residual palmar reflex beyond four or five months of life can interfere with manual dexterity and manipulatory activities.

Speech may also be affected, since a continuing relationship between hand and mouth movements (Babkin reflex) can impair the development of independent fine motor control of the muscles at the front of the mouth. Clear articulation may be just one casualty of this, and the child may have a history of needing SALT.

It should also be acknowledged that although individual reflexes are described for theoretical purposes as discrete entities, there can be a relationship between them during development. André Thomas and his co-workers (1954) found that it was possible to inhibit the Moro reflex by first stimulating the palmar reflex. When the Moro reflex is activated by shaking the head, the arms, hands and fingers will normally extend. If the palmar reflex is stimulated first by placing an object in the palm of one of the hands before eliciting the Moro response, the Moro reaction only occurs in the arm on the side of the open hand (opposite side). If an object is placed in both hands, the Moro reaction seems to be inhibited in the arms bilaterally.

Subconsciously, we sometimes utilise this effect. When about to undertake an unpleasant or difficult task, or in anticipation of a temporary painful stimulus such as an injection, we may clasp and unclasp our hands. Stress balls may be effective as a result of the same principle.

These observations indicate that early reflexes can operate in two ways: either in a chain reaction, or with one reflex having an inhibitory effect upon another. It is these principles that underlie the programmes upon which reflex stimulation and inhibition remedial techniques developed at the INPP are based.

Asymmetrical tonic neck reflex

Emerges:	18 weeks in utero
Birth:	Fully present
Inhibited:	About 6 months of life

Rotation of the baby's head to one side will elicit reflexive extension of the arm and leg on the side to which the head is turned, and flexion of the occipital limbs (Figure 1.5). The asymmetrical tonic neck reflex (ATNR) has an active part to play from the time of its emergence in utero until approximately six months of life. During life in the womb, the ATNR facilitates movement (the kick), develops muscle tone and provides vestibular stimulation.

The ATNR in utero provides a mechanism for motion which stimulates the balance mechanism and increases neural connections. It should be fully established by the time the foetus is ready to be born and is thought to play a part in the birth process. Labour should not begin until the foetus has reached maturity. Several mechanisms are involved in the onset of labour. One is the foetus's release of a hormone into the mother's bloodstream which stimulates contractions of the uterus. Another is the foetal position, which exerts pressure on the cervix. Ideally, mother and baby then act as cooperative partners in the birth process.

Owing to the size and shape of the mother's pelvis relative to the dimensions of the baby's head, the baby has to make two 90° turns to navigate down the birth canal. It is thought that the ATNR together with the neck-righting reflex of the body and the spinal Galant reflex afford flexibility and motility to the shoulders, hips and lumbar region, which assist in rotation. The baby's active participation in this is probably linked to the presence of a full asymmetrical tonic neck reflex that can assist restitution of the shoulders in the final stage of being born. The birth process in return reinforces the ATNR (and other reflexes) so that they are firmly established and active during the first months of life.

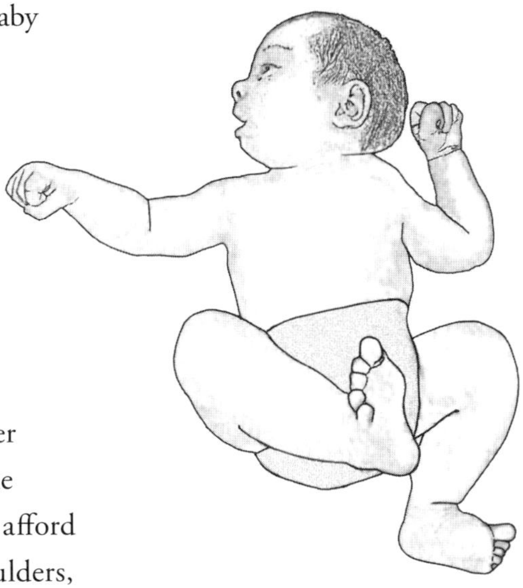

Figure 1.5: Asymmetrical tonic neck reflex.

During the neonate period, the turning of the head to one side, which occurs when the ATNR is activated, should ensure a free passage of air if the baby is in the prone position. The ATNR also helps to increase extensor muscle tone, trains one side of the body at a time and provides the basis for later reaching movements.

Although the true function of primitive reflexes in the first months of life is not fully understood, it is likely that certain reflexes are crucial for survival in the first months of life. Underdeveloped Moro and asymmetrical tonic neck reflexes, for example, may be a factor in sudden infant death syndrome (SIDS) – the Moro reflex because it provides an instant arousal mechanism and the ATNR because it should prevent the baby from lying face down when placed on their tummy (Goddard 1990; 1991; 1996).

DeMyer (1980) describes the ATNR as the first eye–hand coordination to begin. Other authors have explained how:

> It is present at the time that visual fixation upon nearby objects is developing, and it seems that the nervous system is making sure that the appropriate arm stretches out towards visualised objects. As the hand touches the object, the seeds of awareness of distance (at arm's length) and eye–hand coordination are sown. (Holt 1991)

Babies are naturally near-sighted at birth and the visual world they experience is nothing like the way we understand the visual world as adults. Infants have to learn how to see or to make sense of the stimuli provided from the eyes to the brain. This is a multisensory process in which activation of the ATNR causes the eyes to follow the movement of the arm, helping to extend baby's focusing distance from near point to arm's length and back again, and from central vision to peripheral vision and back to central vision again. In this way, movement of the head activates a process whereby the head turns, the arm extends, the eyes follow, the hand may accidentally come into contract with an object (touch) and all of this is combined with additional feedback derived from alteration in relative tension in the muscle spindles and joints (proprioception). This multisensory experience activated through the medium of movement is like a very first lesson in eye–hand coordination and helps the infant to develop perception of distance, space, timing and adjustment between different visual distances and points of focus. The reflex is merely a primary mechanism to facilitate the start of this process, which will take many more months to become refined.

By six months of age, the ATNR should have fulfilled its main functions and the developing brain should release further movement patterns that contain the inhibitor of the ATNR, enabling the development of more complex skills and mature patterns of response and volitional behaviour.

The continued presence of a ATNR will interfere with numerous functions. For example, it is impossible to crawl on the stomach with a fluent cross-pattern movement if the ATNR persists. Crawling and creeping are important for the further development of hand–eye coordination and the integration of vestibular information with other senses. Myelination of the central nervous system is enhanced during these processes.

The child who still has an ATNR when they learn to walk may find their balance is insecure. Movement of the head to either side will result in straightening of the limbs on that side, upsetting the centre of balance and resulting in homolateral movement. If the child walks with the left hand swinging forward as the left foot moves forward, and with the right hand moving at the same time as the right foot, the result will be a robot-like walk. This walk alerts other children to the fact that there is something different and makes the child an easy target for teasing. In sports, tasks such as throwing and kicking a ball will appear awkward.

Conversely, elite athletes may access a naturally inhibited reflex such as the ATNR to enhance performance of specific skills. Examples of these include fencers when they adopt the en garde attitude, shooting in basketball, and discus throwing. The difference between elite athletes who utilise early reflexes in this way and individuals with NMI is that the former is master or mistress of their reflexes, only releasing them momentarily to support a specific skill, whereas the individual with NMI is the servant of reflexes that interfere with the smooth acquisition of a range of skills.

Retention of the ATNR can result in difficulty in crossing the midline from one side of the body to the other when the head is turned to the affected side. In infancy this may hinder the transition from merely grasping to manipulating an object with both hands and interfere with learning to pass objects from hand to hand. This skill is normally acquired at about 28 weeks but if the ATNR persists it can become an invisible barrier to crossing the vertical midline. The entire body will want to execute tasks using one side at a time when the head is turned to the affected side, and thus bilateral integration is impeded.

In later childhood, the ATNR can act as an impediment to establishing a preferred hand, leg, eye or ear and, if there is no dominant side, there will tend to be a slight hesitancy in the child's movements. Gazzaniga (1973) proposed that unilaterality of brain functioning is important in order to have a central organisation point in the brain for processing incoming information. Kohen-Raz (1986) suggests that the establishment of a preferred side (by seven or eight years of age) is a prerequisite to being able to learn to read and write with fluency, while Delacato (1959) observed that:

> The neurological differences between man and slightly lower forms of animals are not cellularly important. The basic difference between man and the animal world is that man has achieved cortical dominance wherein one side of the cortex controls the skills in which man outdistances lower forms of animals. This whole phylogenetic process is recapitulated ontogenetically with each human being. In the event that there is some obstruction to this ontogenetic recapitulation, communication and language dysfunctions occur.

Although this is now considered to be a simplistic and outdated view, a link often does exist between immature postural control, neurological dysfunction, cross or mixed laterality and the fluent expression of the higher cognitive skills of speech and reading.

Eye movements may also be affected, since the child may find it difficult to cross the midline when the head is turned to the affected side. When such a child is asked to follow an object as it is moved slowly in front of them along a horizontal line, there will be a slight hesitancy as the object is moved from one side of his nose to the other. This same hesitancy may also cause the eyes to jump when reading, so that letters, or in some cases whole words, are skipped.

In the classroom, handwriting will be the most obvious casualty of a residual ATNR. When the head turns to direct or follow the movement of the hand the arm will want to extend and the fingers to open. This will make holding and manipulating a writing implement for any length of time tiring and require additional effort and conscious attention. The effect can be as if an elastic band has been attached to the pencil and then tethered to the comer of the table so that the child is having to counteract an invisible force. They may learn to compensate by using an immature pencil grip or by using excessive pressure or an altered sitting position, but the physical act of writing will require additional concentration often at the expense of cognitive processing.

Trying to write and to express ideas at the same time (cognitive process) with an ATNR is rather like being stuck for ever on your third or fourth driving lesson; you know the procedures involved, but you have to pay attention to every stage. If you try to do too many things at one time or someone distracts your attention away from the procedures involved, you stall the engine.

This can affect both the quality and quantity of handwriting. Letter formation may be erratic and writing may slope in different directions from one side of the page to the other or deteriorate as one gets further down the page. The child may rotate the page by as much as 90 degrees when writing or sit in a position that enables them to write with a straight arm in an attempt to accommodate the effect of the reflex. The mechanics involved in writing do not become automatic and the need for continued cognitive control of what should become an automated skill can use up cognitive energy ideally reserved for the expression of knowledge and ideas in written form. This can result in a significant discrepancy between oral and written performance.

Symptoms suggestive of a residual or retained ATNR:

- upright balance may be affected as a result of head rotation to either side
- homolateral instead of normal cross-pattern movements, e.g. when walking, marching, skipping, etc.
- difficulty crossing the midline
- poor ocular pursuit movements, especially at the midline
- mixed laterality (e.g. switching which hand is used for writing or batting a ball)
- poor handwriting, reluctance to write and poor expression of ideas on paper
- visual-perceptual difficulties, particularly in symmetrical representation of figures

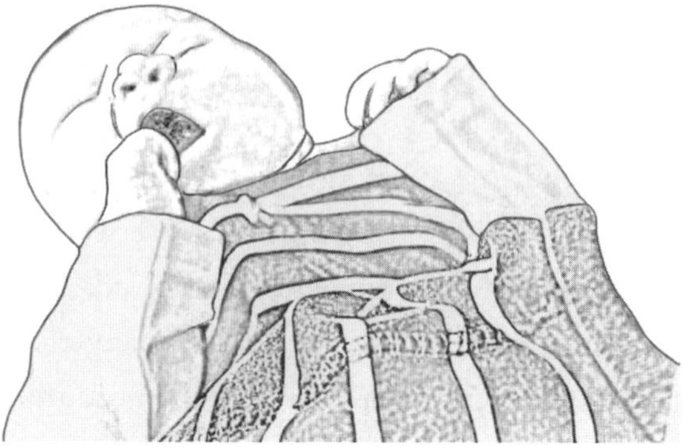

Figure 1.6: Rooting reflex

Rooting reflex

Emerges:	24–28 weeks in utero
Birth:	Present
Inhibited:	3–4 months of life

Searching, sucking and swallowing reflexes should be present in all full-term babies (Figure 1.6). These instinctive abilities also form part of the group of 'grasp' reflexes, which develop in utero.

Light touch of the cheek or stimulation of the edge of the mouth will cause the baby to turn the head towards the stimulus (rooting action) and to open the mouth with extended tongue in preparation for sucking. This reflex may be elicited at all four quadrants of the mouth and thus is sometimes referred to as the 'cardinal points reflex'.

The combination of rooting and sucking reflexes ensures that the baby turns towards the source of food and opens his mouth wide enough to latch on to the breast or bottle. The sucking and swallowing movements that follow are vital for early feeding.

Odent (1991) stated that the rooting reflex is at its strongest in the first couple of hours after birth, and if the baby does not receive gratification for their rooting attempts shortly after birth the reflex will weaken. Righarde and Frantz (2005) compared the behaviour of neonates in the minutes immediately after birth, grouped according to whether the mother had received pain-relieving medication (which passes through to the baby shortly before birth) and/or whether the baby had been separated from the mother before the first feed. The majority of neonates born to unmedicated mothers who were placed on the mother's abdomen as soon as possible after birth spontaneously crawled to find the breast and began to feed. Infants who had been born to medicated mothers made small attempts to root or search for the breast but soon gave up because they were too exhausted and had difficulty latching on. Premature babies who have had to be incubated can frequently be seen rooting for the first couple of days of life, but when they are unable to receive the appropriate response the rooting reflex starts to diminish. In some of these children the reflex can still be elicited in weakened form long after it should have been inhibited.

The strength of the rooting reflex may come and go according to when the last feed was taken. It disappears temporarily after the infant is satiated, to reappear only after some time has elapsed. Conversely, it can appear as a vacuum activity without the external stimulus of touch in the hungry infant, who will turn their head in all directions seeking sustenance.

Peiper suggested that primitive reflex activity leads an infant into the next stage of a conditioned reflex and he cites the rooting reflex as an example of this:

> When we touch the region of the infant's mouth, reflexes are elicited that turn the head, and move the lips so that the touching object is drawn into the mouth. This life preserving function is innate, but the ability to turn to the nipple or the bottle when it appears in the field of vision is not. This is rapidly learned. From the rooting reflex there develops a conditioned reflex that at the sight of the breast or the bottle turns the head to the correct position in space. (Peiper 1963)

Retained or residual oral reflexes result in continued sensitivity to tactile stimuli in the reflex-sensitive region and in the ability to seal the lips, resulting in a tendency to gape and retain an immature swallow pattern that leads to dribbling.

The infant may have difficulty when solid foods are introduced, since a persistent suck reflex influences the position of the jaws and can prevent the tongue from developing the mature combination of movements necessary for chewing and swallowing.

Swallowing, feeding, speech articulation and manual dexterity may all be casualties of a combination of residual or retained oral reflexes in the older child. As Roberta Shepherd (1990) says:

> The development of normal swallowing and of normal coordination between respiration and oral function are all essential elements in the development of speech. It is thought that the muscular action involved in feeding is an essential preparation for babbling and speech.

Manual dexterity may also be affected, since immature sucking and swallowing movements are sometimes linked to a Babkin reflex associated with a persistent link between movements of the mouth and the hands, which in infancy naturally elicits hand clasping and unclasping during suckling.

The stimulus for the Babkin reflex consists of deep pressure applied simultaneously to the palms of both hands while the infant is in an appropriate position, ideally supine. The stimulus is followed by flexion or forward bowing of the head, opening of the mouth and closing of the eyes. The reflex can be demonstrated in the newborn, thus showing a hand–mouth neurological link even at this early stage. It fades rapidly, and normally cannot be elicited after four months of age. Elicitation of the reflex after this age indicates a cerebral lesion (Holt 1991).

Like many other reflexive reactions, the effect of the Babkin reflex can be seen in either direction, in this case from hand to mouth or from mouth to hand.

Long-term effects of retained rooting and sucking reflexes:

- hypersensitivity around lips and mouth
- tongue may remain too far forward in the mouth, which makes it difficult to swallow and chew certain foods, so the child may dribble (lack of mature swallowing movements may lead to increased arching of the palate – 'cathedral palate' – and the need for orthodontic treatment later on)
- speech and articulation problems
- poor manual dexterity

Spinal Galant reflex

Emerges:	20 weeks in utero
Birth:	Present
Inhibited:	3–9 months of life

If the baby is held in the ventral or placed in the prone position, gentle tactile stimulation of the back to one side of the spine will result in hip flexion (outward rotation) to 45 degrees on the side of the stimulus. It should be present with equal strength bilaterally (Figure 1.7).

Although Galant eventually gave his name to this reflex, it had been described by Bertolotti in 1904 as a *réflexe dorsolombaire* (cited in Peiper 1963). Galant observed that stimulation of the skin of the lumbar region resulted in a quick contraction of the dorsal muscles. The response disappeared by two years of age. In 1912, Noica found *une réflexe de la masse musculaire sacrolombaire* to be present in most children but rarely in adults. In 1917, both Veragruth and Galant described similar reactions in normal infants, which Veragruth also found to be present in some mentally ill adults.

When the dorsal skin near and along the vertebral column is stroked, the infant forms an arch with his body; the concavity of the arch is directed toward the stimulated area, and by arching in the opposite direction the infant evades the stimulus. (Galant 1917)

Isbert and Peiper found the response to be more extensive than described by Galant:

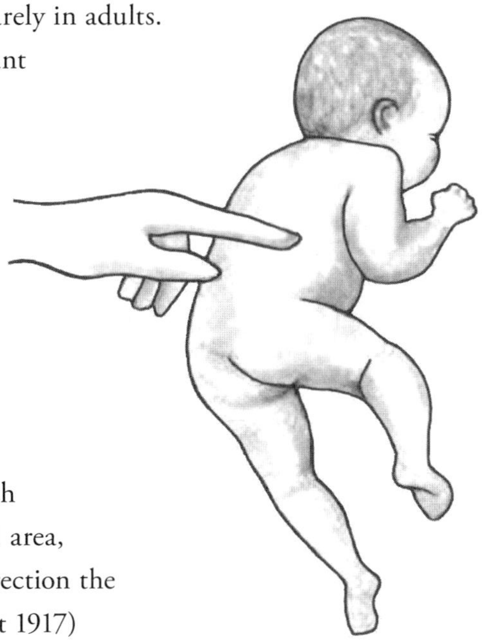

Figure 1.7: Spinal Galant reflex

> Application of the stimulus results in flexion of the pelvis backward and the ipsilateral leg is extended at the knee and the hip joint is flexed… frequently the head position can be changed by stimulation of the anterior surface of the trunk: Stimulation of one side causes turning of the face to the stimulated side. (Cited in Peiper 1963)

The last observation seems to provide evidence of the chain reaction that can occur from one reflex to the next, that is, activation of the spinal Galant reflex sometimes extends into an ATNR.

If both sides of the spine are stroked simultaneously from the pelvis to the neck, the Pulgar Marx reflex is elicited. This response involves:

> … flexion of both legs, lordosis of the spine, elevation of the pelvis, flexion of the arms, lifting of the head, loud crying culminating in apnoea and cyanosis, emptying of the bladder, and relaxation and bulging of the rectum with bowel movement; after the reflex has fully developed there is general hypertonia lasting for a few seconds. (Pulgar Marx 1955)

Not all features of the reflex are present each time it is activated. The Pulgar Marx reflex should be inhibited by two to three months of age. This response is rarely seen in older children with specific learning difficulties. At the INPP, traces of it have been found in several children who were given a diagnosis of Asperger's syndrome and in some children with a history of continued daytime soiling above age five.

Little is known about the functions of the spinal Galant reflex, except that it may take an active role in the birth process. Contractions of the vaginal wall stimulate the lumbar region, stimulating rotational movements of the hip on one side, similar to the head and shoulder movements of the ATNR. In this way, the reflex may help the baby to manoeuvre its way down the birth canal. The Pulgar Marx reflex may contribute to lumbar lordosis in the second stage of labour, assisting exodus.

It has been suggested that the Galant may act as a primitive conductor of sound in utero, allowing sound vibration to travel up through the body in the aquatic environment of the womb, and so enabling the foetus to 'feel' sound, or helping sound vibrations to travel up the spinal column.[5] Some weight was added to this hypothesis by a study carried out by Butler, Hall and Hadley which investigated the effect of auditory integrative training (AIT) on abnormal primitive and postural reflexes. AIT is a system of sound therapy developed by Guy Berard for treating a range of listening- and language-related problems. Butler Hall (1998) found that the spinal Galant reflex was consistently reduced in children as a result of AIT training, which suggests that there is a functional relationship between the spinal Galant reflex and hearing (see Chapter 4).

Another interpretation offered is that the spinal Galant reflex is a legacy of our evolutionary heritage from a time when we had a tail.[6] A tail or tail-like movement is useful during uterine life for moving in the womb. It might also be useful for balance during the time that a child is creeping and crawling (the quadruped stage of development) and for helping to synchronise upper and lower body movements on one side, but it becomes redundant when the erect posture is achieved when the front of the body and the arms are freed from supporting quadruped locomotion.

If the spinal Galant reflex remains beyond the neonate period, it can be elicited by light pressure in the lumbar region. Simultaneous stimulation down both sides of the spine can activate the related Pulgar Marx reflex, which will cause the infant to urinate. A retained or residual spinal Galant reflex is found in many children who continue to wet the bed after the age of five years. Beuret, working with adults in Chicago, found the spinal Galant reflex to be present in a high percentage of patients suffering from irritable bowel syndrome.[7]

For the child in the classroom, the spinal Galant reflex can make it difficult to sit still. This is the 'ants in the pants' child who wriggles, squirms and constantly changes body position, since the elastic of a waistband or simply leaning against the back of a chair may activate the errant reflex. Understandably, the child may dislike clothing that is tight around the waist. The reflex may also interfere with concentration and short-term memory, firstly because postural control provides a physical basis for attention and, secondly, because a constant irritant vies for attention. This is rather like having an insect bite that you know you should not scratch but which you cannot ignore.

If the Galant reflex remains present on one side only, it can affect posture, gait and any other form of locomotion. This can result in the illusion of a limp or contribute to the development of a scoliosis over time. It may also interfere with the full development of the later amphibian and segmental rolling reflexes, affecting fluency of movements used in a range of physical activities or sports.

Possible symptoms of a retained spinal Galant reflex:

- fidgeting
- bedwetting
- poor concentration
- poor short-term memory

Tonic labyrinthine reflex

Emerges:	Flexion in utero
Birth:	Present in flexion and extension from birth
Inhibited:	From approximately 4 months of life (see below for extended period of integration and inhibition)

The Moro and tonic labyrinthine reflexes are closely linked in the early months of life. Both are vestibular in origin, and both are activated by stimulation of the labyrinths, movement of the head through the transverse midplane and alteration of position in space. In the neonate, the tonic labyrinthine reflex (TLR) is elicited by movement of the head forwards or backwards through the transverse midplane (flexion and extension) above or below the level of the spine (Figure 1.8). It is thought that flexus habitus (the characteristic flexed posture of the foetus in utero) is the earliest manifestation of the TLR in the forward position. The TLR in extension is thought to emerge partially as the baby's head extends to pass through the cervix as the birth process begins. The reflex should be present from the time of birth when extension of the head below the level of the spine elicits an increase in extensor tone in the legs.

The TLR should be fully developed in both positions from birth. Inhibition

Figure 1.8:
Tonic labyrinthine reflex
a) Flexion b) Extension

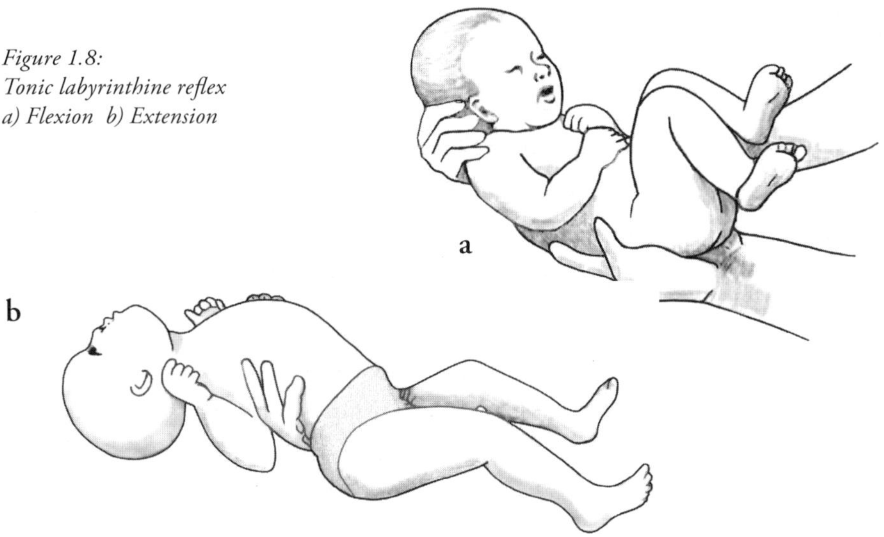

of the TLR forwards should be accomplished by four months of life. Inhibition of the TLR backwards is a more gradual process, involving the emergence of several postural reflexes and taking up till age three-and-a-half years to be completed.

Being born introduces the baby to an entirely new set of challenges. Hitherto, they have been in an enclosed aqueous environment, in which the effects of all sensory stimuli are cushioned and the effect of gravity is reduced. The TLR provides the baby with an early primitive method of response to the problem of gravity before they have developed the muscle tone necessary to support the head. Movement of the head through the midplane results in extremes of flexion or extension through the length of the body, influencing muscle tone from the head downwards. By six months of age, the response should be modified as head control develops with the emergence of the oculo- and labyrinthine head-righting reflexes. Head control is an essential prerequisite for the development of all later functions and should be the prime facilitator of early movement, tonus and balance (cephalo-caudal law).

The TLR exerts a tonic influence upon the distribution of muscle tone throughout the body, probably helping the neonate to straighten out from the flexed posture characteristic of the foetus and the newborn. Balance, muscle tone and proprioception are all trained during this process.

If the TLR fails to be inhibited at the correct time, it can trip the vestibular system in its relationship with other sensory systems, resulting in mismatch between the signals relating balance to and from the body via the vestibular–proprioceptive (vestibular–spinal) feedback loop. The child who has a retained TLR when they start to walk cannot acquire true gravitational security (Ayres 1989), since head movement will influence muscle tone, destabilising the control of balance. Lacking a secure reference point in space, a child may experience difficulty in judging space, distance, depth and velocity. A sense of direction is based upon knowing physically where we are; if our point of reference is unstable, then the ability to discriminate up from down, left from right and back from front may also be impaired. This is similar to a condition described by cosmonauts in space. In the early days of space travel, when cosmonauts were put into a gravity-free environment they started to write from right to left, to reverse numbers and letters and to produce mirror writing – a condition described as 'transient space dyslexia' – and thereby demonstrated the significance of gravity and balance for spatial and directional awareness.

Continued TLR activity can impede the development of the head-righting reflexes. If head control is lacking, control of eye movements can also be impaired, since the eyes operate from the same circuit in the brain – the vestibulo-ocular reflex arc. This loop is functionally linked to postural stability (vestibular–spinal loop). If one loop in the tripartite vestibular–proprioceptive–ocular circuit is out of synchrony with the rest, it will affect the smooth operation of the others (Figure 1.9)

If vestibular–proprioceptive–visual mismatch exists, balance can be affected by discrepant visual information and vice versa, undermining the functioning of centres involved in the control of eye movements that are needed to support visual perception. For the child, this is how their internal world has always been, so they will assume that their experience and perception of the world is the same as others', even though this may not be the case.

The TLR may also prevent the child from being able to creep on their hands and knees if extension of the head results in extension of the legs. The symmetrical tonic neck reflex (STNR) can also remain locked in the system in a futile attempt to override the TLR, preventing creeping on hands and knees.

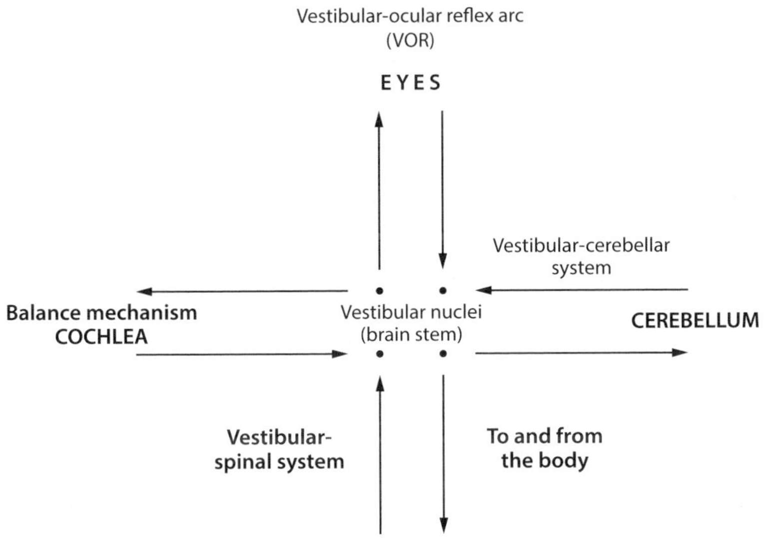

Figure 1.9:
Functional links of the vestibular–cerebellar system in relation to posture and eye movement.

Crawling and creeping fulfil both training and inhibitory processes. Both crawling and creeping facilitate the integration of sensory information in a new relationship with gravity (quadruped) as vestibular, visual and proprioceptive systems all start to operate together for the first time.

It is thought that the process of creeping entrains and enhances a sense of balance, a sense of space and a sense of depth.[8] It is through crawling and creeping that the raw materials of seeing, feeling and moving are synchronised for the first time to provide a more complete picture of the environment.

Prolonged influence of the TLR can have implications for many other areas of functioning. Balance and movement control can be affected. Standing for any length of time may be tiring and posture may have to adjust in an attempt to accommodate the reflex. If the TLR is residually present in flexion, posture may tend to be stooped or there may be a tendency to stand with the head poked forwards. The child may appear to have low muscle tone and seem either lazy in posture and 'attitude' (TLR flexion) or stiff, awkward and inflexible in their movements (TLR extension),[9] particularly when walking, running or jumping. Poor muscle tone may make holding the arms up for any length of time tiring, and so certain physical activities (sports) are avoided.

There may be a fear of heights, since head movement up and/or down momentarily destabilises balance and also visual processing as a secondary consequence. A residual TLR is often a factor in adults who present with long-term symptoms of agoraphobia with associated visual-perceptual problems such as figure–ground effect.

Figure–ground effect organisation is a type of perceptual grouping that is vital for recognising objects through vision. In Gestalt psychology it is known as 'identifying a figure from the background'. For example, black words on a printed page are seen as the 'figure' and the white sheet as the 'background'. A similar situation occurs in focusing at different distances. When one focuses on an object at a near distance, the point of focus should be clear and the background blurred. When one shifts visual attention to the far distance, the distant point of sighting should be clear and near distant stimuli should become blurred. In this way background and foreground do not vie for visual attention. When this system is not working well, visual perceptual misrepresentations can occur. One example often described by adults is fear of walking across a slatted surface such as a bridge where the water or ground can be seen through the gaps. When the visual system does not allow the separation of foreground (solid surface) from background, the brain perceives that the surface is not safe to cross. This faulty information can be sufficient to alert the freeze/fight/flight response and no amount of logic can persuade the brain, misinformed by the visual system and alerted to danger by the limbic system, that it is safe to cross.

Here it should be stressed that the TLR is not necessarily the cause, but rather it may act as an underlying mechanism that can offset the functioning of higher systems. This is because it will continue to influence the functional relationship between the head and the body, which is essential to support the automatic functioning of many other systems.

Symptoms suggestive of a strongly residual TLR forwards:

- poor posture – stoop (flexion)
- hypotonus (weak muscle tone)

- vestibular-related problems, e.g. poor sense of balance, propensity to get car sick
- dislike of sporting activities, physical education classes, running, etc.
- oculo-motor dysfunctions
- visual-perceptual difficulties
- spatial problems
- poor sequencing skills
- poor sense of time

Symptoms associated with a strongly residual TLR backwards:

- poor posture – tendency to walk on toes
- poor balance and coordination
- hypertonus –stiff, jerky movements because the extensor muscles exert greater influence than the flexor muscles
- vestibular-related problems, e.g. poor sense of balance, tendency to motion sickness
- oculo-motor dysfunction, e.g. visual-perceptual difficulties, spatial perception problems
- poor sequencing skills
- poor organisation skills

Symmetrical tonic neck reflex

Emerges:	6–9 months of life
Inhibited:	9–11 months

The STNR has a relatively short lifespan. Present for a very short period of time at birth, it returns as a transient reflex between six and eleven months of life (there is some variation in the literature on the precise timing). It helps the baby to defy gravity by pushing up from the floor on to hands and knees (quadruped position) from the prone position and is thought to assist in aligning the occipital and sacral regions of the spine in the quadruped position before the infant learns to stand and walk (Figure 1.10). The STNR may, like the stepping reflex, be temporarily

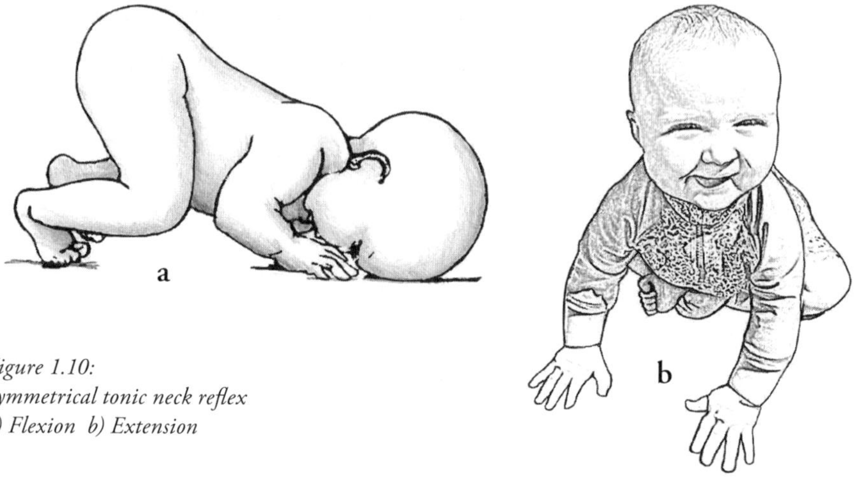

Figure 1.10:
Symmetrical tonic neck reflex
a) Flexion b) Extension

present after birth to help the neonate to push their way up the mother's tummy to find the breast. Videos of alert newborn babies, whose mothers have not received artificial analgesia during labour, show the baby crawling towards the breast using what appears to be a combination of the stepping reflex (pushing with the feet) and STNR (flexing the legs to push the body forward) (Righarde and Frantz 2005).

Capute and colleagues (1981) suggest that the STNR may be not a true reflex, but a stage of integration/inhibition of the TLR. Whereas the TLR elicits an increase in extensor or flexor tone through the entire length of the body in response to flexion or extension of the head, the STNR separates the reaction in the middle of the body, causing the top and bottom sections of the body to respond in opposite directions: head flexion elicits flexion in the upper half of the body and increased extensor tone in the lower half; head extension elicits increased extensor tone in the upper half and flexion in the lower half. To make this easily accessible to students learning about reflexes for the first time, Peter Blythe would say in jest that, whereas retention of the ATNR created a vertical midline barrier in the functioning of the two sides of the body, retention of the STNR created a midlife crisis at the waist (horizontal midline).

The STNR certainly helps to modify the TLR by blocking the influence on muscle tone at the horizontal midline of the body, providing a bridge to the next stage of locomotion – creeping on hands and knees. However, although it helps the child to acquire the quadruped position, it will interfere with forward progress in this position if it remains strongly active. The baby's control of muscle tone (and therefore support for the crawling position) will be at the mercy of their head position, potentially interfering with the ability to move effectively because during this period of development the position of the head influences the degree of extensor or flexor tone in the limbs (Bobath and Bobath 1955). Gesell describes progression through the early postural reflexes thus:

> At 20 weeks the supine infant can roll over on his side by rotating the upper portion of the body and then flexing the hips and throwing the legs to that side (segmental rolling reflex). This accomplishment represents the first gross shift in body posture. At 28 weeks, the child can attain a crawling position (full arm extension and amphibian reflex) and sustain the weight of the upper portion of the body by one or both arms. He can bring one knee forward beside the trunk but cannot raise his abdomen. Locomotion begins at about 32 weeks. The child pivots about by means of his arms. He succeeds in raising himself to the crawling position at 36 weeks (symmetrical tonic neck reflex) but cannot progress on his hands and knees until 44 weeks. It is at this stage that the contralateral arm and leg movements begin. (Gesell 1947)

The STNR seems to divide the effect of the TLR at the pelvis for a short period of time – just long enough to allow the infant to defy gravity, adopt the quadruped position and learn how to use the upper and lower sections of the body independently. However, locomotion in both the quadruped and biped positions involves synchrony between the upper and lower sections of the body and it is thought that the rocking motion used by many infants just before they learn how to creep on hands and knees helps to integrate the STNR, synchronise functioning of the sacral and occipital areas and enable the child to move on to the next stage of creeping.

Children who retain the SNTR may omit the stage of creeping on hands and knees. They may 'bear walk' on their hands and feet, shuffle on their bottoms or simply pull themselves up to standing and walk. Those who do creep may do so in an unusual fashion: the hands may be rotated outwards to lock the elbows and/or the feet may be raised. In this way, the child still learns to creep but with the STNR imprinted into the creeping pattern and experience, resulting in an unsynchronised pattern, since the timing of movements in the upper and lower sections of the body do not quite match.

There can be many reasons, environmental, developmental and neurological, why a child does not creep. One girl who had been adopted at three years of age had suffered severe environmental deprivation in the first three years of life. She had neither space nor opportunity to crawl. When asked to creep as part of a neurodevelopmental assessment at seven years of age, she did so with her hands rotated to the 6 o'clock position and her feet up in the air. She also had a retained STNR.

Similarly, children who have had little opportunity to play on the floor in the first eight months of life may bypass the developmental stages of crawling and creeping because they have not had sufficient time and experience to develop motor skills in the prone position, which help to develop head and upper trunk strength from the prone position and precede the ability to creep. Others may have been provided with more interesting cognitive entertainment such as an iPad while seated in a baby chair and the cognitive stimulation will have detracted from time spent exploring movement experience.

Blythe suggested that the symmetrical tonic neck reflex (STNR) helps to complete a sequence of eye training.[10] Bending of the legs as a result of head extension encourages the infant to fixate their eyes at far distance. Bending of the arms in response to flexion of the head will encourage a return to focus at near distance, thus training the eyes to adjust between far and near distance.[11] The ATNR begins by extending the baby's ability to focus from about 17cm (7in) at birth to arm's length on either side. As the ATNR is being inhibited in the first six months of age, visual acuity is extended to distant objects. The STNR then brings the vision back to near distance once more, improving visual accommodation or fusional reserve. It remains for the process of creeping on hands and knees to further develop the visual skills the infant has learned so far and to integrate them with information from other senses.

Creeping is one of the most important movement patterns in the prolonged process of teaching the eyes to cross the midline. In addition to looking ahead, babies also learn eye–hand coordination from following movement of the hands with the eyes. At times, the eyes focus from one hand to another, the hands acting as moving stimuli. This occurs at the same relative visual distance a child will use to read and write a few years later on. This ability will be essential to the ability to read without losing the words in the middle of the line and to visually follow the moving hand when writing. It is also through creeping that the vestibular, proprioceptive and visual systems connect to operate together for the first time in a new relationship with gravity. This period of development and locomotion coincide with the development of depth perception.

The 'visual cliff' is a test given to infants to see if they have developed depth perception. A platform is covered with a cloth and then a solid piece of transparent material is placed on top of the platform and extends beyond the platform to form a bridge. An infant is placed on the platform with their mother standing on the other end of the clear bridge. The mother encourages the infant to come towards her. If the child crawls off the platform on to the clear bridge, they do not yet have depth perception. If they stop when they get to the edge of the platform, look down and either are reluctant to cross or refuse to cross, then the child has depth perception.

In an article on how crawling and walking infants see the world differently, Kretch and colleagues explain how locomotor development affects opportunities for learning. Here, the term 'crawling' refers to creeping on hands and knees.

> The onset of crawling is a major milestone, and crawling experience facilitates psychological advances. Crawling allows self-initiated access to the larger world (Campos et al., 2000; E. J. Gibson, 1988; Piaget, 1954), which is linked with improvements in cognitive skills such as spatial search (Horobin & Acredolo, 1986; Kermoian & Campos, 1988), position constancy (Bai & Bertenthal, 1992; Bertenthal, Campos & Barrett, 1984), optic flow perception (Anderson et al., 2001; Higgins, Campos, & Kermoian, 1996; Uchiyama et al., 2008), and memory retrieval (Herbert, Gross, & Hayne, 2007). The changes brought about by independent mobility also have implications for social development: Crawlers display more attachment behaviours and are more adept at following a gaze/pointing gesture than pre-crawlers. (Kretch et al., 2014)

When comparing crawlers and walkers the researchers also found that crawling infants could see the floor ahead of their hands whereas walkers could not see the floor in front of their feet. Crawlers therefore had an advantage in planning movements ahead and avoiding obstacles. Rosanne Kermoian and her colleagues conducted a study at Reed College in 1988 and found that many cognitive skills, such as object permanence and space perception, are learned during the creeping period – and not until then.

Pavlides and Miles (1987) observed that a high percentage of children with reading difficulties had omitted the stages of crawling and creeping in infancy. Here it should be stressed that when a child does not crawl or creep in infancy it does not follow that they will go on to develop specific learning difficulties. Neither can it be claimed that all children with specific learning difficulties failed to crawl or creep in earlier life. What can be said is that there is a high coincidence of these groups, that some of the 'higher' cognitive perceptual skills needed to support reading and writing tend to be immature. Crawling and creeping are thought to be instrumental in helping some of these skills to develop through the process of quadruped locomotion, during which aspects of hand–eye coordination and visual accommodation are entrained.

Studies of the Xinguana Indians have revealed that they, like people of other tribal cultures, possess remarkable visual acuity at far distance but have not developed a written language of their own. The Xinguana can fire a dart from a blowpipe with deadly accuracy over several hundred metres, but they cannot read or write. In the jungle terrain in which they live, the children spend most of their first year carried upon their mother's body. The ground is fraught with danger from poisonous insects, snakes and plants. Consequently, the children are never allowed to learn to crawl or to creep on the ground. Following his observations of the Xinguana's way of life, Veras remarked:

> And since that time, we've been around the world and have yet to find a truly primitive people who permit their babies to be on the ground... Not only is creeping an important level of development in a child's mobility, it is also terribly important in the child's visual development. In all the primitive people we have seen, the children are never allowed to creep, and none of them can focus their eyes on anything closer than arm's length. They are all far sighted. We believe that when a child creeps, his near-point vision is developed. (Veras 1975)

Anecdotal information from other sources also suggests that physical experience in the first year of life may influence the development of visual skills and visual perception. I once heard a vision therapist from South Africa describe how infants tend to be carried on the mother's back in the first year of life. This restricts central vision ahead but allows plenty of scope for developing peripheral vision. It was her contention that this had an influence on visual attention later on, attention being more easily drawn to peripheral visual stimuli at the expense of being able to maintain visual attention on central stimuli. In theory, this could affect skills like visual attention when driving.

Bein-Wierzbinski (2001), using an infrared computerised eye-tracking machine, found the STNR to be a factor in a group of children tested for aberrant eye movements. She found that whereas other reflexes were associated with difficulty with horizontal tracking, the STNR was linked to problems with vertical tracking. After a reflex stimulation/inhibition programme had been followed, control of eye movements generally improved markedly as the reflexes matured and improvements in vertical eye tracking movements correlated with inhibition of the STNR. Vertical tracking is necessary to align columns correctly when one is carrying out arithmetical calculations.

In the older child, the influence of the STNR may be seen in a stooped posture, severe slouching, or bending of the arms when sitting at a desk, since bending the head to look down will cause the arms to bend or collapse. This is the child who ends the lesson almost lying on the desk in order to write.

A child with an STNR may be a clumsy child who has difficulty coordinating hand and eye movements, dreads physical education classes and is a disaster at ball games. They may lose sight of the ball in motion and by the time they have perceived it at near distance again it is too late to hit or to catch it with any degree of accuracy. Basic skills such as eating may be messy, since the hand never quite seems to be in the right place to find the mouth. Posture at the table, also, will be poor. (The latter is something that often returns in old age when there is either structural or functional degeneration. As eyesight, posture and/or functioning of the nervous system decline, the STNR, as one of the latest early reflexes to be inhibited, may be the first to be disinhibited.)

In a study carried out by Miriam Bender (1976), a retained STNR was found to be present in 75 per cent of a group of learning-disabled children who were compared with a similar group with no learning disabilities. At the Bender Institute, O'Dell and Cook (1996) found a retained STNR to be a significant factor in children with attention deficit disorder (ADD) and attention deficit hyperactive disorder (ADHD). Both groups improved markedly when the STNR was inhibited as a result of a specific movement programme.

Symptoms suggestive of a strongly residual STNR:

- poor posture
- tendency to slump when sitting, particularly at a desk or table
- simian walk
- 'W' leg position when sitting on the floor
- poor hand–eye coordination resulting in 'messy eater' and/or 'clumsy child' syndrome
- difficulties with readjustment of binocular vision (cannot change focus easily from whiteboard to desk)
- slowness in copying tasks
- difficulty learning to swim, or unsynchronised movements when swimming at the surface (often children with a retained STNR swim better underwater, where the effect of gravity is reduced and the weight of the water keeps the body level)
- attention loss owing to discomfort sitting in one position

Summary

Primitive reflexes are a particular type of reflex that emerge during life in the womb, are fully developed at the time of birth in a healthy baby born at full term and are inhibited by higher centres in the developing brain in the first six months of life.

Chapter 2

From Primitive Reflex to Postural Control

If it is the primitive reflexes that lay the foundations for later functioning, then it is the postural reflexes that provide the support for other systems to operate efficiently. The transition from primitive reflex reaction to postural control is not an automatic one. There are no set times at which the later reflex asserts control over the earlier one; there is a gradual process of interplay and integration during which several reflexes operate together for a short period of time.

Investigation of postural mechanisms began as early as 1824 when Flourens noted disturbances of movement and posture in a pigeon when its vestibular canals were destroyed. Postural reflexes provide the basis for the development of a repertoire of voluntary movements and adaptive responses at a subcortical (subconscious) level to be called upon at any time in response to changes in position or the environment.

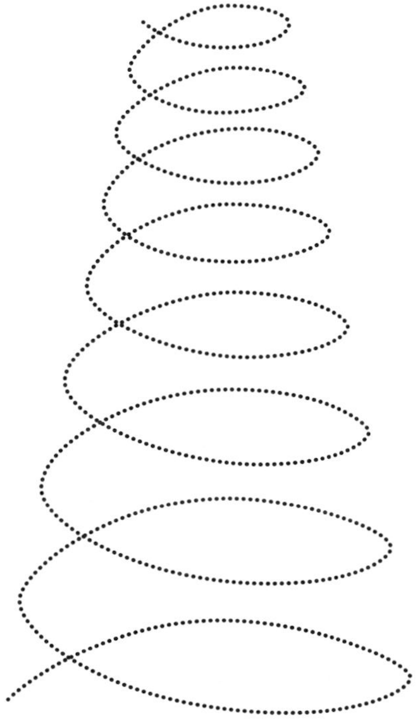

Figure 2.1:
Interweaving spiral illustrating relationship between primitive and postural reflexes in the first year(s) of life.

This period of growth, change and elaboration operates rather like an interweaving spiral (Figure 2.1) through which nature ensures that primitive survival patterns are still accessible until such time as more mature postural reactions are in place.

As certain movement sequences are practised over and over again, more mature patterns of response can supersede primitive reflexive response. Postural reflexes may better be described as movement and stabilisation reactions. They are those reflexes that provide the basis for the development of voluntary movements and adaptive responses that should be available at a subcortical (subconscious) level at any time in response to positional or environmental change.

The postural reflexes

Postural reflexes with one exception are mediated from the level of the midbrain. Their appearance signifies the active involvement of higher brain structures over brainstem activity and is a sign of increased maturity in the central nervous system. Some postural reactions are educationally significant; others are more important to facilitate fluency of movement and adaptive responses. They comprise two groups categorised by Fiorentino (1981) as:

- righting reflexes (quadruped)
- equilibrium reactions (bipedal)

Both are concerned with posture, movement and stability. The righting reactions emerge at three to twelve months and should remain present throughout life until disease or old age intervenes. They enable the child to adjust and maintain their head and trunk in a specific position when the body position is altered in any way. Their emergence facilitates movement through rolling, crawling and creeping and later will support the stability and fluency of coordinated gross motor movements. Movements made as a result of reflex actions help to myelinise the neural pathways involved in a way similar to laying down the core of a road network. Reflex actions are only the outline; subsequent development and experience extend, elaborate and refine the network.

Righting reactions consist of the oculo-head-righting reflex, the labyrinthine head-righting reflex, the amphibian reflex, Landau reflex and segmental rolling reflexes.

Postural control and the coordination of movement

Mature or conscious postural control is initiated in the motor cortex but is dependent upon lower centres to coordinate and execute those movements in various stages of complexity.

Starting from the lowest level:

1. Spinal level – comprises simple reactions controlled only by nerve cells in the spinal cord which ensure that, as one group of muscles contract, the opposing set relaxes.
2. Brainstem and midbrain – act to keep muscles in a state of readiness maintaining muscle tone. The primitive and postural reflexes are mediated at the levels of the brainstem and midbrain.
3. Basal ganglia and thalamus – coordinate each movement in cooperation with the cerebellum. The cerebellum then regulates and fine-tunes the progress of coordinated actions.
4. Cerebellum – ultimately responsible for regulating the postural reflexes (Bloedel and Brachfa 1997). Holt (1991) suggested that the cerebellum depends upon the postural reflexes to make fine motor skills automatic (Figure 2.2).

Equilibrium reactions do not appear until connections to the cortex are more firmly established. They first become evident at approximately three to six months of age and persist throughout adult life. They comprise the protection and tilting reactions that are elicited if balance is lost or the centre of gravity is altered. They include the startle (also known as 'Strauss') reflex and the parachute reflex.

It used to be thought that, educationally, equilibrium reactions are not of immediate significance and that absence of equilibrium reactions simply provided an indication of immaturity in the functioning of the central nervous system. The impact of underdeveloped equilibrium reactions was more likely to affect general coordination and social skills based on body awareness. This is because the child can appear clumsy and uncoordinated; the body language they communicate to others can bring teasing and result in the child feeling isolated from the group. Organisational skills could also suffer, because when

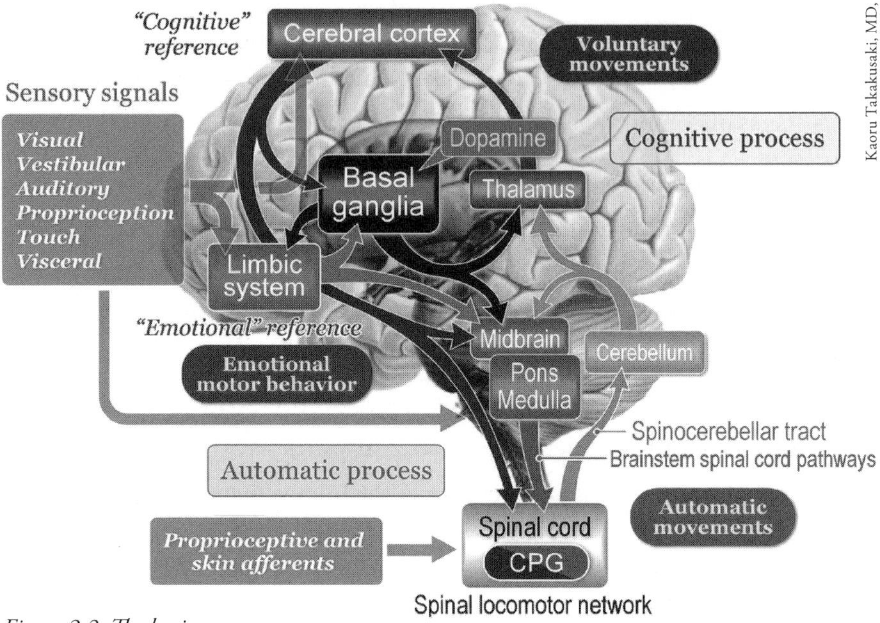

Kaoru Takakusaki, MD, PhD
Functional Neuroanatomy for Posture and Gait Control

Figure 2.2: The brain.

balance is impaired resultant disorientation can interfere with spatial awareness, processing of external sensory stimuli, and concentration.

More recently, the significance of both the Strauss and parachute reflexes has become of interest in relation to startle reactions and anxiety. This is because the parachute reflex provides a defence when there is loss of balance. Loss of balance elicits a startle reaction (Strauss reflex); if the parachute reaction is not available, then the system will access a less mature startle reaction – theoretically, the Moro reflex, although it is possible that an even more primitive reaction may be elicited. This profile has implications for adults presenting with anxiety disorders when insecure control of balance as an underlying factor has been neither investigated nor identified as a possible precondition.

Startle patterns

The Strauss or adult startle reflex develops as the Moro reflex is inhibited at about four months of age. The child tenses their muscles, blinks, uses their senses to scan the environment to seek out the source of potential danger and then makes a cortical (conscious) decision about how to react. This mature startle response may be seen as the result of the completion of three developmental stages:

Withdrawal reaction

This is thought to be a vestige of a very early startle reaction, which is active before the developing embryo has any means of defending itself.

> Sensori-motor behaviour begins a long time before birth. Initially the muscle fibres develop separately from the nervous system. At about 7½ weeks these muscles begin to come under the influence of the nervous system through the formation of the earliest crude reflex arcs. (Galley and Forster 1987)

These authors go on to describe how:

> The motor response at this stage is a crude mass movement of the head, neck and trunk away from the stimulus. One week later, when more reflex arcs have been formed, more areas of the body join in this mass response. Only when the structures involved have undergone a period of further maturation will these movements become more differentiated.

By 13–14 weeks, the foetus can turn with his head and lip movements towards the stimulus rather than withdrawing from it.

Reflexes that produce a response to tactile stimuli are the first to develop prenatally, starting in the oral region between five and seven-and-a-half weeks after conception. As described above, these oro-facial cutaneaous reflexes are characterised by a withdrawal reaction and it is thought that this early, crude withdrawal may be linked to later, more complex reflexes, including the fear paralysis reflex (FPR).

The FPR exists throughout the animal kingdom and results in an immediate shutdown or shock reaction characterised by immobility, slowing of the heart rate, change in blood pressure, cessation of breathing, a highly alert cortical state and extreme fear. A similar response can be seen in animals such as rabbits who freeze in one position when startled and remain motionless until the threat is removed. Although this response may aid survival in the animal kingdom, where immobility and suppression of metabolic activity make prey less detectable to predators (feigned death), it is not an effective adaptative response to everyday human social situations or to the modern technological world.

It has been hypothesised that the FPR, as described by Kaada (1986), may have its developmental origins in this early withdrawal response (Goddard 1989a; 1989b). Kaada suggested that the FPR may be linked to the mammalian diving reflex and that the associated cortico-electrical activity in the brain observed when the FPR is activated resembled brainwave states seen in rapid eye movement (REM) sleep and sleep paralysis.

Paradoxical sleep, also known as 'REM sleep', is a distinct phase of sleep during which there are bursts of nerve impulse activity from the brainstem and intense activity in the forebrain and midbrain. It is characterised by dreaming (visualisation) and the absence of motor function with the exception of the eye muscles and diaphragm. This lack of motor function and the accompanying low muscle tone probably enable us to travel in our dreams without physically acting out the content of our dreams. Sleep disorders such as bedwetting and sleepwalking occur during non-REM or slow wave sleep (SWS), when muscle tone is present.

Sleep paralysis occurs when a person awakens without first emerging through several stages of sleep. Simply put, the conscious brain is awake before muscle tone is restored and so the person is unable to move. Although this state usually only lasts for a few seconds, it can be associated with extreme fear. Kaada (1986) described one of the characteristics of induction of the FPR as:

> A condition of helplessness and hopelessness; there is no solution available, the animal is in an inescapable, overwhelming situation with which it is unable to cope.

Activation of the diving reflex results in immediate slowing down of the heart rate (bradycardia) and is thought to be a physiologically protective oxygen-conserving mechanism that keeps the animal alive during submergence by slowing down the metabolism and, in so doing, protects the brain from the deleterious effects of oxygen deprivation. Landsberg (1975) suggested that the diving reflex could act as either an oxygen-conserving mechanism or the start of a pathophysiological asphyxial response. In other words, if it is activated for too long the results may be fatal. Kaada suggested that this might be an important factor in SIDS.

Although the link between these reflexes, which have a temporary life-preserving function in extreme situations in later life, and the earliest withdrawal reactions seen in the embryo has not been proven, an oversensitive withdrawal reaction is a characteristic of a number of disorders and may play a part in the presentation of symptoms in some cases of selective mutism, post-traumatic stress disorder (PTSD), stage fright, autistic spectrum disorder (ASD), panic attacks and agoraphobia. In PTSD this may result from extreme threat and/or a prolonged situation of hopelessness and helplessness, in which this atavistic reflex can continue to be triggered by environmental and psychological events and memories long after the period of trauma has passed. Similarly, children who have suffered extreme neglect or abuse in early childhood before expressive verbal language developed may continue to react with an FPR to stimuli or events that remind them of the original trauma. In ASD, hypersensitivity in one or several sensory systems may act as a catalyst. Panic attacks and agoraphobia may develop for a number of reasons, but Kaada linked his work on the FPR to observations made by Klein suggesting that:

> Panic attacks in agoraphobia and panic disorders in adults, which like the fear paralysis and sudden infant death syndrome (SIDS) are, in part, genetically determined (Torgerson 1983), are due to having too low a threshold for the release of an innate built-in separation fear mechanism. (Klein 1980)

In these examples environmental triggers or memory (in addition to immediate environmental stimuli) can elicit a deep-seated freeze response in the absence of a real and present threat to life. It is also possible that under extreme and prolonged situations of hopelessness and helplessness, such as hostage-taking, torture and incarceration, volitional use of the FPR, which is also associated with activation of pain-suppressing mechanisms, may help the victim to access a physical and psychological space in which they can temporarily disassociate from reality. If this defence mechanism becomes too well developed, it can continue to obstruct recovery long after the original trauma has passed. In other words, the body has a memory and, even though cognitive centres in the brain have a strong desire to recover, feelings can continue to elicit a response that has long since become maladaptive.

It was just such a situation that led a therapist working at a torture and trauma recovery unit to seek out the INPP method in the 1990s. His hypothesis was that if the body continues to utilise reactions developed in response to trauma, then cognitive and psychological methods alone will not be enough to bring about recovery. It will also be necessary to work with the body.

If this were the case in early development, then it would be essential for nature to have installed an accessible reverse or 'override' mechanism. This appears to be one of the functions of the Moro reflex. Whereas the characteristic of the withdrawal reaction is to shrink away from the stimulus and slow down the metabolism, the Moro reflex activates the sympathetic division of the autonomic nervous system, which results in immediate arousal (Figure 2.3).

When fully developed, the Moro reflex belongs to the group of reflexes whose characteristic is to clasp or to embrace (rooting, suck, palmar and plantar reflexes). It develops gradually, comprising two stages: the first part emerges nine to twelve weeks after conception and consists of movement of the arms and legs outwards (abduction) and extension of the head with momentary freeze (a withdrawal response); after birth, it is accompanied by an intake of breath and arousal. It is only as the second part of the Moro reflex is developed (by 32 weeks after conception) that withdrawal is overcome by closing the arms and legs (adduction), flexion of the head and, after birth, release of breath. The hypothesis mooted was that a full Moro reflex is necessary in the first months of life to inhibit and integrate the previous withdrawal response and protect the infant from an overactive withdrawal reaction to non-threatening startling situations (Goddard 1989; 1990).

If the earlier reflex remains overreactive, then the reflexes can, in theory, operate in a reverse chain reaction, placing the infant at risk, rather than protecting it from noxious stimuli. The withdrawal, Moro and mature startle (Strauss) reactions thus have the potential to operate in either direction in a chain response. If the more mature response is fully developed, it should act as the primary responding mechanism and thereby prevent the initiation of the more primitive responses; in other words, a higher, more adaptive protective system of response is in control. However, the Moro reflex is sensitive to vestibular stimulation and the Strauss reflex works in cooperation with more

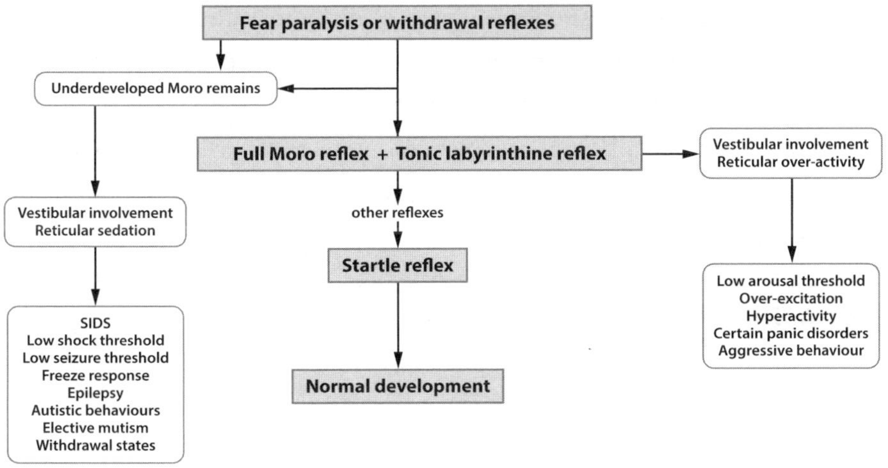

Figure 2.3: Model showing different pathways probably involved in activation of the fear paralysis and Moro reflexes.

mature reactions involved in postural control; immature postural control could therefore, in theory, undermine the mature startle response and result in a more primitive startle reaction to destabilisation of balance or posture.

Moro reflex

This is a primitive overreaction to startlement, which results in stimulation of the sympathetic nervous system – arousal, increase in heart rate, immediate rise in blood pressure, rapid shallow breathing, and flushing of the face, accompanied by anger or distress.

Strauss reflex

The adult startle reflex emerges alongside the development of postural control. It was described by Strauss in 1929 as:

> … flexion of the legs and trunk, forward flexion of the head, raising and forward movement of the shoulders, forward raising and inward turning of the arms, pronation of the forearms, closing of the hands, lid blinking, facial grimacing and contraction of the abdominal muscles.

It should develop at about four months of age as the Moro reflex is inhibited, although for a time the two reactions may coexist. It is thought that cortical analysis of the required response is involved in the mature startle pattern but is not a feature of the Moro reflex reaction. Hence, the individual with a Moro reflex tends to react first when it is elicited and then think afterwards.

Even in adults, all responses remain potentially available, but, once inhibited, the earlier ones should lie dormant, only to be awakened in situations of extreme danger or complete helplessness or hopelessness.

Postural control

Postnatal motor development takes place in a cephalo-caudal (head to toe) and proximo-distal (centre-outward) sequence. The development of postural reflexes reflects this pattern. The first task a child must accomplish is mastery of head control and muscle tone, before further postural control and a full range of flexible, adaptive voluntary movements can be achieved. Control is gained in the prone position before the supine. By six weeks of age, the child can raise their head in line with their body when lying prone and can maintain the position for several seconds. By 12 weeks, they can lift their head well above the general body line and keep it there for several minutes. By 12 weeks, also, their legs are no longer flexed and their pelvis is flat on the surface when lying prone. By 16 weeks, the child can press down with their forearms to lift their head and upper torso, stretching their limbs and is able to made 'swimming"' movements in this position (Figure 2.4).

Righting reactions

Righting reactions to gravity result from somatosensory, visual and proprioceptive influences acting together when the three inputs are available and functioning appropriately (Figures 2.5 and 2.6). With the exception of the oculo-head-

Figure 2.4: 'Swimming' when supported in the prone position.

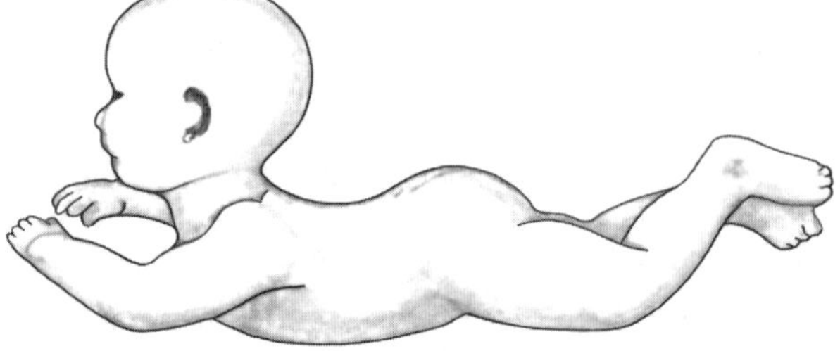

righting reflex, for the most part they are integrated in the nuclei of the midbrain.

This gradual sequence of head control in the first two to four months of life heralds the development of the oculo- and labyrinthine head-righting reflexes. Together these ensure that the head maintains a midline position (perpendicular to the ground when upright) despite movement of other parts of the body, whether actively or passively induced. In other words, the head makes an equal and opposite adjustment to the displacement of the body so that the head remains in a central position. The oculo-head-righting reflexes operate as a result of visual cues, while the labyrinthine head-righting reflexes depend upon vestibular input. The two should synchronise to supply accurate data upon which head position is adjusted. If they fail to develop fully, or only one develops adequately, balance, controlled eye movements and visual perception can all be impaired. This is because under optimum conditions the position of the head relative to the supporting base provides the vestibular system with a stable platform from which centres involved in the control of eye movements take their cue. If this reference point is level and stable, then eye movements are smooth and well controlled; if the platform is tilted or unstable, then control of eye movements may be affected. Madaule (1993) described the effects of

Figure 2.5:
Head lag in supine position at one month of age.

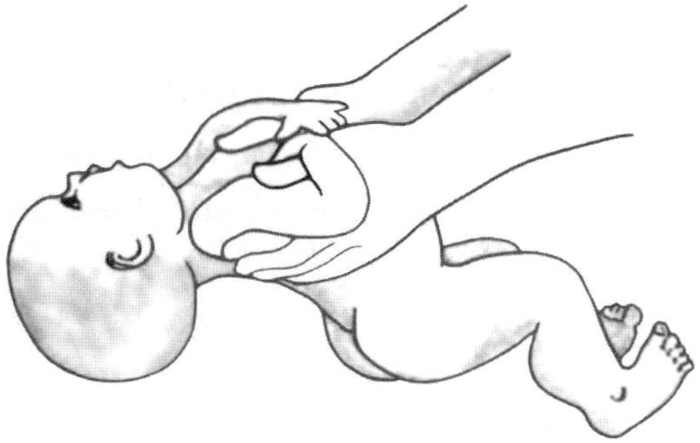

Figure 2.6:
Head control in line with the body at three months of age (supine).

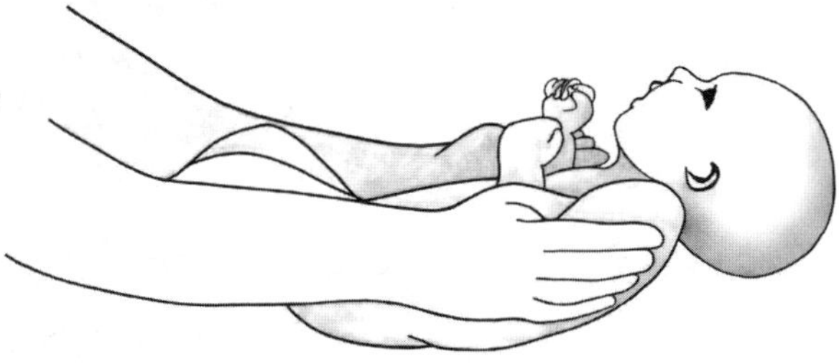

unstable eye movements on reading as being like trying to read while standing on the thwart of a small rowing boat on a choppy sea.

Muscle tension in the neck and shoulder region combined with poor posture may also be symptoms of underdeveloped head-righting reflexes, since the 44 pairs of muscles in the neck responsible for holding the head up have to work harder to maintain head control without the support of automatic righting reactions.

During normal development, there is a lag in attaining head control in the supine position, and so the infant will be approximately five months of age before they can raise their head and hold it for some time above the level of the spine in that position.

Labyrinthine head-righting reflex

The labyrinthine head-righting reflex is elicited by tilting of the body and/or stimulation of the otolithic organs in the inner ear. The reflex comprises compensatory contraction of the neck muscles to keep the head level. Normal position can be described as 'head vertical, mouth horizontal' (Crutchfield and Barnes 1993). This reflex is barely evident in the neonate but develops rapidly in the first weeks of life as neck muscles strengthen and the relative size of the head in relation to the body decreases. The ability to begin to right the head develops from two months of age.

Oculo-head-righting reflex

The oculo-head-righting reflex is initiated by visual cues and is dependent upon the functioning of the cerebral cortex. It maintains the head in a stable position

Figure 2.7: Head-righting

a) Body moves back, neck extends and head moves forwards

b) Body moves forwards and head tilts back

c) Side to side

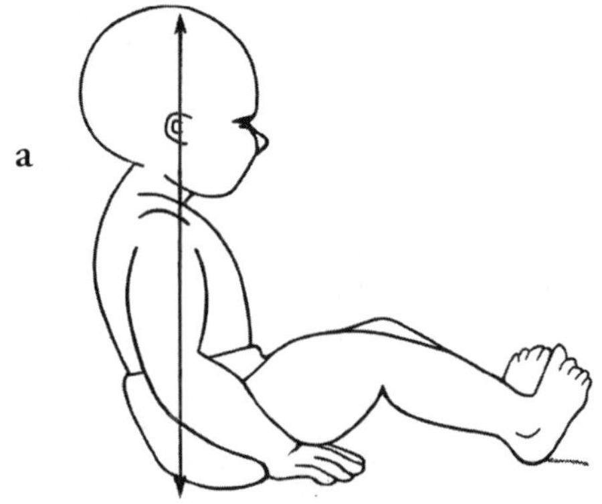

and the eyes fixed on visual targets despite other movements of the body. This is necessary for visual fixation and sustained visual attention. The oculo-head-righting reflex may also be elicited by a combination of visual and vestibular stimulation, stretching of the neck muscles and/or movement of visual images on the retina.

In normal development, the visual abilities to fixate and to follow are enhanced as stability of head posture is achieved. If oculo-head-righting reflexes are underdeveloped, visual fixation and visual pursuit can be impaired. This can then affect reading ability, reading comprehension and spelling (Figure 2.7).

Landau reflex

The Landau reflex has a relatively short lifespan, emerging around three months of age, reaching its peak at about five to six months as the head-righting reflexes are becoming established and being inhibited by the age of approximately three-and-a-half years. The Landau reflex elicits extensor tone throughout the body in the prone position if the child is suspended in the air with support under the abdomen.

Development of the Landau reflex helps to increase muscle tone when prone (Figure 2.8). Simultaneously it acts as an inhibitory influence upon the TLR in flexion, increasing head-righting reactions and muscle tone in the torso. It enables the child to elevate not only the head but also the chest and is an important prerequisite for more advanced movements involving the arms and hands in the prone position later on. At three-and-a-half years of age, by which time the child should be secure as a mobile biped, the Landau reflex should no longer be necessary. Its continued presence in later life suggests

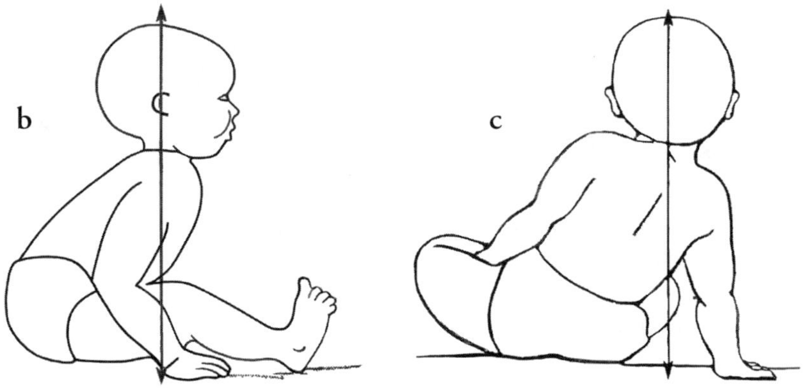

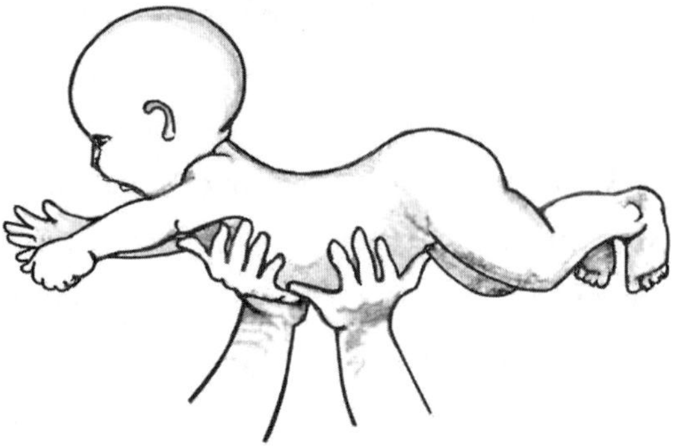

Figure 2.8: Landau reflex.

underlying primitive reflex activity, particularly retention of the TLR, and will affect development of balance and of voluntary alteration of muscle tone in rapidly changing conditions – for example, a child may run with stiff awkward movement in the lower half of the body and find hopping, skipping and jumping difficult because they cannot easily flex the leg muscles if the head is extended.

Neither the Landau nor the STNR is a true primitive or postural reflex in the theoretical sense. The Landau reflex is not present at birth and therefore cannot be categorised as primitive. Neither remains present for the rest of life and therefore neither is a true postural reflex. Both seem to act as important bridge reflexes that have an inhibitory effect upon the TLR, help to integrate the transition from some primitive reflexes to postural reactions, strengthen muscle tone and assist in supporting the development of vestibular–ocular motor skills.

Figure 2.9: Amphibian reflex in prone position.

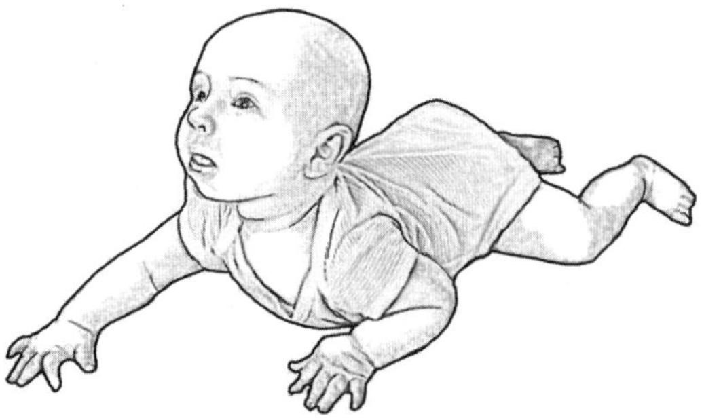

Figure 2.10: The four quadrants of the body: Upper/Lower/Left/Right.

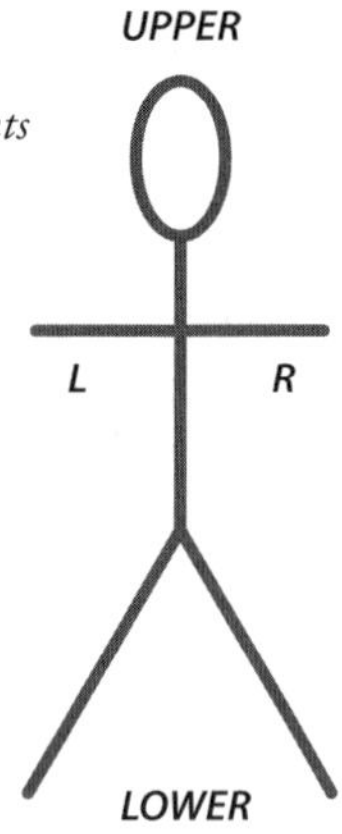

Amphibian reflex

The amphibian reflex develops between four and six months of life, first when prone, then when supine. Elevation of the pelvis elicits automatic flexion from the hip to affect the knee on the same side (Figures 2.9).

Flexion of one leg irrespective of head position permits an increase in mobility and marks an important stage for the development of crawling on the tummy. Hitherto, flexion or extension of the legs bilaterally has been influenced by head position and by the activities of the ATNR and TLR. The amphibian reflex denotes significant inhibition of the ATNR and partial integration of the TLR. Freedom from these constraints permits the independent movement of the legs and arms which is essential for crawling, creeping and gross muscle coordination later on and enables the child to move one quadrant of the body independently of the other three (Figure 2.10).

An underdeveloped amphibian reflex in the prone position will impede cross-pattern crawling and may contribute to hypertonus in later life, interfering with activities dependent upon gross muscle coordination, such as in physical education and sports.

Segmental rolling reflexes

The segmental rolling reflexes are a later modification of the 'neck on body and body-righting reactions'. Whereas the neck and body-righting reactions align the trunk with the head when either is rotated or turned, the segmental rolling reflexes are strictly rotational responses – 'one part of the body initiates the rotation and other parts follow in a segmental fashion' (Crutchfield and Barnes 1993). When well developed, this facilitates maximal performance with minimal effort as one part of the body initiates movement and the other segments follow through sequentially.

The earlier neck-on-body-righting reactions act if the head is righted but the body is tilted out of alignment. This results in the thorax righting and initiates a wave of stretch reflexes that pass down the body, righting the abdomen and the legs.

The body-on-body-righting reaction occurs if the infant is laid on their side and pressure is applied to the side of the body. This initiates reflex righting of the body (even if the labyrinths have been destroyed). If the head is turned, the body will follow in line with the head in a 'log roll'.

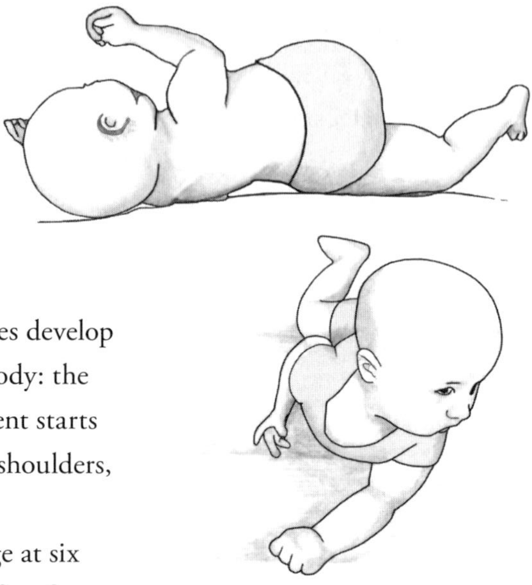

The segmental rolling reflexes develop from two key positions in the body: the shoulders and the hips. Movement starts at the head, then follows to the shoulders, thorax and pelvis, or vice versa.

These reflexes start to emerge at six months of age to allow rolling, first from supine to prone at six months, then from prone to supine at eight to ten months, followed by sitting, four-point kneeling and eventually standing. As the child becomes practised and adept at these activities, the reflex becomes redundant for progress from lying to standing, but should be accessible through life to facilitate changing positions and to give fluidity to movements such as running, jumping, downhill skiing, etc. (Figure 2.11).

Figure 2.11: Segmental rolling reflex:
a) Supine to prone;
b) Prone to supine.

Equilibrium reactions

The establishment of postural righting reactions is only the beginning of postural control. Once the righting reactions are operating, equilibrium reactions start to develop from about nine months of age. Equilibrium reactions are elicited by stimulation of the labyrinths; they are compensatory in nature in response to changes in the centre of gravity and should become available to modify the patterns of righting reactions.

Equilibrium reactions are primarily protective in nature; they occur in response to a sudden alteration in position or when balance is lost. They depend upon visual stimulation, and it has been suggested that they are linked to the mature startle or Strauss reflex (Fiorentino 1981).

The parachute reflex may be elicited if the infant is held in the air and then tilted forward towards the ground. The arms extend as if to protect the head and trunk from the full force of impact. If the infant is held upright and dropped rapidly towards the ground, the lower limbs first extend, then tense, then abduct. The reflex is a protective one.

At approximately six months of age, the sideways parachute or 'propping' reflex also emerges. This is essential if a child is to learn to sit, since it remedies any loss of balance in the sitting position through a compensatory movement of the arm on the side to which the child is falling, propping the trunk and preventing the infant from toppling over. This reflex should be present during the child's early attempts at standing, cruising and walking.

Equilibrium reactions affect our ability to maintain balance, particularly moving balance. They are necessary for a child to maintain control of movement while in action (running, jumping, hopping). Children who lack equilibrium reactions tend to be clumsy, to fall over more often than their peers and to have difficulty with movements that require sudden shifts in direction (Pyfer and Johnson 1981) (Figure 2.12).

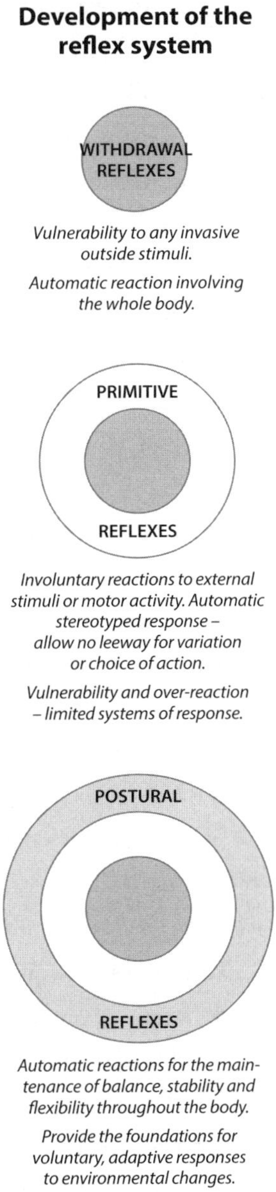

Figure 2.12: Development of the reflex system

Combined effects of immature reflexes

If a higher level of response is unavailable, an organism will respond regressively with the next most mature response it can muster. If, for example, a child has underdeveloped righting or equilibrium reactions, there is no effective mechanism to protect them against falling when balance is lost; loss of balance may then elicit the Moro reflex as the final defence available because the higher systems needed to maintain balance and postural control have failed. In this situation, the Moro reflex may persist because higher adaptive and protective systems are unavailable, rather than as the primary trigger mechanism. Under either condition, 'gravitational security' – A Jean Ayres's (1989) term to describe the sense of competence and confidence in a gravity-based environment – will be compromised.

Lack of gravitational security can result in generalised insecurity and greater susceptibility to anxiety – both often typical in children with coordination problems and poor postural control. The effect may also be seen in adolescents and adults who appear to have compensated for underlying postural problems but who start to experience emotional difficulties when placed under increased academic or emotional stress. These may be individuals who manifested learning-related problems for the first time only when they reached higher education, where the education system is less structured and greater flexibility in learning styles and a wider range of life skills are required.

Whereas there is documented evidence that retained primitive reflexes underlie difficulties in the learning of basic skills such as reading, writing and copying, less attention has been paid to the role of postural reflexes in providing a functional link between postural control, cognitive functioning and academic performance.

Lawrence J Beuret (2000), who worked in Chicago with adolescents and young adults who had neurodevelopmental problems, observed that members of this older age group (college students) sometimes present a profile in which the primitive reflexes have been inhibited but the postural reflexes have not developed fully (Beuret 2000). These individuals appear to have compensated well and therefore have not been diagnosed with a specific learning difficulty in childhood, issues only emerging relatively late in development – sometimes well into adolescence or beyond. They might have benefited from motor training or sensory integration intervention at an earlier age and often have slipped through the net of services that should have picked up a problem in the primary school years.

The specific symptoms this group shows are typically problems in:

- adaptation
- applying known concepts (problem-solving)
- linking
- multi-processing
- sequencing
- coping with large volumes of information (information overload)
- history of underachievement, 'could do better', often masked by studying hard and support such as tutoring
- unwillingness to engage in new tasks or challenges

All of the above are skills that become essential at higher levels of education.

Additional related problems in this older age group may include:

- history of fine motor disturbances
- low energy levels that mimic depression but do not respond to medication
- lack of torso flexibility (truncal integration)
- difficulty carrying out complex movement patterns such as those required in martial arts or dance routines (often they will comment on having to 'think through' each movement sequence and have difficulty adapting to rapid changes in routine)

The effect on a child of having underdeveloped postural reflexes is the environmental and social equivalent of having an underdeveloped vocabulary. Often an individual can cope as long as the rules remain the same and it is possible to use previously learned skills. If the rules required by a situation change, the child will have to 'learn and practise' the new rules because they are unable to adapt to meet the altered circumstances. This can result in feelings of personal and social awkwardness, a tendency to avoid activities that require immediate adaptation, and a greater propensity to suffer from 'overload' anxiety.

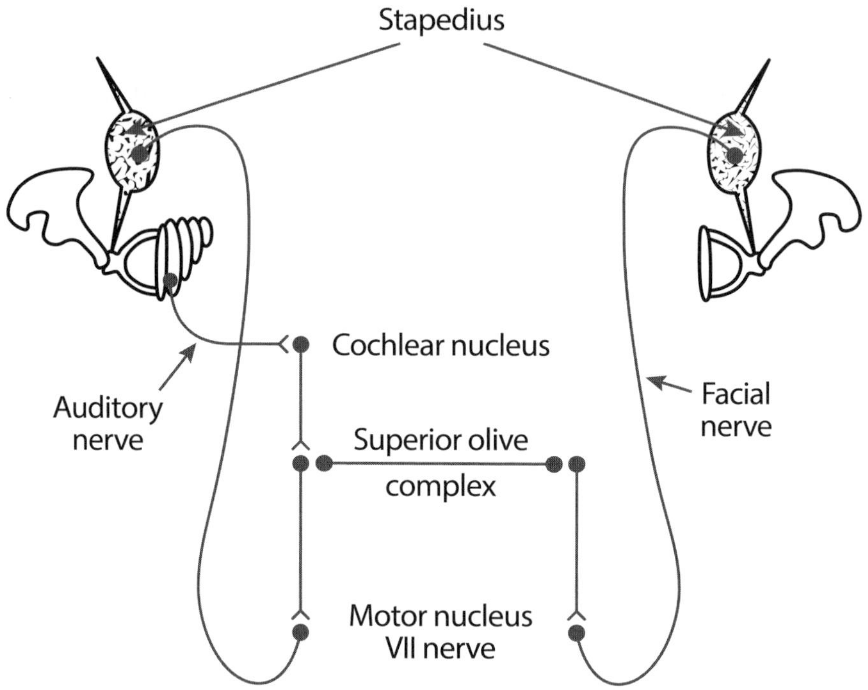

Figure 2.13: Mechanisms involved in the acoustic stapedius reflex.

Reflex maturation – a continuing process

There are many other reflexes, besides the postural reflexes outlined previously, that have an impact upon both motor and sensory functioning. One example of a later, non-postural reflex is the acoustic stapedius reflex. The stapedius muscle of the inner ear is attached to the stapes and is the smallest muscle in the human body. If there is a loud noise, the acoustic stapedius reflex should activate involuntary contraction of the stapedius muscle immediately after the sound (usually noises louder than 80–90 decibels [db]). The effect is to dampen the sound that is actually heard by as much as 20db or more, thereby protecting the inner ear from noise damage. The reflex should also occur just before a person vocalises, to reduce interference from the sound of one's own voice (Figure 2.13).

The acoustic stapedius reflex starts to operate between two and four months of age, at the same time as the Moro reflex is being inhibited. The hypersensitivity to sound observed in many children and adults who still have traces of a Moro reflex may be because the continued presence of the Moro reflex has prevented the acoustic stapedius reflex from developing fully. Equally, lack of an acoustic stapedius reflex might activate a Moro startle response because there is no adequate protection against loud noise. This may also be a factor in children who seem to be abnormally timid and avoid situations where there are loud noises. They hate balloons – they might pop – and detest fireworks. Often they talk as if they were afraid of their own voice. Certain methods of sound therapy can probably help to develop this reflex, which may be one reason why some autistic children respond well to AIT (see Chapter 4).

Reflexes and sensory processing cannot be separated. Figure 2.14 illustrates

Figure 2.14: Reflex connections to the sensory systems.

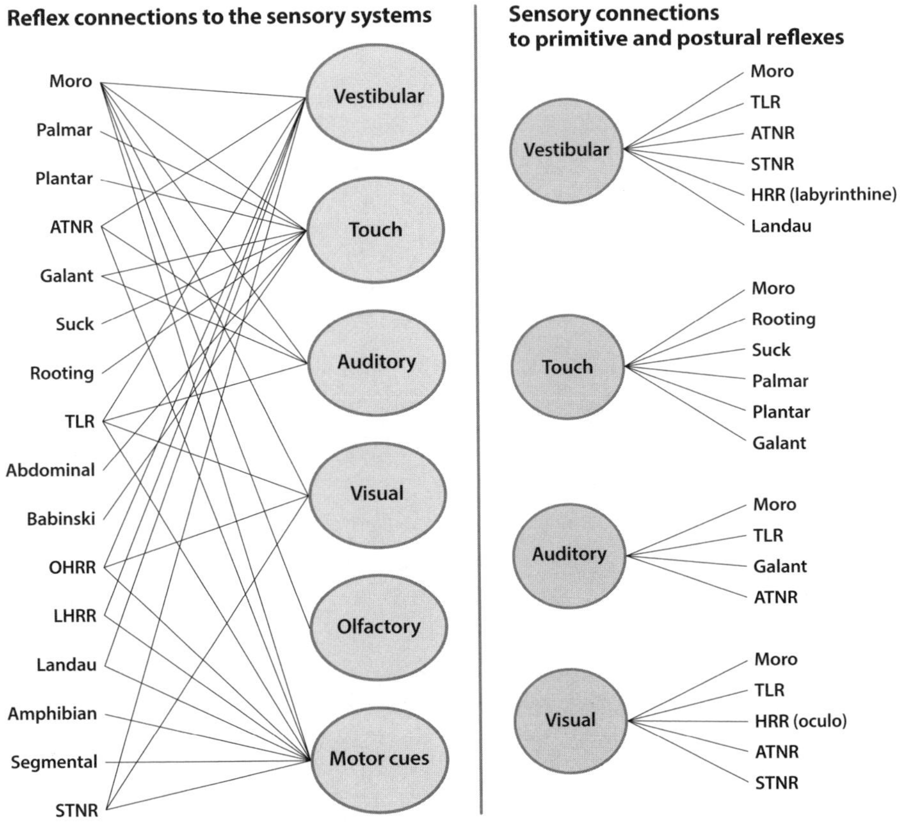

just some of the connections between primitive and postural reflexes and the senses.

In functional terms, the postural reflexes form part of a main highway of connections between the motor cortex and the muscles. If part of that highway is still under construction, it can interfere with the rapid flow of information along that route. Alternative routes are available, but these may not be as efficient or as direct as the main pathway.

Chapter 3

Brain Development

Absent or underdeveloped postural reflexes have long been accepted as contributory factors in coordination problems and associated disorders, such as dyspraxia, 'clumsy child' syndrome, and apraxia. With this in mind, motor-training programmes have been devised to encourage the development of postural reflexes to improve coordination and balance. Some of these, such as what became known as the Doman–Delacato programme, are based on the concept that brain organisation has an impact on learning problems and can be modified by repeating early developmental movements. In other words, just as the brain controls the body, so also can the body inform and entrain the brain.

Other techniques, such as those employed in sensory integration (Ayres 1989), are based upon the concept that stimulation of the postural reflexes through sensory–motor stimulation can encourage the development of more mature patterns of response and will also suppress underlying primitive reflex activity. General improvement in balance and coordination demonstrates the value of such programmes, particularly when postural reflexes are underdeveloped and primitive reflexes are largely inhibited.

However, if the primitive reflexes are still strongly active, stimulation of postural reflexes alone will rarely reap concomitant changes in the areas of fine muscle coordination, oculo-motor functioning, perceptual processing and academic performance. This may be because, although general motor-training programmes strengthen postural control and coordination, they fail to inhibit those retained primitive reflexes that continue to impede the processing of information in the brain. In order to understand why this may be the case, we need to examine some of the mechanisms in the brain and how they develop during the first year of life.

Establishing a hierarchy

The brain comprises many separate entities that are all interlinked and interdependent. At birth, connections to the superficial layers of the cortex are only tenuously made, but in the first few months and years of life the developing child must form millions of new connections between nerve cells. These connections will provide a network of communication or neural circuitry of almost unimaginable complexity upon which future behaviour and learning will be based. The layering of the connections between motor areas is sometimes viewed as a hierarchy of systems involving multiple levels of control.

Let us start from the lowest (most primitive) level.

Spinal level

Spinal mechanisms provide a point of contact between the nervous system and the muscles. Simple reflexive movements controlled only by nerve cells in the spinal cord ensure that as one group of muscles contract, the opposing set relax. An example of a simple tactile elicited reflex can be seen in the case of the sea slug, which reacts automatically with a withdrawal response if an unexpected blast of water is aimed at its abdominal cavity. Spinal reflexes can be modified by higher levels in the brain.

Brainstem

The brainstem is situated at the top of the spinal column and houses the nerve pathways that carry impulses between the brain and the body. It is part of the central nervous system and is responsible for the neurons that control heartbeat, blood pressure, breathing and also the signals to swallow, laugh, sneeze, etc. It constitutes a primitive structure shared by mammals, fish and reptiles. The function it fulfils is so fundamental that injury to the core of the brainstem results in death. The brainstem also contains the point at which the nerve tracts between brain and body cross over to the opposite side. The brainstem includes the pons and medulla oblongata. Primitive reflexes are mediated at the level of the brainstem, while the postural reflexes with the exception of the oculo-head-righting reflex are controlled from the midbrain.

Midbrain

The midbrain serves important functions in motor movement (mediation of several postural reflexes) as well as movements of the eye, and in auditory and visual processing.

Linked to the brainstem is the reticular formation, which is responsible for maintaining consciousness and arousal.

Reticular activating system

The reticular activating system (RAS) is the brain's own floodgate system for conducting sensory signals, either allowing them to pass through to alert higher brain systems or dampening the signals, according to the circumstances. It plays an important part in maintaining consciousness and in the regulation of the sleep–wake cycle and therefore also affects waking alertness and the ability to pay attention.

Both conscious and automatic control of the sensory motor system depend on the constant, though fluctuating, interactions between all the different centres – including the cerebellum – that comprise the central nervous system (Figure 3.1).

Figure 3.1: Hierarchical structure of the brain – areas involved in sensory, motor and hormonal functions.

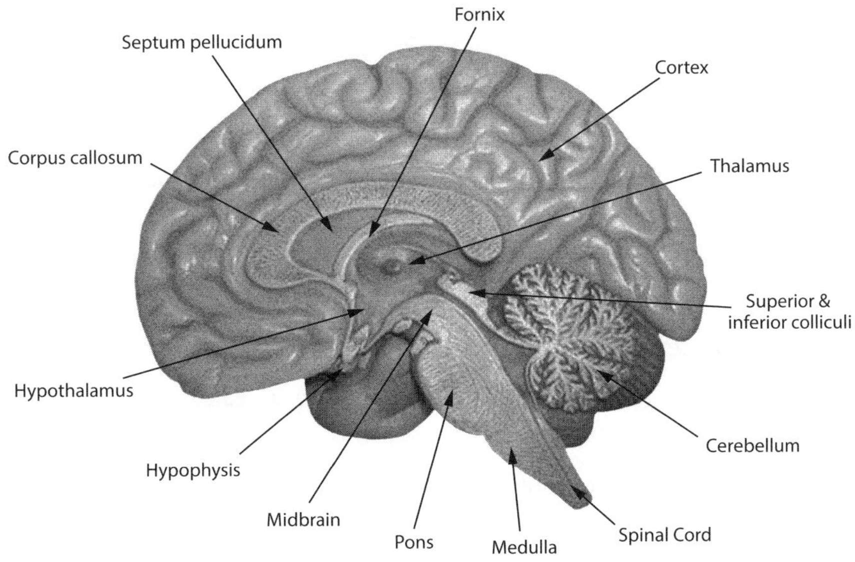

Thalamus

The thalamus is a twin-lobed mass of nerve cells at the top of the brainstem. It acts as an important relay station for sensory and motor fibres. It both sends and receives impulses from the cerebellum, reticular system, neural ganglia and the cortex. All of the senses, with the exception of smell, are filtered through the thalamus before they reach their specialised regions in the cortex, and it therefore plays a vital role in supplying information upon which the interpretation of sensory stimuli will depend.

Hypothalamus

The hypothalamus is situated slightly below the thalamus and acts as the synthesiser of the hormones involved in temperature control, water balance, hunger and sexual behaviour. These hormones are then funnelled into the pituitary gland, where they are stored or released into the bloodstream. These two centres together with the hippocampus and amygdala are labelled the seat of the 'limbic system', which man has in common with other mammals.

Limbic system

It is from the limbic system that feelings of passion, drive, fear, anger and grief are all generated. If the brainstem represents survival, then the midbrain and the limbic system represent what we call instinct and largely controls our metabolism, our feelings (physiological sensations of emotion) and our metabolic reactions to the outside world. The amygdalae comprise a pair of small almond-shaped regions deep in the brain which help to regulate emotion and encode memories – especially when it comes to more emotional memory.

Hippocampus

The hippocampus (named for its resemblance to a seahorse) is thought to be principally involved in storing long-term memories and in making those memories resistant to forgetting, though this is a matter of debate. It is also thought to play an important role in spatial processing and navigation. The limbic system as a whole is involved in the hormonal chemistry of laying down memories, which may be one reason why children seem to learn better when they relate physically and emotionally to the material. It is also why the memory of past traumatic events can reawaken the physical sensations of fear and distress associated with the original event.

Gaddes suggested that some behaviour results directly from reflexive or spontaneous stimulation of the hypothalamus and related structures, combined with inhibitory learned processes emanating from the cerebral cortex: 'Too much hypothalamic stimulation with too little cortical (or intellectual) control presumably results in the socially obnoxious child who disregards the rights and wishes of others. The reverse pattern may result in the overcontrolled, inhibited, unimaginative child' (Gaddes 1980). This sounds remarkably similar to the two profiles that are characteristic of the Moro-directed child described in Chapter 1.

Basal ganglia

The basal ganglia are a group of nuclei at the base of the cerebral cortex which help regulate body movements (Figure 3.2). The basal ganglia are responsible for the organisation of involuntary and semi-voluntary activity, upon which consciously willed movements are superimposed. They receive input from the cerebral cortex and then influence movement by affecting the output of the motor cortex. The basal ganglia and the cerebellum are involved in various aspects of planning and monitoring of movements but have no outputs of their own to the spinal cord. They are prominently involved in adjusting ongoing movements and should maintain the balance between inhibitory and facilitating influences. When a particular part of the basal ganglia (the striatum) is damaged, as occurs in Parkinson's disease, inhibition of involuntary movement is impaired and there is continuous tremor when the patient is at rest. In normal development, activities that at first need practice should eventually be absorbed into the automatic repertoire of the basal ganglia together with the cerebellum. Learning to play the piano, to drive a car or to ride a bicycle would fall into that category.

Cortical control

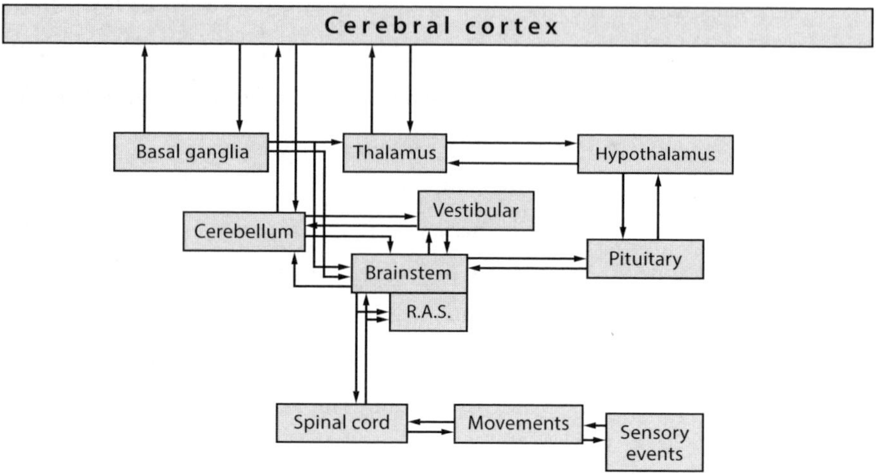

Figure 3.2: Functional links between cerebral cortex and lower brain centres involved in sensory, motor and hormonal response.

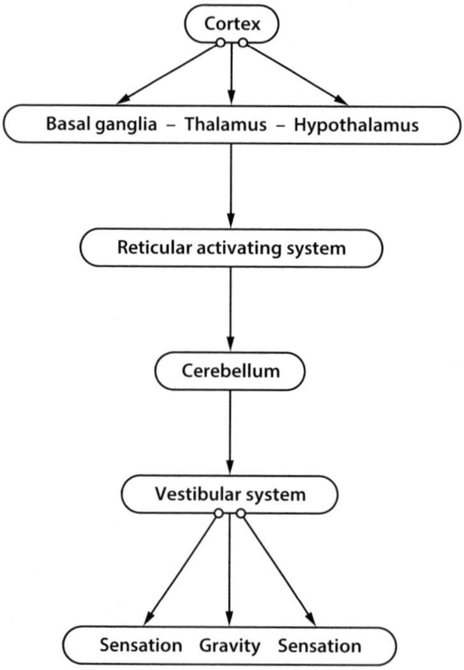

Figure 3.3: Major brain areas centres involved in postural control and arousal.

Cerebellum

Connected to the brainstem, but not a part of it, is the cerebellum. Its name means 'the little brain'. Whereas the cerebral cortex enables us to perform all the higher functions that are unique to humankind, the cerebellum governs the fine-tuning of our every movement (Figure 3.3). Although it can initiate nothing by itself, the cerebellum deals with impulses from the motor centres in the brain and from the nerve endings in the muscles. Incoming impulses outnumber efferent impulses three to one, for it is the cerebellum's job to sift and to fine-tune relevant information to refine motor output. Impulses to the cerebellum are directed from the vestibular system, the eyes and the muscle joints of the lower limbs and trunk (proprioceptors). Ultimately, the cerebellum is responsible for regulating the postural reflexes and muscle tone (Bloedel and Brachfa 1997) and thereby for maintaining the body's equilibrium.

If the cerebellum is damaged, control of movement becomes fragmented, with movement output unable to match intent. The principal signs of cerebellar dysfunction include ataxia – unsteadiness or incoordination of limbs, posture and gait. This disorder arises from inadequate control of the force and timing of movements and leads to abnormalities in the regulation of speed, range and rhythm and in the ability to start and stop movement at a set point. This results in overshooting of the target. Cerebellar problems can affect numerous functions, including the control and regulation of speech (dysarthria), muscle tone, and the ability to carry out rapid alternating movements (dysdiadochokinesia).

For over a century, the cerebellum has been seen as a motor organ. A growing body of research now suggests that the cerebellum is involved in far more than the regulation of various aspects of motor learning. Studies of patients with cerebellar atrophy imply that it also plays a part in visuo-motor learning and adaptation, planning, strategic thinking, time processing (Ivry and Keele 1989) and associative learning. Further evidence from studies that have used functional imaging (PET [positron emission tomography] and MRI [magnetic resonance imaging]) supports the hypothesis that the cerebellum acts in concert with other structures as part of a frontal–subcortical system devoted to the storage and organisation of timed sequential behaviour (Hallett and Grafman 1997), associative learning (Leiner et al. 1986; 1993), word generation (Posner and Raichle 1994) and rapid shifting of attention from one task to another (Courchesne et al. 1994).

Some studies have found the cerebellum of certain autistic children to be smaller than normal; it has been suggested that this may lie behind the autistic child's tendency to become fixated on certain stereotyped activities and their inability to shift attention to appropriate external stimuli. Another interpretation is that the autistic child has inadequate filtering mechanisms to shut out unwanted sensory stimuli, and is therefore overloaded by too much sensory information, and that repetitive stereotyped activities are a way of shutting out the external world, focusing on an inner world that may not be unlike a dream state, thereby reducing the anxiety produced by sensory overload.

Nicolson and Fawcett (1994) concluded that the cerebellum appears to be involved in the 'automisation' of basic skills related to motor competency, phonological processing and visual perception – skills found to be deficient in individuals diagnosed with dyslexia. These are problems that are also present in children who have a cluster of abnormal primitive and postural reflexes (Figure 3.3).

The cerebellum and development

The cerebellum is situated at the back of the brain, above the brainstem and below the cerebral cortex. Like the neocortex, it is more highly developed in human beings than in any other species; it accounts for 11 per cent of the brain's weight. From birth to four years of age, it grows at a faster rate than the cortex, attaining 80 per cent of its adult size by two years of age and completing a major period of myelination by four years of age. It continues to develop at a slower rate up to 15 years of age and beyond.

Its period of most rapid growth and maturation occurs at the time that early motor patterns are being learned. As early motor patterns are learned and practised, they are filed away in the basal ganglia and cerebellum, to be accessed when required. The cerebellum assimilates the actions involved in complex and habitually used movements, and then releases sequences of movements on command, modifying parts of the sequence to match output to intent. This is the motoric equivalent of building up a dictionary of frequently used phrases. The cerebellum is particularly involved in the learning stages of a new skill. As a child becomes more adept at a skill, cerebellar activity decreases.

The cerebellum learns by doing; practice improves performance as a result of synaptic connections being repeatedly fired and the involved neurons adapting their function to become more efficient – Hebb's (1949) observation that neurons that fire together wire together – eventually resulting in maximum efficiency for minimum energy output.

Like the brain as a whole, the cerebellum is organised in three layers. At the base is the archicerebellum. This is an evolutionary outgrowth of the vestibular system, from where certain fibres pass directly to the cerebellar cortex, while the majority relay information via the vestibular nuclei and the reticular activating system in the brainstem. The palaeocerebellum receives action potentials from the skin, joints and primary endings of the neuromuscular spindles (tactile and proprioceptive connections). The neocerebellum has developed together with the cerebral cortex in mammals. It has achieved its greatest size in primates; its evolutionarily most recent part, the neodendate of the dentate nucleus, is present only in humans. The neocerebellum plays a major part in the control of hand and mouth movements and is therefore also involved in speech, articulation and the fine control of manipulative skills, including handwriting.

Leiner et al. (1986) argued that it is the unique enlargement of the neodentate region of the cerebellum that has enabled humans to improve the performance of any other part of the brain to which it is linked as a result of two-way neural connections. The INPP has found that a high percentage of children who have abnormal primitive and postural reflexes also demonstrate difficulties with dysdiadochokinesia of the fingers, hands and feet, a skill that is also regulated in part by the cerebellum.

Development of cerebellar connections

When a child is born, the different regions of the brain are functional but not fully linked. How does the young child develop and integrate these systems in the first years of life?

In prenatal development the vestibular system is remarkable for its precocious development, being in place eight weeks after conception, functional at 16 weeks and myelinated at the time of birth. It is the only one of the sensory systems to be mature at birth with functional connections to and from the cerebellum, but in the first few months of life it must learn to interact effectively with the other sensory systems (touch, proprioception, vision and hearing), which mature rapidly from the time of birth to form major connections to the cerebral cortex. The relative maturity of the vestibular system at birth does not immediately endow an infant with good control of balance. This is a skill that must be learned through experimentation, experience and practice in cooperation with the entire sensory-motor system.[12] In terms of acquiring mastery of postural control, this is like being given a grand piano at birth. Neither piano nor child can reveal their potential without regular practice over an extensive period of time.

The archicerebellum matures early in foetal life but it will take until between 15 months and four years of age for the first stage of neocerebellar connections to the cerebral cortex to be laid down.

One of the ways a child learns to calibrate these different systems is through movement – through utilisation and practice of movement patterns over and over again. First, through spontaneous and reflexive movements in which movement experience acts as a primary medium for the integration of sensory information from multiple sources. Later, this becomes more refined and elaborate as voluntary control over an increasing range of movements develops in tandem with postural control. Movement feeds information to the brain, helping to develop a sense of body map, of spatial awareness and body schema in relation to the self and to the environment. The dual processes of maturation and environmental opportunity operate in concert to facilitate this process. The cerebellum can then utilise the information to modify and refine subsequent motor activity on the basis of a repertoire of known actions. A reflex stimulation/inhibition programme may improve cerebellar functioning by stimulating postural reflexes upon which the cerebellum relies.

Hallett and Grafman (1997) suggested that 'the role of the cerebellum in timed sequential cognitive processing may be analogous to its role in motor processing and suggests a mechanism by which cognitive events become sequenced and temporally labelled'. As early as 1944, Snider and Stowell found that the tactile, visual and auditory centres of the cerebellum are linked to corresponding areas in the cerebral cortex. This led them to conclude that 'the cerebellum is equally involved in the coordination of touch, hearing and sight as it is with movement… it is an accessory control system imposed upon the basic ascending (sensory) and descending (motor) circuits of the motor system'.

This observation opens up many possibilities for remedial intervention. A reflex stimulation/inhibition programme may improve cerebellar functioning by maturing the postural reflex system on which the cerebellum partly relies to function efficiently.

Levinson introduced the use of anti-motion-sickness and antihistamine medications for the treatment of dyslexia and some phobic disorders. Many anti-motion-sickness medications affect the functioning of the vestibular–cerebellar circuit and connections to the reticular activating system. Levinson (1991) described children with vestibular–cerebellar problems as 'upside-down kids' because their perceptual and metabolic systems often react to certain types of medication in reverse. Not only do their symptoms show evidence of cognitive directional confusion, such as letter and word reversal when writing and spelling, but many of them are hypersensitive to specific medication, sometimes responding to tranquillising drugs with hyperactivity and becoming sedated after administration of stimulants. By fine-tuning the operation of these circuits, Levinson claims to have evidence of alteration in cognitive functioning and behaviour.

The smooth operation of the motor system is dependent upon the entire central nervous system, both motor and sensory. Voluntary and semi-voluntary movement develop through practice but are not possible without pre-existing postural patterns that are already established by the basal-reticular system. As the child approaches maturity, the order of command should function from the top downwards – the cerebral cortex influencing and modifying the

Phylogenetic	Major connections	Type of function
Archicerebellum	Vestibular	Posture (subconscious)
Paleocerebellum	Spinal Cord Sensory	Progressive movement e.g. walking, running etc.
Neocerebellum	Cerebral Cortex via Pons	Fine muscle coordination, particularly of the hands & mouth
Dentate Nucleus	Association Cortex	- word association - mental imagery of movement sequences (ideation) - practice-related learning - error detection - judging time intervals & velocity of moving stimuli - rapidly shifting attention between sensory modalities - cognitive operations in 3D space
The above results were obtained using PET scans (Leiner, Leiner and Dow, 1993)		

Table 3.1: Organisation and major connections in the cerebellum.

action of the basal ganglia, which in turn modifies centres of the brainstem, which then modifies the spinal cord reflexes. At every level there is feedback of information to the centres, and the cerebellum acts as a vital regulator in this feedback network (Table 3.1). Dysfunction at any level can potentially release centres below from the influence of those above. Equally, the failure of lower centres to be inhibited may prevent higher centres from maintaining control. The chain of command should resemble the diagram in Figure 3.4.

Cerebral cortex

Finally, at the top of the inverted brain pyramid is the cerebral cortex, comprising two hemispheres that are linked together by the corpus callosum. Although some tasks are shared by both hemispheres, the left and right sides of the cerebral cortex have specialised functions to perform but are dependent upon each other for the execution of those tasks, hence the significance of the corpus callosum between them (Figure 3.5).

Feedback of information

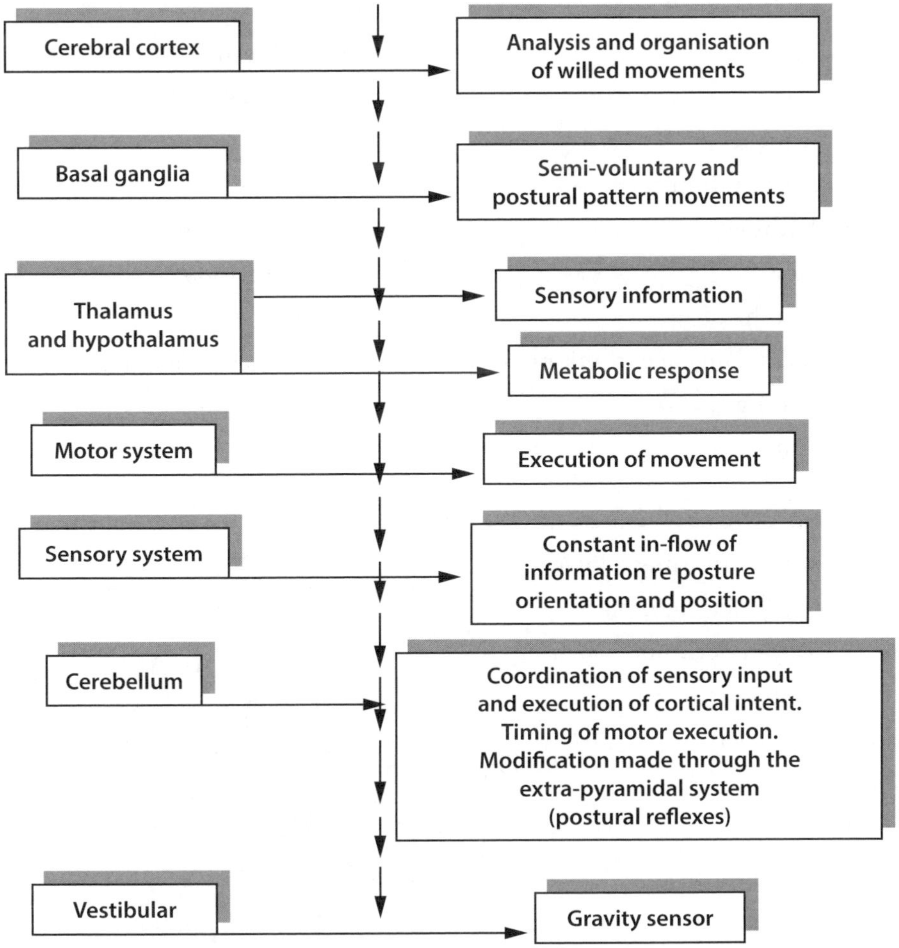

Figure 3.4. Function and feedback.

Hemispheric specialisation

The brain's two hemispheres function differently. This first came to light in the 1960s as a result of the research of psychobiologist and Nobel Prize winner Roger W. Sperry.

The left brain is more verbal, analytical, and orderly than the right brain, while the right brain is more visual, holistic, intuitive and creative with a less organised way of thinking. As a generalisation, specific left and right brain abilities can be categorised as:

Left brain
- Logic
- Sequencing
- Linear thinking
- Arithmetic
- Facts
- Speech
- Verbal language (thinking in words)
- Writing
- Time

Right brain
- Intuitive
- Visual
- Holistic
- Number patterns
- Imagination
- Feelings
- Non-verbal language
- Drawing/pictures

Irrespective of whether someone is performing a logical or creative function, input is received from both sides of the brain. For example, the left brain specialises in the verbal aspects of language, but the right brain is involved in understanding context and tone (non-verbal). The left brain handles arithmetical and sequential aspects of maths, but the right brain helps out with memorisation and retrieval of number patterns (multiplication tables for example), comparisons and rough estimates.

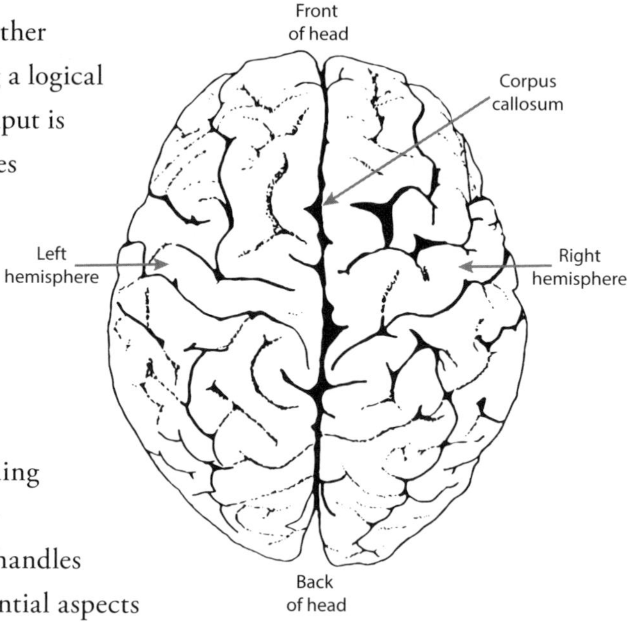

Figure 3.5: Two hemispheres, one brain.

There can be some individual variation in where specific skills are located.

For example, a small percentage of left-handed individuals have a dominant centre for language in the right brain.

In addition to mediating specific skills, the right hemisphere of the cortex seems to play an important part in the learning of new tasks. In a sense, it is the practice ground for some new skills that will eventually gravitate to the left hemisphere for the purposes of applying analysis, logic and detail. When a certain level of understanding or attainment has been reached, one side of the brain can become the specialist for that task, the other side providing a supporting role or simply taking a back seat. This dual process of learning is prevalent in the first seven years of life.

Right hemisphere reading is based on visuo-spatial and holistic skills – for example, whole words or the 'look–say' method. Left hemisphere reading involves decoding of individual symbols, word building from letters, and phonological processing.

In initial reading, the balance of brain activity favours the right hemisphere, whereas advanced readers favour the left hemisphere. Thus, there is a moment in the learning-to-read process at which the balance in the brain tips from right to left at approximately the age of 6½–7½ years (Bakker 1990).

This is the same age at which a major period of myelination and linking takes place between the vestibular apparatus, the cerebellum and the corpus callosum. It is, then, no quantum leap to suppose that a child's reading readiness is closely linked to their neurodevelopmental age in terms of how the brain processes information. Developmental age may not necessarily equate to chronological age and, ideally, teaching methods should take a child's processing and motor abilities into consideration.

When damage occurs to specific regions of the left hemisphere, it can result in severe speech and language problems. One young man seen at the INPP had been in a ghastly car accident in his early twenties and suffered severe left hemisphere damage as a result. With difficulty, he was able to describe what it felt like for him: 'I no longer see sound as I used to. Sound for me is a flat map; there are no hills and valleys although I know there once were. I know what I want to say but the words are like Everest and I cannot see the top.'

His speech was flat, monotone, stuttering and without cadence. He was attempting to use the sublanguage centre of the right hemisphere to communicate, and the result was like an adult making first attempts to speak in a foreign language. His mother tried to help him use what remained intact of his left language centre by pointing to the inch markers on a ruler for each word he wanted to say. This had the effect of itemising and slowing down the individual elements of speech, helping him to locate and articulate individual words rather than try to convey the whole of what he wanted to say. Although the damage was primarily to the left side of the brain, his speech also lacked the musicality (tonal variation, phrasing and cadence) usually associated with the right side. As the clinician working with him, I was reminded that although certain functions are located in specific parts of the brain, function is never simple and damage to one area can also impact on the functioning of all other areas that cooperate with it.

Many children who are right-handed, left-ear dominant demonstrate some form of language difficulty either in speech or in written spelling. Galaburda et al.'s (1978) research on the brains of children with dyslexia showed that a high percentage have abnormally small left hemispheres, suggesting either compromised left hemisphere development from the outset, or underdevelopment through lack of use.

Specific learning difficulties associated with verbal skills can also be culturally specific. Much of Eastern philosophy is also based on right hemisphere thinking, such as the ability to perceive past, present and future as coexisting simultaneously. When we dream, we also do this, so that logically disconnected events can be brought together and viewed through a visuo-spatial, holistic representation unconstrained by the laws governing the physical world.

Many individuals with dyslexia appear to favour right hemisphere methods of learning. When reading, writing and spelling, they have difficulty applying left hemisphere techniques such as phonological decoding. Steffert (1997) suggested that there may be two distinct types of learners: 'sign minds and design minds'. She found that, among a group of art and design students, many had a history of difficulty with written expression. They had found it easier to express themselves through pictorial or three-dimensional media and had struggled with essay writing. She contended that they may have had undiagnosed features of dyslexia.

On the other hand, Portwood stated that dyspraxia (developmental coordination disorder) is primarily a right hemisphere dysfunction involving difficulty with spatial skills and the ability to visualise, ideate and execute controlled voluntary movement.[13]

Corpus callosum

The corpus callosum contains millions of nerve fibres that facilitate communication and instantaneous feedback between one side of the brain and the other. If, for example, the two sides of the cortex were chemically or surgically separated, and the patient asked to pick out two previously identified faces in a large crowd such as in a football arena, each side would use a different method. The left side of the brain would laboriously search every face one by one in logical sequence until it found the face it was looking for. The right brain would scan the sea of faces until it alighted on the target, but the owner of the brain would not be able to tell us their name, since connection to the language centre in the left hemisphere has been severed. Communication between the two sides is of vital importance.[14]

If the corpus callosum fails to pass information fluently from one side to the other, the child may have difficulty decoding certain types of information or linking known facts to new situations and solving problems. This is because problem-solving involves the specialist faculties of both sides of the brain requires information to be communicated between them in both directions. Inadequate transmission from left to right or from right to left via the corpus callosum can obstruct the completion of sequential processes or result in a mental block in the ability to recognise or articulate solutions. One side of the brain may not be given the opportunity to recognise that it knows the answer and become stuck at one point in the process.

The corpus callosum also acts as a screening device, at times shielding information between the two sides of the cortex and thereby reducing interference from information that is irrelevant to the situation. If the corpus callosum fails to inhibit the transmission of information from one side of the brain to the other when the active involvement of one side is not needed, the result can be too much interference and lack of hemispheric specialisation. The latter is sometimes a problem in children and adults diagnosed with ADD who are faced with too many possibilities and then struggle to make decisions.

Functional hemispheric specialisation is associated with the development of lateral preference and is generally established by about eight years of age.

Lateral preference

Lateral preference may be observed in the establishment of a preferred side of functioning in the use of the body. Ideally, by the age of eight years, if a child is right-handed they should use the right hand, foot, eye (far and near distance) and ear for the majority of skilled tasks; in left-handed children, the picture is reversed, with the possible exception of an advantage to having a right ear preference, since the right ear provides the most efficient route from the ear to the main language-decoding centre in the brain for the majority of people.

The continued presence of the ATNR can interfere with unilaterality of brain function. (Gesell and Ames 1947; Telléus 1980). This may be seen in homolateral (one-sided) patterns of movement and a functional midline barrier to the execution of cross-pattern movements (hand, eyes or feet). It can also affect organisation in the processing of sensory information within the brain.

Unilaterality of brain function may be likened to two people in the front of a car – one acting as the driver and the other as the map reader. If both people are focused on their job and trust the skills of the other, the map reader directing the driver when needed and the driver concentrating on vehicle and road, the journey should be relatively easy and stress free. If on the other hand, each constantly interferes with or distracts the other, with the map reader criticising the driver or drawing their attention to the scenery, or the driver questioning or ignoring the directions of the navigator, the journey will become chaotic, prolonged and more stressful. In other words, when one person (or side of the brain) is able to carry out its specialist function and lead on that task with the support of the other, functioning is efficient.

Kohen-Raz (1986) linked the establishment of a preferred side of functioning to maturity in postural control, which he believed to be an important precursor to reading readiness.

Difficulties with dysdiadochokinesia – difficulty in the execution of rapid alternate movements – can be symptomatic of lack of cerebral dominance. Until the cerebellum has mastered control of fine muscle movements so that the child can perform the finger opposition test without difficulty, independent movement of each side of the body will not have been established and cerebral dominance will not have been established.

In the cerebellum the greatest period of growth and of maturation is between birth and 15 months, exactly the period when the adjustments from primitive reflex to postural control are being made. Maturation continues at a slower rate until the age of seven or eight years, when the final linking takes place between the vestibular apparatus, the cerebellum and the corpus callosum. It is generally accepted that occasional letter, number and word reversals in reading and writing are normal until the age of approximately eight years. Continued reversal after this age may not be merely symptomatic of a dyslexic type of problem; they may also be suggestive of vestibular/cerebellar immaturity with implications for many other areas of functioning. Although immaturity in the functioning of the vestibular–cerebellar system can exist for a number of reasons, underdeveloped head-righting reflexes can be one indication of such immaturity (Figure 3.6).

Relationship between brain development and the integration of primitive and postural reflexes

The cortex is the seat of intellect, of decision-making and of controlled response, but it can only do its job easily and effectively if the reflexive action of the lower centres becomes integrated, freeing higher centres in the cortex to focus on executive functions.

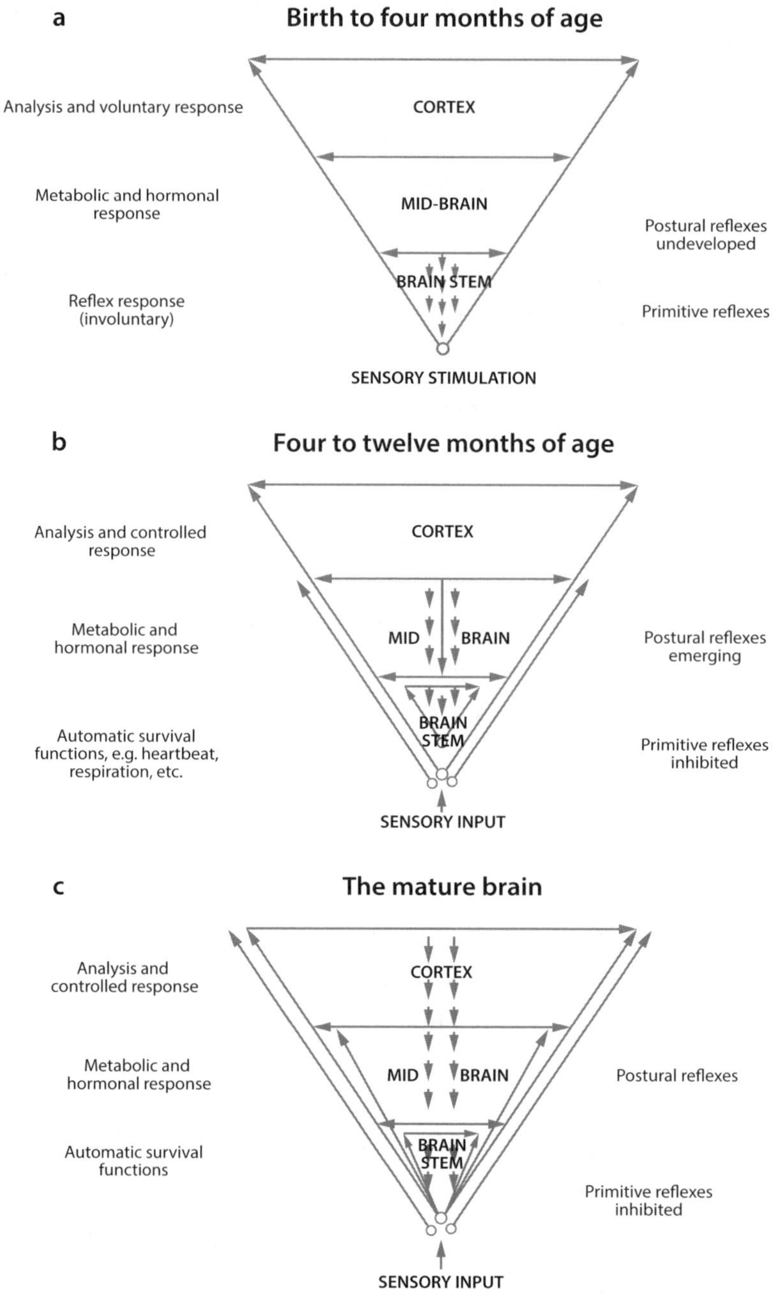

Figure 3.6: Relationship between increased cortical control, level of reflex response and other systems in the first two years of life.

The term 'triune brain' was used by Paul MacLean (1978) to describe the brain as comprising three levels. Each level corresponds to a stage in evolution. The brainstem, for example, was said to symbolise the 'reptilian brain', because it is shared by all vertebrates from reptiles to humankind. In their early weeks of life, the neonate is a totally brainstem-dominated creature, and the movements they make are reptilian in character – head lift, squirming and rolling in a gravity-bound world. The midbrain represents MacLean's 'mammalian brain' and takes the young infant through the stages of rolling, crawling, sitting, creeping and standing. Finally, the cortex takes control, enabling us to stand and to move with independent use of the hands, and eventually to grow into rational, logical linguistic and altruistic human beings. All levels remain with us, but lower brain regions should become subordinate to higher centres. Although this theoretical construct is now considered simplistic and outdated, the course of development in both the brain and postural and motor capabilities does follow this pattern.

Fiorentino (1981) linked the primitive and postural reflexes to three stages in the development of mobility – apedal, quadruped and bipedal – each one signifying a new stage in the recapitulation of our evolutionary heritage and the active involvement of higher systems of the brain (Figure 3.7).

During the process of primitive reflex inhibition and postural reflex development, the infant recapitulates stages of evolution. The stages of brain maturation and the movements made are inextricably linked, the one being a reflection of the other. Continuous development of neural pathways is facilitated through such movement sequences:

> Practice and repetition of movement patterns result in them being absorbed into the individual's repertoire of skills, probably also resulting in physical changes taking place in the neurons concerned, so that the flow of impulses along a specific pathway is facilitated. Repetition enhances facilitation and adeptness. (Draper 1993)

This theory forms the basis for the physical remediation programmes developed at the INPP.

Levels of development

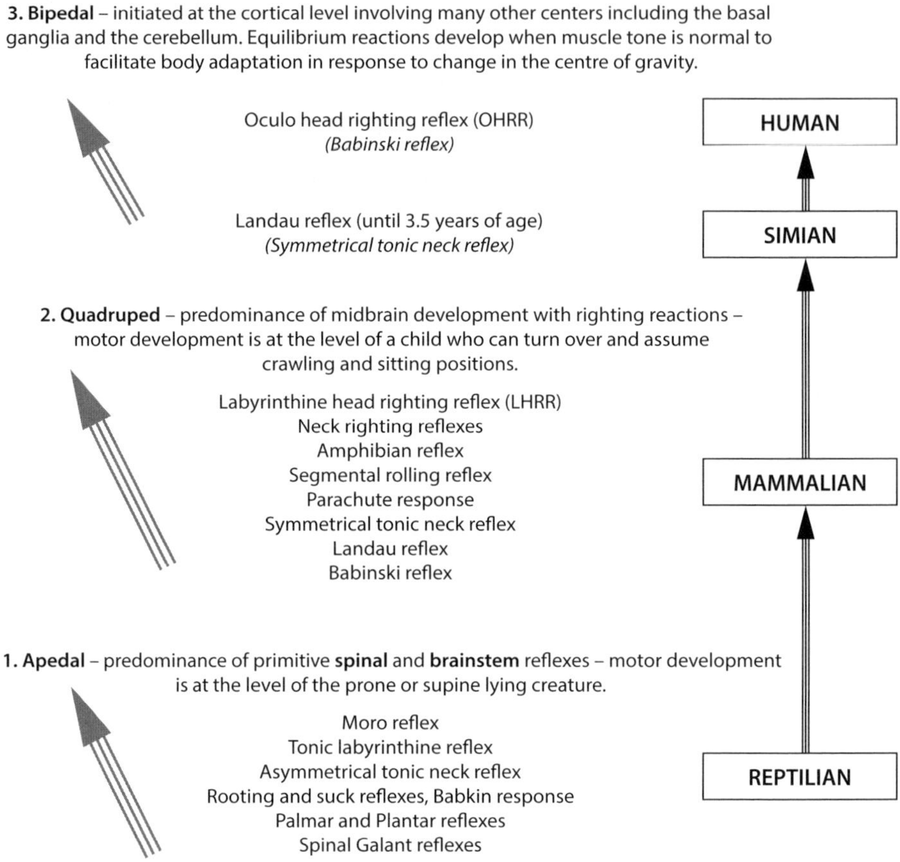

Figure 3.7: Levels of development.

In summary, the motor responses of the newborn infant are extensions of those established during foetal life and reflect in part the immediate needs of the developing foetus and infant. The motor activity of the neonate does not involve true volitional activity and reflects a lack of inhibition of the segmental apparatus of the nervous system by higher neural centres. As the central nervous system slowly matures during infancy and childhood, inhibitory influences begin to work. Primitive reflexes are gradually inhibited by higher brain centres and integrated into developing patterns as higher brain centres are differentiated.

Although the conventional view has been that absence, delay, persistence or reappearance of certain reflexes in their crude form at key stages in development may indicate neurological disorder, there can also be mild variation in reflex responses in infants and behavioural state.

Research over the last 30 years (McPhillips and Sheehy 2004; Goddard Blythe 2005; González et al. 2008; Andrich et al. 2018; Ivanović et al. 2018; Gieysztor et al. 2018; Goddard Blythe et al. 2021) has indicated that primitive reflexes can persist to a lesser degree or be elicited under specific conditions in pre-school and school-aged children and in adults, indicating immaturity in the functioning of the central nervous system which may continue to impede specific functions linked to learning outcomes and emotional regulation.

Primitive reflexes may also be released voluntarily in later life to enhance specific skills. Fukuda (1961) observed use of the ATNR in fencers taking up the en garde attitude and in elite discus throwers. High divers may momentarily reactivate the STNR as they emerge from a foetal position in descent before they straighten up to enter the water. This voluntary or trained release of earlier primitive movement patterns is very different from the unsought continued presence of these patterns.

Examples of the relationship between primitive reflexes and brain function

The following list are examples only of how, in theory, the persistence or underdevelopment of individual reflexes may be linked to specific brain functions. These examples should be viewed not as absolute connections (1 + 1 = 2) but rather as functional links or possibilities that may be expressed or suppressed in various ways.

Asymmetrical tonic neck reflex:

- may interfere functionally with the establishment of a preferred side of functioning, resulting in ambilaterality or cross-laterality
- hand–eye coordination in crossing the midline with implications for handwriting and written expression

Hierarchical connections between the brain, reflexes and functioning

Integrated in	Reflex	Stimulus	Response	Receptor
Spinal cord and medulla	Stretch reflexes	Stretch	Contraction of muscle	Muscle spindle
Spinal cord	Positive supporting reaction (magnet)	Contact on sole of foot/ body (or upper-hand body)	Foot extended to support	Proprioceptive flexors
Spinal cord	Negative supporting reaction	Stretch	Release of positive support reaction	Proprioceptive extensors
Medulla	Tonic labyrinthine reflex	Gravity	Contraction of limb extensor (hands/ knees table position)	
Medulla	Tonic neck reflexes (ATNR STNR)	Head turned: 1 to side 2 up 3 down	1 Extension of limbs on side to which head is turned 2 Leg flex 3 Arms flex	
Midbrain	Labyrinthine head-righting reflexes	Gravity	Head alignment	Otolithic organs
Midbrain	Neck-righting reflexes	Stretch of neck neck muscles	Righting of thorax, shoulders, then pelvis	Muscle spindle
Midbrain	Body-on-head righting reflexes	Pressure on side of body	Righting on head	Exteroceptors
Midbrain	Body-on-body righting	Pressure on side of body	Righting of body even when head held sideways	Exteroceptors
Cerebral cortex	Optical head-righting reflexes	Visual cues	Righting of head	Eyes
Cerebral cortex	Placing reactions	Various visual, exteroceptive and proprioceptive cues	Foot placed on supporting surface in position to support body	Various
Cerebral cortex	Hopping reactions	Lateral displacement while standing	Hops, maintaining limbs in place to support body	Muscle spindles

Table adapted from Ganong (1997) and Galley & Forster (1982)

Table 3.2: Hierarchical connections between the brain, reflexes and functioning.

Tonic labyrinthine reflex:

- balance and postural control
- secondary effect on oculo-motor control (eye movements), potentially affecting visual perception

Symmetrical tonic neck reflex:

- upper and lower body integration, potentially affecting truncal or core stability
- hand–eye coordination (hand to mouth)
- body awareness, body schema

Moro reflex:

- hyper-arousal
- hypervigilance
- lowered threshold to stress
- stimulus-bound effect in one or several sensory channels, affecting how information is processed in stressful or multisensory environments

Head-righting reflexes:

- needed to support congruence in the functioning of the vestibular-proprioceptive and visual systems and the corresponding neural circuits

As mentioned in previous chapters, these reflexes are not necessarily the underlying cause of the presenting problems but may reflect an impairment of sensory processing or other neural pathways.

Increased cortical control of neurological function in humans proceeds rapidly in the first year of life, coinciding with the development of postural control. As Delacato (1959) observed, humankind's unique development diverging from other species has been the achievement of vertical posture – which has enabled us not only to stand and move on two feet but to have free use of the hands, oppose the thumb and forefinger, carry out tasks using one side of the body at a time (hand, foot, eye and ear), supinate and pronate the hand and develop cortical hemispheric specialisation of function. Other animals possess a cortex, but it was Delacato's belief that 'man's final and unique developmental progression takes place at the level of the cortex, and is lateral (from left to right and from right to left)' and that the cortical dominance made possible by the vertical organisation of bipedal posture has enabled humans 'to out distance lower forms of animal' in the development of higher skills. He also maintained that, before a child can achieve lateral organisation, they need time in their first eight years of life for the development of bilateral skills so that when they have achieved a certain competency in vertical posture and bilateral skills they will be ready to choose a preferred side.

Although this view is now considered to be outdated and simplistic, the achievement of vertical postural control in humans remains fundamental to how other systems operate: balance, coordination, control of eye movements, visual perception and orientation are all linked to stability in bipedal posture. Primitive and postural reflexes existing at key stages in development provide indications of functional maturity in the the attainment of postural control. These reflexes can be used as 'tools' to identify signs of immaturity, 'clues' to the type and level of intervention needed and 'measures' with which to evaluate change.

Chapter 4

The Senses

Interoceptor and exteroceptor systems

Long before a child reaches school age, they will have begun to learn. Learning begins at conception and should continue in unison with the body throughout the course of natural life. All learning takes place in the brain, but it is the body that acts as the vehicle through which knowledge is acquired. Brain and body work together as a function of the central nervous system, but both are dependent upon the senses for all information about the outer world. This information derived from external sensory systems (vision, hearing, touch, taste and smell) must be integrated with information from internal sensory systems (vestibular and proprioceptive together with a general sense of the internal state of the body) to provide the basis for coherent perception and emotional regulation.

Interoception can be conscious and non-conscious and encompasses the brain's process of integrating signals received from the body into brain subregions involved in the representation of the physiological state of the body. This is important for maintaining homeostasis and may potentially affect self-awareness. Misrepresentations of internal states, or a disconnect between signals from the body and the brain's interpretation and prediction of those signals, have been suggested to play a part in some mental disorders such as anxiety, depression, panic disorder, eating disorders, ADHD and ASD.

Exteroceptors are afferent nerve endings that sense stimuli originating from outside the body, such as pain, temperature, touch, vibration and sound, visual stimuli, taste and smell.

When a child reaches school age, it is generally assumed that the basic systems necessary for academic learning are established and that good teaching, combined with the child's willingness to learn, will enable them to succeed. In order for them to be able to do so, at least three supporting systems have to operate effectively:

- reception of information via the senses
- the processing of information in the brain
- response to that information via the efferent system

We have seen how the reflex system can affect performance at the levels of motor control, processing and response, causing brainstem reactions to direct the response without full involvement of higher levels of the brain. Equally, incoherent sensory input may reawaken reflex activity that would otherwise be inhibited, setting up a vicious circle of scrambled sensation and immature response.

It has long been accepted that defects in vision and in hearing will impede the learning process, but they are generally investigated in isolation by a professional expert in the relevant field. Frequently, the child is only examined for deficit in one area and further investigations into what a child sees, what they hear or how they experience touch are not carried out.

When I studied fine arts at university, we spent an entire term on the processes of visual perception and how the artist may view the world differently from people without artistic talent. In *The World Through Blunted Sight*, ophthalmologist Trevor-Roper (1987) suggested that defects in eyesight have probably played an important part throughout history in determining the activities people have willingly engaged and succeeded in and the skills and professions that may be built on the individual's unique combination of talents and defects. He suggested that myopia (short sight) predisposes a child to pay attention to near distance activities such as reading, writing, playing a musical instrument, and craftwork, whereas the child with hyperopia (long sight) will naturally tend to enjoy sports that involve more use of far distance vision. He went on to suggest that changes in artistic style over a lifetime could also be linked to the development of visual defects.

This hypothesis was followed up by another ophthalmologist, James Ravin, who believed that the softness in style characteristic of Renoir arose because he was near-sighted, that Monet's later impressionist style could be linked to the development of cataracts and that Degas, who began as a painter with a very detailed academic style, evolved a looser impressionistic style as his vision deteriorated, switching to pastels, which are easier to work than oil, dry quickly and do not require fine lines.

When a member of my family who is an artist had his cataracts removed, for several weeks he could not believe the 'whiteness of white'. As the cataracts had developed slowly over several years, whites had become cream and other colours had lost their true brightness, which over time had become reflected in the tones he selected for his paintings. He painted the world as he saw it, and the colours he used during that period tended to be dingy and autumnal irrespective of the season. Following surgery, his colours came alive. In other words, the ways we see, hear, feel, smell and taste the world define not only our experience of the world but also how we express our inner interpretation of those sensations.

Similarly, differences and distortions of hearing may enable someone with perfect pitch to become a consummate singer or musician, while even mild hearing impairment can distort speech sounds, affect spatial awareness and interfere with social interaction. What a child perceives is therefore just as important as whether they can see or hear – in supporting all aspects of learning in the classroom. We cannot assume that a child's perceptual experience of the world is the same as ours. At best, we expect there to be consistency between individuals in major elements of discriminating shape, form and intensity so that we are able to communicate using a common language of human experience. As deviations from these common types of experience increase, the likelihood of difficulties with specific aspects of learning, communication and emotional regulation also increases.

Visual and auditory hypersensitivity, for example, can be just as much of a handicap to learning as can impairment in these areas, and in some cases both hyper and hypo can coexist in a child (Delacato 1974). Vision and hearing interact with the vestibular system, but the optometrist, occupational therapist and the audiologist work in separate departments and may never know that they both see the same child whose primary problem is located in the inner ear.

When a system is overloaded, the child can go into a defensive reaction in which they seem not to respond to obvious stimuli. This may be misinterpreted as being undersensitive, when in fact it is a protective mechanism resulting from oversensitivity. It is sometimes described as 'paradoxical' behaviour.

None of the senses develops or operates in isolation. Each one is reinforced, modified and influenced by information from the others. Our language and our interpretation accept cross-sensory reference as fundamental to our understanding of the world. Hearing has been described as a 'specialised sense of touch'; we 'taste with our nose', 'feast with our eyes', 'see with our fingers' and, according to Tomatis (1980), 'read with our ears'. We accept balance between the different aspects of our lives as fundamental to health and to well-being, and yet the senses of balance and proprioception are perhaps the forgotten sixth and seventh senses of the 21st century. An understanding of the senses and how they complement one another is essential if we are to understand and to help the child who cannot always 'make sense' of the world and therefore has difficulty succeeding through the standard channels of education.

Balance and the vestibular system

Balance is fundamental to functioning in a gravity-based environment. It is the first system to be fully developed, becoming operational at 16 weeks in utero and is myelinated at birth, having provided the foetus with a sense of direction and orientation inside the womb. It is in place to help sense and elicit forces that counteract gravity, which the child will only experience in its full force for the first time at birth.

Every living creature shares one relationship throughout wakefulness and sleeping: a relationship with gravity. Gravity provides us with our centre, whether it be in space, in time, motion, depth, or sense of self, acting as the spatial nucleus from which all operations become possible. Problems in the balance system will have repercussions for all other areas of functioning. Such problems affect the sensory systems, because all sensation passes through the vestibular mechanism at brainstem level before being transmitted elsewhere for integration and analysis.

The vestibular system operates closely with the reflexes to facilitate balance. It is located in the inner ear, and its job is to monitor and make adjustments to any movement of the head or the environment.

> As we move and interact with gravity, sensory receptors in the ear are activated, and impulses appraising the central nervous system about the position of the head in space are directed to various parts of the brain and down the spinal cord. It is believed that sensory impulses from the eyes, ears, muscles and joints must be matched to the vestibular input before such information can be reprocessed efficiently. If that is true, what we see, hear and feel makes sense only if the vestibular system is functioning adequately. (Pyfer and Johnson 1981)

The vestibular system has two main parts:

- three fluid-filled semicircular canals set at right angles to each other
- two fluid-filled sacs (otoliths)

Hair cells line the inside of both organs. Any movement of the body, particularly the head, sets up motion of the fluid in the canals and the sacs, stimulating the hair cells. Movement of the hair cells triggers the release of nerve signals that provide the brain with information about the direction, angle and extent of the movement so that appropriate muscle adjustments may be made. Certain hair cells are particularly sensitive to gravity, informing the brain of any deviation from the upright position. Signals from the vestibular system then pass along the vestibular nerve to the cerebellum.

The cerebellum has been called 'the moderator between sensation and brain level response' (Levinson 1981), since it coordinates information from the inner ear with other parts of the body. It regulates our responses to where we are in space and what position we are in, whether standing, sitting, running, climbing, somersaulting or whatever. If information from the vestibular system is out of alignment with information from the other senses involved in the perception of motion (vision and proprioception), motion sickness results. Astronauts can experience a unique form of this when placed in a gravity-free environment where their sense of centre is lost and they rely heavily on tactile and visual stimuli to retain a sense of location.

It has long been recognised that sensory deprivation, particularly disorientation, will result in emotional and physical distress. In extreme cases it has been used as a method of interrogation and torture, producing irreversible insanity within a very short period of time. The unfortunate victim would be blindfolded and placed in a suit that covered them from head to toe (depriving them of external tactile stimuli) and white noise was then played into the ears through a headset. If this did not yield results, the victim would be placed in a centrifuge and spun for several minutes with devastating effect. Very few such victims ever recovered their sanity.

The vestibular is possibly the oldest and the most primitive of the sensory systems. It is believed that the human ear is an outgrowth or development of one of the earliest vertebrate complex sensory end organs – the lateral line receptor. The lateral line receptor probably had its beginning in the armoured fish of the Silurian period over 400 million years ago. Movements of the hairs situated in the sensitive areas of the lateral line receptor are used by fish to detect chemicals and electrical fields in the surrounding water and thereby alert them to approaching obstacles, food and predators.

During the course of evolution, this region has become more complex in mammals and has developed into the labyrinthine portion of the inner ear that houses the organs of balance and of hearing. In embryonic development the upper portion of the labyrinth forms three hollow semicircular tubes each arranged at right angles to each other which will eventually form the basis for the control of balance. After birth, it can detect movements of the head from the motion of the fluid inside these three small tubes. Each tube responds to motion in a different plane in relation to gravity, sometimes described as 'pitch', 'roll' and 'yaw'.

The lower half of the labyrinth stretches into a long tube that coils to form a shell-like structure. There is the cochlea, the hearing apparatus, which functions by detecting sound vibrations. Both organs, together with the jaw, facial muscles, swallow mechanism and organs of speech production, are evolutionary developments from the gill bars of our fish ancestors. The lateral line receptor has also formed projections to the brainstem which provide the structural foundation for the cerebellum (Larsell 1947). The cerebellum of higher species plays a dominant role in sensory–motor integration and coordination but is heavily dependent upon reciprocal interaction with vestibular centres.

In mammals the ear has become more highly developed than in other animals, dividing into the two main structures mentioned above:

- the vestibular apparatus, or balance mechanism
- the cochlea, or auditory apparatus

Although these are often viewed as separate systems by specialists, they share a common chamber and fluid (endolymph) and transmit information using the same cranial nerve, the VIII cranial or vestibulo-acoustic nerve. This common pathway means that hearing can potentially be influenced by information passing to and from the vestibular portion and that the vestibular system can be influenced by sound. Ménière's disease, for example, is a disorder of the inner ear which is characterised by episodes of vertigo, tinnitus, hearing loss and a sensation of blockage in the ear. The cause of Ménière's disease is unclear, but symptoms are believed to be the result, in part, of increased fluid build-up in the labyrinth of the inner ear, which thus affects both balance and hearing.

Both portions of the inner ear are involved in the perception of relative position in relation to motion. Madaule (1993) stated that it is the vestibular portion alone that monitors slow movement, but we also use the auditory component to judge the position (orientation), direction, speed and timing of any form of motion that has a frequency of more than 20Hz (hertz), by calculating the speed and distance to each ear.

Steinbach (1994) suggests that 'sound is not sound' but is the physical expression of movement or vibration. The ear acts as a receptor and transmitter of vibrations over a specific range of frequencies, to be interpreted by the brain. Defects in vestibular functioning may affect thresholds of auditory system sensitivity, and problems in the auditory apparatus may result in the vestibular system working overtime to compensate.

One reason for this inequity in how sensory systems operate together may be that the vestibular system provides no special sensation of its own. It communicates through affecting levels of sensitivity in other sensory systems, which in turn affect levels of arousal and physiological reactions. For example, the first conscious signal of motion sickness may be a heightened sense of smell preceding headache or drowsiness. A heightened sense of smell may then become associated with feelings of nausea, the smell of a car subsequently being enough to induce feelings of motion sickness. This is an example of a secondary associative response. If the vestibular system is artificially overstimulated by excessive spinning, then for a few seconds afterwards vision will be blurred and the entire visual world appears to be moving. In other words, we only become aware of functional problems with the vestibular system through symptomatic changes in other systems.

Both the vestibular system and the reflex system are closely aligned to the visual system, acting as the substrata upon which oculo-motor and visual-perceptual skills are built. Impulses from the vestibular system to the brainstem affect equilibrium reactions, with motor nerves that control eye movements and with nerves that lead to the somatosensory portion of the cerebral cortex.

De Klein and Magnus (1924) believed that, functionally, the vestibular system is inseparable from the proprioceptive, visual and motor systems in the acquisition of developmental reflexes and of postural control. Together with the cerebellum it is involved in the maintenance of equilibrium, the direction of eye gaze and the maintenance of a plane of vision dependent upon head position. These functions are achieved as a result of modification by the vestibular system of underlying muscle tone and neuromuscular reflexes. Mismatch between the vestibular, visual and proprioceptive systems can produce sensations of vertigo, motion sickness, and hallucinations in relation to position and motion experience, which then lead to anxiety.[15]

Vestibular control underpins balance, poise and, according to Hubbard (1971), provides the foundation for 'the relationship of body image and motion which endlessly reflects changes in the social, moral, professional and personal life of an individual'. Paul Schilder (1933) believed that 'organic changes in the vestibular apparatus might be highly significant in the etiology of certain neuroses and psychoses', a concept later followed up by Blythe and McGlown (1979), Levinson (1989) and Blythe (1990). While Levinson treated the symptoms of vestibular–cerebellar dysfunction with anti-motion-sickness medication, Blythe went on to develop vestibular and reflex inhibition programmes to treat the symptoms of agoraphobia and panic disorder in adults: problems with balance and immaturity in the functioning of the central nervous system were detected using a range of tests that assessed gross muscle coordination and balance, immature primitive and postural reflexes, oculo-motor dysfunction and visual-perceptual difficulties.

Adequate vestibular input is essential for the automatic control of balance, posture and controlled voluntary action. Shaskan and Roller (1985) suggested that 'a newborn's body tone, its fear of falling, the Moro reflex and the neck-righting reflex may all be expressions of the sequential development of the central nervous system and its relative normalcy or pathology'.

Signals to and from the vestibular system in the inner ear pass through four nuclei – the vestibular nuclei – in the pons of the brainstem. The vestibular nuclei serve as a junction for messages passing between the balance mechanism and the body via the vestibular spinal system, and for signals passing between the balance mechanism and the eyes along the vestibulo-ocular reflex arc (VOR). A further connection links both systems to the cerebellum, whose task is to modulate and regulate communication and from all of these centres so that movement output is smooth and controlled.

The relationship between the vestibular, visual and somatosensory systems and their connection to arousal and attention are beautifully described by Allan Hobson in *The Dreaming Brain*:

> The intermediate brainstem serves not only as a way station for reflex information from spinal cord to cortex (and vice versa) but as a mode selector for both structures determining the ratio of stimulated to spontaneous neuronal information processing.

> In evolution, the brainstem was one of the first structures to be added to the purely segmental spinal cord. In many primitive animals, the brainstem was all there was. It enabled organisms to achieve control of such special sense organs as eyes and to coordinate the increasing number of motor acts that developed as animals became more specialised with respect to limb functions. Thus, the brainstem contains within it the neurons that move the eyes and neurons capable of coordinating those eye movements with the position of the head and the body. The complex orchestration of head, eye and body position is conducted by the oculo-motor, reticular and vestibular systems of the brain. (Hobson 1988)

Hobson goes on to say that attention and arousal demand precise control of eye and head position:

> Lorento de No (1933) showed that every change in head position is immediately and accurately translated by the vestibular system into an appropriate change in eye position. Also participating in this neuronal calculation are the cerebellum and the reticular formation. We know that Lorento de No's circuit is spontaneously activated in rapid eye movement (REM) or dreaming sleep so that head, eye and body position signals are internally generated. Thus when lying immobile in bed one has dream sensations of running, turning, and even flying. (Hobson 1988)

Berthoz (2000) explained how even our thoughts and dreams are an internalised simulation of action. In other words, movement experience and action build up a physical equivalent of a lexicon in the brain through which we are able to imagine (visualise) scenarios even in the absence of full conscious awareness or physical interaction in real time. Visualisation is based in part on historical physical patterns of movement experience.

Oosterveldt (1991) explained that balance is not something we have; it is something that we do. It is a constant process of adjustment to prevent falling over. Even the process of walking – something we take for granted until injury or degeneration interfere – is a process of moving from stability to instability (two feet to one) and then placing the leading foot on the ground to regain stability again. The vestibular and reflex systems act as interdependent systems in the control of posture and movement at a subconscious level. Vestibular dysfunction can alter the level of reflex response, and immature reflex responses can impede the functioning of the vestibular system.

The vestibular system has connections to:

- the autonomic nervous system – digestion, etc.
- the visual system (90 per cent of cells in the visual system respond to vestibular stimulation)
- the sleep and waking cycles
- REM dream sleep
- the perception of weight (King and Schrager 1999)

Inappropriate vestibular signals may elicit primitive reflex reactions, but equally, aberrant reflex activity can impede the activities of the vestibular system. If a child is to utilise the information provided by their senses effectively, sensory information must be integrated and congruent.

Signs suggestive of vestibular dysfunction include:

- poor balance
- delay in postural and motor milestones such as head control, sitting, crawling and walking
- poor muscle tone
- motion sickness beyond the age of puberty
- dislike of heights, swings, carousels, escalators and lifts (hypersensitive), or, conversely, no fear of heights, seeking physical thrills (hyposensitive)
- easily disoriented, poor sense of direction
- clumsiness
- difficulty remaining still (may actively seek vestibular stimulation through activities such as excessive rocking or spinning)
- difficulties in space perception
- poor organisational skills, scatterbrained behaviour
- cannot work out how to do certain activities, e.g. push/pull

- fatigue, lethargy
- inability to mentally rotate or reverse objects in space, or procedures (can affect such things as the ability to read an analogue clock, which is a spatial ability, or to understand that multiplication and division are the same processes in reverse)

Tactility

Although the vestibular system is the first to be fully developed and myelinated, it is the sense of touch that provides the first observable signs in the embryo of response to outside stimuli. The first response to tactile stimulation occurs at approximately five weeks after conception when the mass cutaneous withdrawal reflexes emerge.[14] Gentle stimulation of the upper lip results in immediate withdrawal from the source of contact by the whole organism. The area sensitive to touch rapidly spreads over the next four weeks to encompass the oral region of the face, then the palms of the hands and the soles of the feet, until eventually the entire body surface becomes responsive to touch. However, the earliest primitive realisation of touch is a defensive one characterised by withdrawal.

During the second and third trimesters of pregnancy, tactile awareness should mature to allow clasping reflexes to develop (palmar, plantar, rooting, suck, Moro, etc.), so that by the time the baby is born, touch is associated with security, with feeding, comfort and eventually exploration. Touch precedes both hearing and vision as the primary channel of learning and touch receptors cover the entire outer surface of the body.

The area in the brain which perceives touch stretches like a headband and is called the 'somatosensory cortex'. It is capable of registering heat, cold, pressure, pain and body position. The most sensitive areas of the body have a correspondingly large representation area in the somatosensory cortex, the lips, hands and genital regions occupying a large section of the somatosensory map. Even the bases of the hair follicles have touch receptors. Since the vestibular apparatus functions through the movement of fluid over hair cells, the sense of touch is also implicated in the functioning of balance, orientation and motion.

Ayres (1989) divided the tactile system into protective and discriminative subsystems. Protective receptors are located around the hair follicles and respond to subtle stimulation such as sound and air waves (vibration) moving across the body. 'They literally tell us where our body ends and where space begins' (Pyfer and Johnson 1981).

Discriminative receptors are located in the dermis and respond when we come into contact with something – either actively or passively. These systems should be mutually exclusive, that is, one shuts down as the other comes into action. The protective system stays in operation until we are touched. Provided the contact is harmless, the discriminative system comes into play as soon as contact takes place.

The child who has an overactive protective system will be 'tactile defensive'. If this is the case, then touch can be neither an instant source of comfort nor a consistent purveyor of information, since defensive reflex responses can be more easily elicited, resulting in a tendency to withdraw from the source of contact before discriminatory receptors can come into play. The 'hypertactile' child may have abnormal perception in all or only some input to the area of the cortex which registers touch. They may have poor tolerance and/or adaptive mechanisms to heat and cold. They may have a low pain threshold for specific types of pain (e.g. pain associated with grazing or piercing the skin) but, paradoxically, a high tolerance to internal pain.

This may be the child who overreacts to injections, grazes and small cuts but who will fail to notice that their legs are covered with bruises. They may dislike any form of physical contact and therefore have difficulty in either receiving or demonstrating physical affection, which makes it more difficult for the mother to establish a warm relationship with the child. They may appear to be inordinately stubborn about the clothes they wear (labels, textures, waistbands, etc.) and the way that they do things. Contact sports may be avoided, and the child may have a poor body image and sense of position in space.

In extreme cases, hypersensitivity may play a significant part in the distortion of body image, which is characteristic of anorexia nervosa. Anorexics feel themselves to be fat and believe that their own body occupies a far greater space than it actually does. Despite all attempts to shrink from within, no amount of weight loss will alter this sensation, since the same amount of skin surface and therefore the same number of receptors remain in contact with the outer world. Because a sensation of this type is mediated at the brainstem, the feeling of discomfort will override any logic that is imposed from the cortex, and no amount of evidence to the contrary will change the anorexic's perception of themself.

Tactile discrimination should be a rich source of information about the environment as well as a medium for (non-verbal) communication and the expression of affection. It can also influence the functioning of the immune system. Studies with rats have shown that offspring handled in the laboratory have better immune systems and gain weight better. Early handling also leads to permanent sensitivity of the part of the brain that controls the stress response, resulting in reduced levels of stress hormones. Studies of premature infants have shown a 45 per cent increase in weight gain among children who are massaged for 15 minutes, three times a day.

Without touch, small children rapidly become disturbed and may attempt to supply themselves with essential sensory information through self-stimulation of other sensory systems. One example of this is the rocking observed among some children abandoned in orphanages where the quality of childcare has been grossly inadequate. Repetitive rocking among institutionalised patients is recognised to be a sign of mental retardation, but it may also occur in children who are attempting to provide themselves with essential vestibular, tactile and proprioceptive information in the absence of sufficient physical stimulation and care. Self-generated vestibular stimulation can also be comforting and is sometimes seen following trauma, extreme distress or neglect. As Blythe repeatedly stressed in his lectures to students, we cannot assume that a specific behaviour is the result of a specific cause; rather, the good clinician must seek to discover what purpose that behaviour serves for the patient. Trying to remove the behaviour without understanding the cause will only achieve limited results.

Most of a child's earliest touch experiences are provided by the parents during breastfeeding, changing and play. Allan Schore (1994) suggests that in the early months the mother acts as the primary facilitator of the forming of connections between different levels in the brain, and the laying of foundations not only for later learning ability but also for emotional regulation and immune response.

By providing well-modulated socio-affective stimulation, the mother facilitates the growth of connections between cortical, limbic and subcortical limbic structures that neurobiologically mediate self-regulatory functions ... the core of the self lies in patterns of affect regulation that integrate a sense of the self across different states of arousal, thereby enabling a continuity of inner experience.

Early handling is an important part of this process. Diamond et al. (1963) describe the mother as 'playing the role of higher brain structures: she is the child's auxiliary cortex'. Sensory and emotional experience derived from handling and engagement play an important part in the process.

Touch is important for a child to develop their body image – sometimes referred to as a 'mental picture' or 'map' of the body. In addition to the potential influence of tactile hypersensitivity in the later development of body dysmorphic issues, which are often present in eating disorders, many children with developmental coordination disorder (DCD) have a poor sense of body image, difficulty locating different parts of their body in space in the absence of visual cues, and inadequate awareness of whole sections of their body. This can be related to a mixture of poor tactile and proprioceptive awareness. When the child draws a picture of a human figure, often the head is drawn disproportionately large with little or no neck (a common feature of drawings by children who have underdeveloped head-righting reflexes). Drawings of large hands and awkward limbs or stance are also indications of impairment of the internal sense of body image and position in space (vestibular, proprioceptive and tactile). Omission of the hands or fingers or abnormally large representation of these may or may not be related to the continued presence of primitive tactile reflexes such as the palmar reflex and Babkin reflex.

a

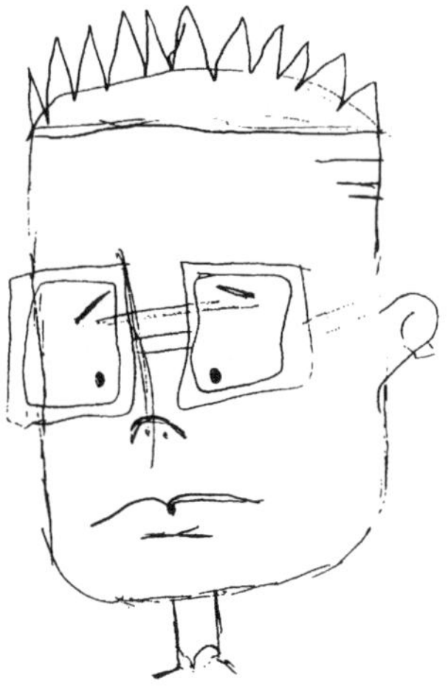

b

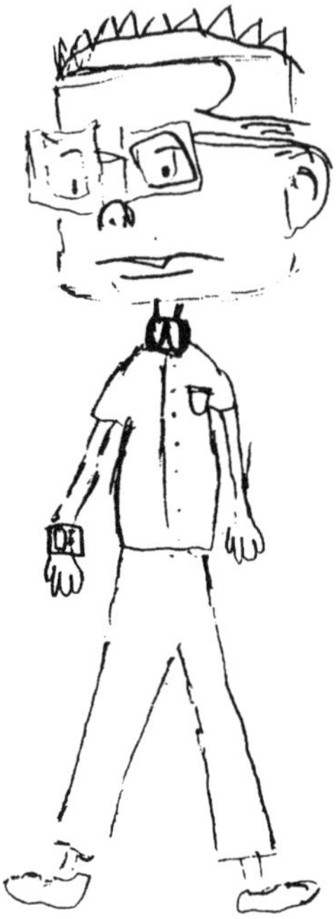

Figure 4.1:
Drawings of the
human figure by an eight-year-old boy:

a) Before starting a reflex stimulation and inhibition programme;

b) After nine months on a reflex stimulation and inhibition programme.

Figure 4.1a is an eight-year-old boy's drawing of a human figure before he started a reflex stimulation and inhibition programme. This boy had a diagnosis of dyslexia and his teacher had suggested to his mother that he also seemed to demonstrate features of Asperger's syndrome. Note the large head (the boy had an unusually large head) and the fact that he has made no attempt to draw the body. Figure 4.1b is a drawing of a human figure after nine months on a reflex stimulation and inhibition programme. Although the head is still drawn disproportionately large, the rest of the body is now also drawn.

One nine-year-old girl, who had been adopted from one of the former Eastern bloc countries at the age of three-and-a-half, had spent the first three years of her life confined to a cot with minimal opportunity for gross movement or weight-bearing on the lower half of the body. At 12 years of age she always drew the human figure without legs. After several months on a reflex stimulation/inhibition programme, which involved carrying out exercises lying on her back and moving her legs through space in slow motion with her eyes closed (providing proprioceptive feedback from the muscles, tendons and joints in the legs), her drawings of the human figure started to include legs.

One test for soft signs of neurological dysfunction is the 'tandem walk': the child is asked to walk forwards slowly, placing one foot in front of another with the heel touching the toe of the other. Children with reflex problems can have difficulty locating their feet without looking at them or placing them with precision. They may, for example, leave a gap, tread on their toes or slide one foot until it abuts with the other. This can be a sign of poor proprioceptive awareness of where different parts of the body are in space, and of overreliance on support from the visual system.

In the early months of life, it is the mouth – through rooting, sucking and exploring with the lips and tongue – that provides the child with their primary source of tactile information. The hands are also involved – initially in palmar movements and the Babkin response– and later in an interplay between hand and mouth, the mouth providing the primary arena for discovery. This is the so-called 'oral' phase of development. As in the growth of prenatal tactile response, postnatal tactile development starts with the mouth and spreads outwards to the hands, the feet and eventually the whole body. If either tactile withdrawal or grasp reflexes remain prevalent beyond their allotted time, they can disrupt the delicate balance between protective and discriminative tactile responses in regions of the body where the reflex is naturally elicited in infancy.

As children grow older, physical contact with the parents diminishes. At puberty the adolescent tentatively seeks tactile stimulation anew with the blossoming of sexual awareness, and thus a cycle of search for contact continues through life. It is perhaps the eight- to sixteen-year-old age group who will suffer most if they have undetected tactile problems, for this is the age when they must seek tactile information for themselves, since parents and teachers no longer supply it with the generosity or abundance that they did during early childhood.[17]

Symptoms of hypertactility:

- hypersensitivity
- dislike of being touched, but may be a compulsive toucher
- allergic skin reactions
- poor temperature control
- low external pain threshold
- body dysmorphia
- dislike of contact sports
- tendency to rely on sensory instead of verbal language

Symptoms of hypotactility:

- hyposensitive to touch
- high threshold of pain
- craving for deep proprioceptive feedback, enjoys contact sports
- may provoke roughhousing or fighting
- compulsive touching
- body dysmorphia
- 'bull in a china shop'

Audition

Hearing, like vestibular sensation and touch, is the result of the reception and transmission of energy through motion and vibration.

The human ear is a compound development that forms during the second half of the embryonic period (four to eight weeks in utero). As the ossicles of the middle ear develop, central nervous system connections are established to the cochlea and the vestibular structures. Myelination of auditory fibres occurs between the 24th and the 28th week in utero, and sound perception develops slowly from this time onwards. At this stage, the ear is tuned to a relatively narrow range of frequency of sounds – specifically to the sounds heard in utero – said to range from 83Hz to 3000Hz (Johansson et al. 1964) or from 250Hz to

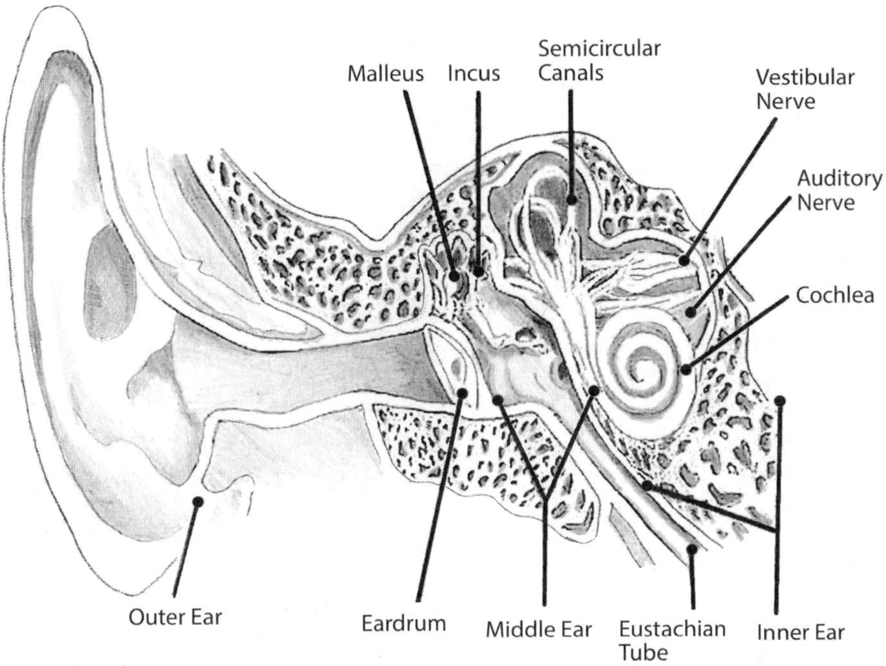

Figure 4.2: The ear.

5000Hz (Lecanuet et al. 1988), depending on gestational age. The foetus also responds to some external auditory stimuli as well. The range of frequencies to which the foetus responds widens with gestational age. As the foetus matures, the intensity of sound needed to elicit a response diminishes.

When sound intensity is measured ex utero the fetus is most responsive to the 500 Hz tone and below. When using intensity assessed in utero, the fetus may be more sensitive to 500 Hz tones and above. The results indicate that foetal response to sound commences in the lower parts of the adult frequency range and expands its frequency range and increases in sensitivity as the fetus matures. (Hepper and Shahidullah 1994).

To put this range of sound frequencies into context, shortly after birth the normal range for hearing is about 20Hz to 20kHz, with most sensitivity in the range 2–4kHz; the normal range of the human voice is about 500Hz to 2kHz with vowels and bass tones falling in the lower frequency range and consonants in the higher frequencies (Figure 4.2). Sounds are often classified as being low, medium or high frequency.

The low frequency range lies between 10Hz and 200Hz. Humans can hear sounds from 20Hz upwards, but the range between the 10Hz and 20Hz can be detected through the tactile system as vibration even though not perceived as sound. Sounds in this sensory bridge between systems can affect the psychological moods of humans. The low-frequency sounds are carriers of the enrichment function, saturation of emotions, and final response. The male voice has the capability of falling in the region of 100 Hz and a large number of musical instruments can produce sounds in this low-frequency range.

The medium frequency range starts from 200Hz and goes up to 2400Hz. During stages of human evolution, the auditory system started to capture the mid-frequency sound range that corresponds largely with the range of human speech. The vocal capability of men, women and a large number of musical instruments falls within this range, including the guitar, piano, keyboard, and wind instruments.

The high frequency range starts from 2400Hz and goes up to 20kHz but there can be individual variation in how far this range extends. For example, a normal human cannot hear any sound above 20kHz, but there are sensitive people who can hear up to 30kHz.

Scientists in New York – using a superconducting quantum interference device (SQID) on subjects listening to music – found that an eerie reflection of

Figure 4.3: Inner ear – hair cells responding to sound

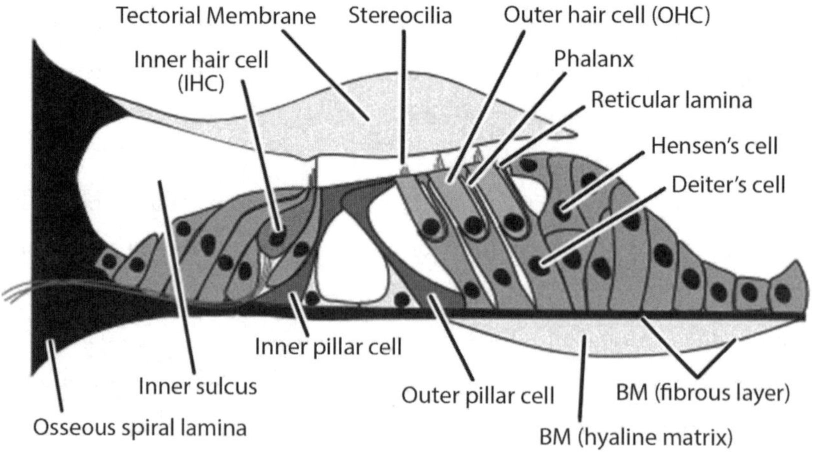

BioMed Research International, vol. 2015, Article ID 727434, 2015. https://doi.org/10.1155/2015/727434

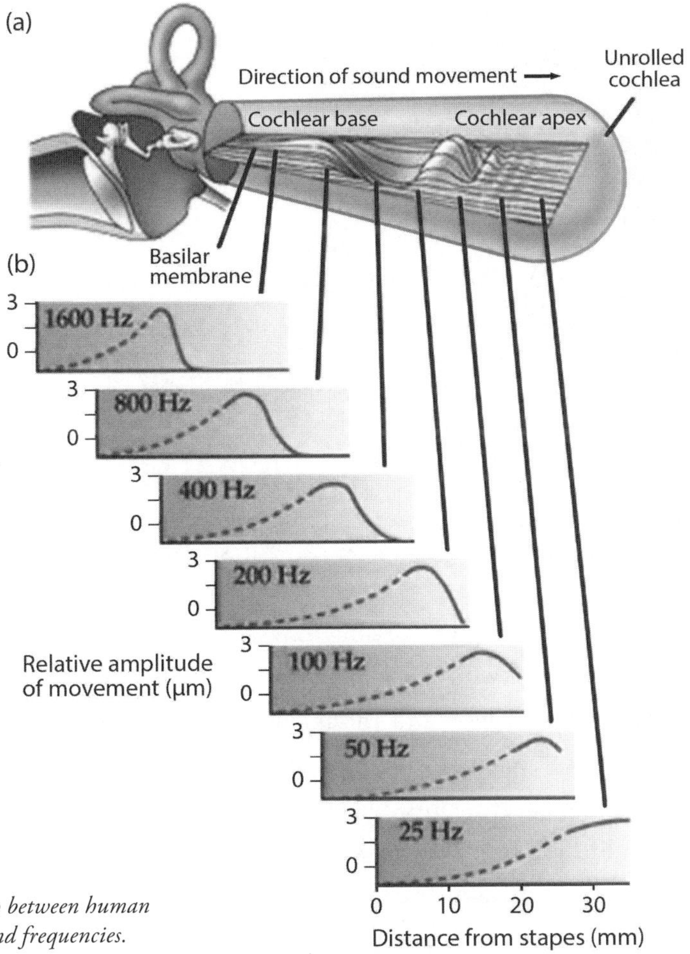

Figure 4.4: Relationship between human ear and sound frequencies.

the black and white keys of a piano was mapped in the brain and responded to the notes that were heard (Figure 4.5). The SQID is used to measure extremely weak signals, such as subtle changes in the human body's electromagnetic energy field. One of the device's most promising uses is in magnetoencephalography (MEG), the process of measuring magnetic fields to enable brain imaging.

'The brain hears loud sounds in a totally different place from quieter sounds, but the areas which register tones are laid out like a keyboard' (S Williamson quoted in Begley 1992). It is possible that failure to register specific sounds at critical stages of language learning may result in part of the mental keyboard

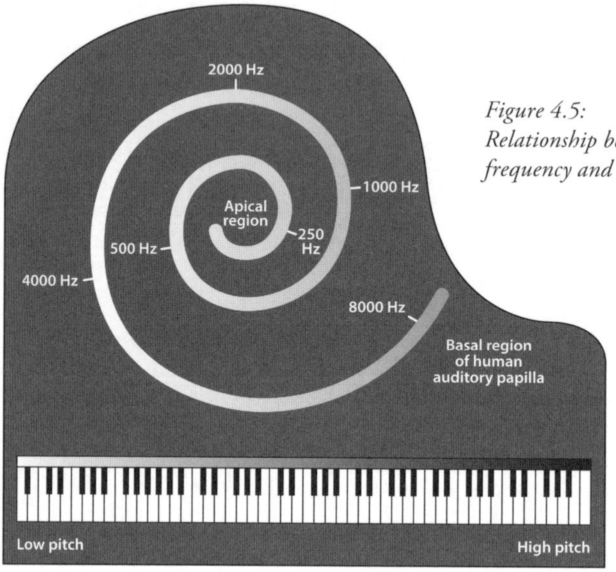

Figure 4.5: Relationship between sound frequency and musical tones.

or sound map being omitted or ceasing to respond (Figure 4.5).

Hearing deteriorates with age, hence a narrowing in the band of frequencies that a person is able to hear and the intensity required to elicit a response. Certain behaviours also tend to change when there is either bilateral, unilateral or frequency-specific hearing loss. Damage to the hearing apparatus can occur at any time in life as a result of exposure to loud noise, infection, neurological conditions, oxygen deprivation and physical trauma.

Learning to listen

For the first few days after birth, the ears of the neonate are still filled with superfluous fluid (similar to the water in the ears after swimming or bathing), with the result that the infant inhabits an auditory no man's land between uterine and extra-uterine sound. Once the fluid has cleared, the neonate ears become receptive to a vast range of sound frequencies, something in the region of 0–20,000Hz and beyond.

During the first three years of life, the child must learn to use their ears and brain together to tune in to the specific frequencies of their own language, in much the same way that a radio is adjusted to select specific stations. At this time, the child has the potential to learn any language if they are exposed to the sounds of that language continuously over a period of time, no matter what language their mother speaks. After the age of six years, when these primary fine-tuning adjustments should have been made, it becomes far more difficult to assimilate a new language and to speak it without a trace of accent.

If a child suffers from frequent ear, nose, throat or upper respiratory tract infections in the first three years of life, hearing can be compromised, not only for the period of acute infection, but for up to eight weeks afterwards. If a child suffers two or three such bouts per year, hearing may be affected intermittently for six months during a single year. If the hearing is tested after the infection has cleared, it may be normal, but the periods of temporary hearing loss that occurred during this critical period for learning to differentiate the specific sounds of speech can have a longer-term effect on a child's auditory discrimination and processing skills, with implications for learning in the classroom later on.

Hearing loss has long been recognised as being an enormous handicap linguistically, educationally and socially. Much less attention has been paid until recently to problems of hearing discrimination among children with learning difficulties or language disorders. Speech may have developed at the correct time, but the more detailed analysis of sounds essential for reading and spelling can be affected. The child cannot hear the difference between similar or blended sounds such as 'ch' and 'sh', 'th' and 'f', or 'p' and 'b'. If the letters sound the same to them, they presume that they should be spelled the same way.

Storr (1993) explains that two essential components are involved in reading – vision and hearing. He describes the 'auditory reader' as someone who is not just a phonetic reader, but is able to read silently using an 'inner voice' that enables them to see and hear the words inside their head, as if they were being seen on the page and read out loud. Poor auditory discrimination skills can interfere with the development of this process.

In addition to intermittent hearing loss in early childhood, insufficient auditory stimulation in terms of social engagement (conversation) with another human being can stunt the development of a child's speech and language skills.

An infant's first language is one of gesture, movement, musical tones and rhythms. We are able to understand the mood and many of a child's needs from changes in posture, facial expression and the speed and quality of their movements. These are elements of non-verbal language that we continue to rely on the for the remainder of life. Mothers quickly learn how to discern when their infant is hungry through the appearance and increase of rooting activity; a distressed infant will tend to throw their head back with an increase in extensor muscle tone, whereas a contented infant in a relaxed state will make balletic movements with their arms and legs as they try to invite engagement. The cooing and babbling of an infant are also essentially musical in nature.

Mothers naturally use a special form of language described as 'motherese' when talking to their babies. Motherese involves exaggerated intonation, slower speech and longer pauses accompanied by animated facial expressions and gestures. This slowing down of speech and enhanced intonation make it easier for the infant to differentiate speech sounds, and the longer pauses give the baby time to process and respond vocally and motorically. Infants are naturally attuned to the sound of the mother's voice before any other, because the tones, rhythm and cadences of her speech are familiar from life in the womb.[18]

Research carried out at the University of Edinburgh analysed early mother–infant interactions. They found that if the mother used short phrases with exaggerated intonation and then paused for a few seconds, the baby would return a perfect answering melodic musical phrase. This musical dialogue would continue for several seconds, provided that the mother included a pause each time. When another adult entered the room, started to talk to the baby, but did not give it time to respond, the infant simply gave up trying to take part in the conversation, as if to say, 'How rude! Don't you understand the manners of good conversation?' In other words, early interaction with an attentive, sympathetic listener who allows time for the child to react encourages the development of preverbal communication.

Inadequate auditory stimulation or an environment in which there is a constant cacophony of background noise in early life can also discourage early listening: the child learns to shut out and ignore certain types of sound from an early age. Similarly, electronic games do not provide the same process as one-to-one human engagement in real time. Although recordings of lullabies and

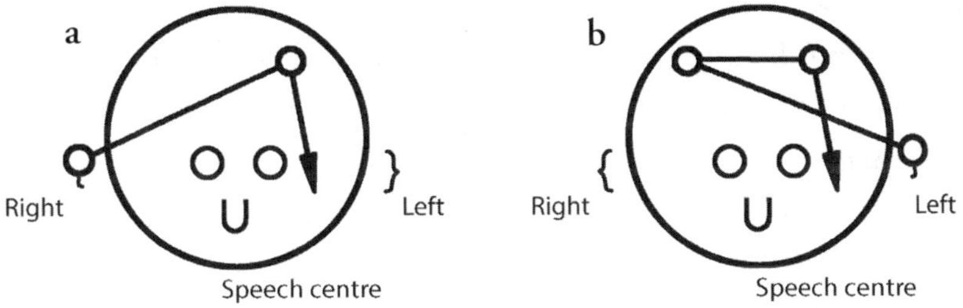

Figure 4.6: Main routes for transmission of sound to the brain: a) Right ear; b) Left ear

nursery rhymes may be useful for entertaining a baby or helping to send them to sleep, they do not encourage dialogue. Recordings are preset. They have no interest in what the child has to say and therefore do not wait for the child to respond and do not take their cue from the child's response.

Hearing too much, or 'auditory hypersensitivity', can be just as much of a problem as hearing deficit. The inability to filter or occlude miscellaneous sound suggests poorly developed listening skills and can have a profound effect upon later learning, language, communication and behaviour. In the last 40 years, research has turned to focus upon the problems of listening, as opposed to problems of hearing. Alfred Tomatis, in France, and Christian Volf, in Denmark, quite independently of each other, were pioneers in this approach. Since then, various techniques have been devised to assess and to retrain the listening skills of individuals with such diverse problems as autism, hyperactivity, dyslexia, depression and, among musicians, imperfect pitch discrimination.

Tomatis also showed that there is a difference in the way that sounds are transmitted to the language-processing centre in the brain, depending on which ear is used as the dominant listening ear. The right ear is the more efficient of the two for receiving and transmitting the sounds of language for most people in whom the main language-decoding centre resides in the left side of the brain. Left-eared children who also have the main language centre in the left side may be at a disadvantage. Sounds heard through the right ear pass directly to the main language centre in the left hemisphere (Figure 4.6a). Sounds heard via the left ear pass first to the sublanguage centre in the right hemisphere and then have to pass through the corpus callosum to the left hemisphere for decoding (Figure 4.6b). This longer route results in a delay of milliseconds, somewhat like the delay experienced on an overseas call while the sounds pass to the satellite and down again. This small delay in timing can alter the sound that the brain actually hears, since the difference in the brain's perceiving a sound as 'd' or 't' is a difference of some 40–60 milliseconds in the timing of the onset and offset of the first and second bursts of sound. The child who is primarily left-eared may also have difficulty processing and remembering a list of verbal instructions, since they may still be decoding the first two instructions when the third is being given. The child who suffers from auditory delay may also appear to be slow or inattentive when spoken to.

Lack of ear preference may further confuse the situation, resulting in sounds reaching the brain in a different order from the order they are arranged phonetically in a word;[19] thus the child who switches ear preference while listening or sounding out a word may find that the sounds processed through the left ear arrive a fraction later than the sounds processed through the right ear, irrespective of their correct order. For example, if the word 'phon/et/ic' were heard using the left ear for the first syllable and the right ear for the latter two,

Table 4.1: Results of Dichotic Listening Test when sounds were played to each ear sequentially.

Left ear	Right ear	Sound heard
Fak	Bat	Mut
Gep	Ris	Gris
Kit	Nur	Nut
Bat	Gep	Net

Source: Adapted from Ganong (1997) and Galley and Forster (1987).

Table 4.2: Number of correct responses on Dichotic Listening Test/20

Ear	Number of correct responses
Right ear	16/20
Left ear	19/20
Right ear ignoring the left	12/20
Left ear ignoring the right	4/20
Right and left ear sequentially	4/20

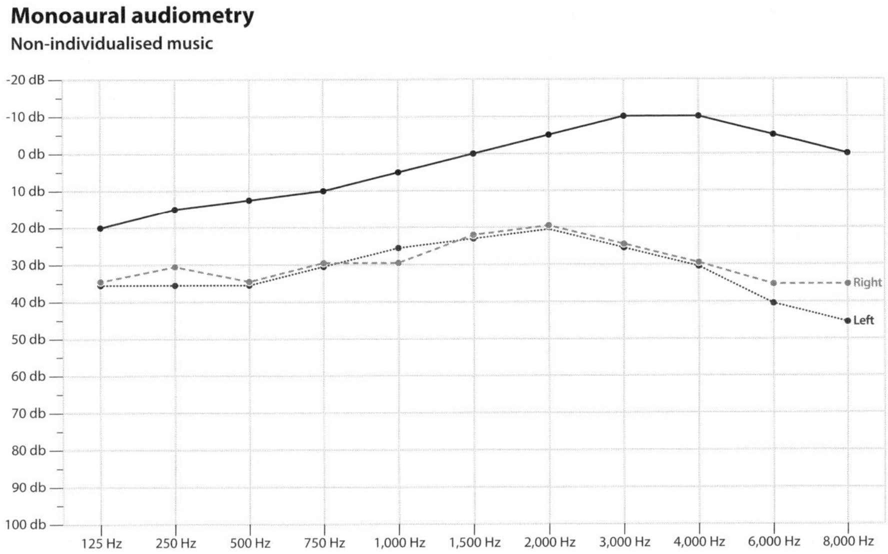

Figure 4.7: Client's audiogram compared with the optimum English-language curve.

it might arrive at the brain as 'eticphon' or even 'etphonic'. Inconsistencies in spelling involving letter, syllable and word reversals are a logical outcome.

Use of a dichotic listening test using Danish-language syllables with English-speaking children demonstrates this effect. When asked to repeat the sounds being played into one ear at a time, children with a lack of ear preference perform reasonably well with each ear. When sounds are played into one ear after the other and they have to repeat sounds going to one ear only, they start to mix or confuse syllables. An example of confusion when sounds were sent to each ear, one after the other, and the child had to repeat both is shown in Table 4.1. In this particular example, there was a marked deterioration in the number of correct responses when sounds were played to both ears rather than to one ear at a time.

This child had a history of frequent ear infections in their early years (at least six infections a year) until grommets were inserted at four years of age. Two subsequent sets of grommets were inserted 18 months later and the adenoids removed. Her hearing was assessed at 12 years of age as a part of an assessment to investigate whether auditory-processing difficulties were contributing to an uneven profile on an educational psychological assessment, which had revealed verbal comprehension scores to be in the high range while performance on perceptual reasoning was average and processing speed and memory skills were in the low range. Audiometric assessment revealed hearing thresholds for both ears to be between 25dB and 45dB throughout the frequency range (Figure 4.7), good enough for the child not to be referred for further medical investigations but, as revealed by the results from the dichotic listening test above (Tables 4.1 and 4.2), clearly inadequate to support functional hearing discrimination and accurate processing.

If a child is to be able to hear words and then to separate specific sounds and distinguish the phonemes and formants in them, they need to have excellent hearing throughout the range of frequencies from 125Hz to 8000Hz. Every language has its unique frequency band, within which fall all the sounds used in that language, with differing sensitivity thresholds. Key stages or windows for learning are well known. If a key stage is missed, the chances of subsequently developing skills in that area are considerably reduced. The window for pre-language is during the first three years of life, when the child learns to filter out unnecessary sounds and tune in to the sounds of their mother tongue so that they can start to hear and reproduce the sounds necessary for speech and later for written language.

When a standard hearing test is carried out, response to a stimulus applied at a volume of 20dB or above is considered normal. Response at thresholds starting from 40–60dB is considered moderate hearing loss; at 60dB and beyond, severe hearing loss. A volume of 40dB would be considered adequate but not ideal for a child to cope in a noisy classroom, from the point of view most school doctors or audiologists whose primary job is to detect hearing deficit. Thus, a child whose hearing threshold falls between 20dB and 40dB will not be considered sufficiently at risk to warrant further investigation or treatment. Nevertheless, this type of hearing can have a profound effect upon the child's ability to discriminate between similar but different sounds.

The chart in Figure 4.8 shows the optimum English-language curve. This curve illustrates the typical volume thresholds (in db) to detect specific speech sounds. The English-language curve requires sensitivity at lower thresholds (<20db) in the high-frequency range to perceive specific sounds such as 'f', 's', 'sh', 'ch' and 'th' which cannot be read on the lips. Vowel and consonant sounds

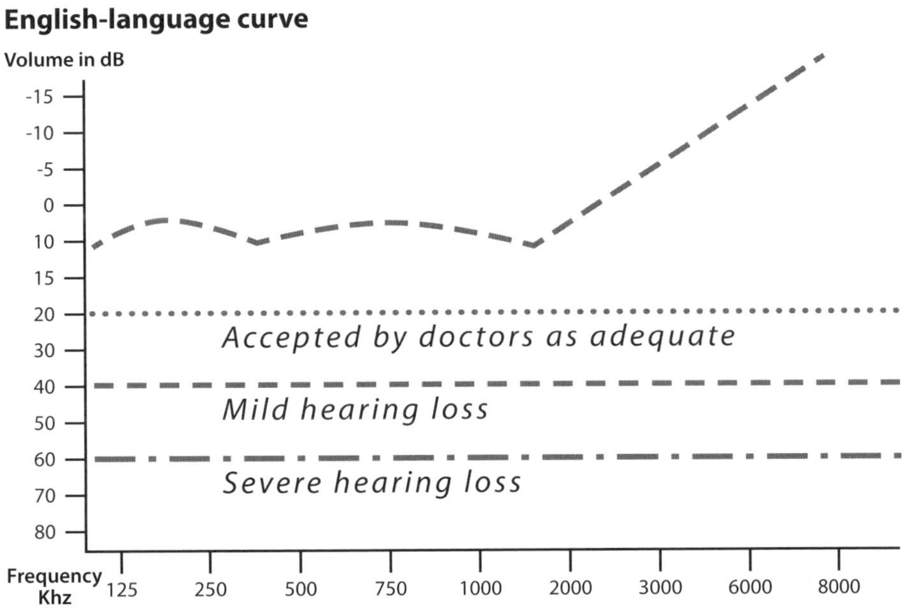

Figure 4.8:
Standard audiogram showing optimum English-language curve and levels of hearing loss.

cross the spectrum of frequencies, and so minor deviations from the language curve may cause specific speech and spelling problems.

The differences on the page between 'b', 'd', 'p' and 'q', is one of directionality, but the decision as to which way the symbol should face is based upon the fact that each letter sounds different. If a child has difficulty in distinguishing a difference between the sound of these letters ('b' and 'p' are close to each other in frequency and are difficult to tell apart on the lips), the rationale for writing each letter one way or the other is meaningless. Similarly, 'f', 'th', 'sh' and 'ch' sounds in English are hard to distinguish if there is any high-frequency hearing loss, and these are letters and blends that are often incorrectly used by children with spelling difficulties and dyslexia.

Some children suffer from hyperacuity, but, as this is not measured in standard hearing tests, the child is again dismissed as not having a problem. Hearing too much can result in enormous concentration difficulties, speech difficulties, overload in noisy environments, and problems with social interaction. Tomatis describes how high-frequency sound is 'energising' whereas low-frequency sound tends to be relaxing or 'enervating'. Clinical tests at the INPP carried out on children with ADHD or diagnosed as being on the autistic spectrum have revealed them to be hypersensitive in the high frequency range of sounds, in some cases still perceiving sounds between 2000Hz and 6000Hz at a volume of -10dB and below. One boy with low-frequency sensitivity was even convinced he had extrasensory perception, since he knew a car was coming round a corner several seconds before anyone else did.

Kjeld Johansen, at the Dyslexia Research Laboratory in Gudhjem, Denmark, devised a system of assessing and treating problems of auditory discrimination and auditory processing. Over 40 years of independent research developed from the original ideas of Christian Volf have resulted in a therapeutic approach that has been statistically proven to be effective. Audiometric tests are carried out to measure monaural thresholds and to determine hearing acuity throughout the hearing range. A dichotic listening test is also used to establish which is the primary ear. Once the tests have been analysed, children are given frequency-specific music to listen to for ten minutes per day. Specific tracks have been made in which all sounds except the frequencies they have difficulty hearing have been filtered out, the volume of specific frequencies is adjusted to compensate for differences in the individual hearing curve, and, if indicated, sounds are biased towards one ear. By listening to pure frequencies unpolluted by extraneous sound, children can start to hear the sounds that they were formerly unable to discriminate against the background of a multitude of frequencies. The music can also be specially adjusted to encourage right-eared listening if this is required. Both frequency range and adjustments are altered at 6–8-weekly intervals, and hearing is rechecked every few months to ensure that improvements are taking place. As the children's listening skills improve, concomitant changes take place in reading, writing, short-term memory, language use and behaviour.

Although there are apparently fewer direct connections between primitive reflexes and hearing than between these and vision, primitive reflexes (particularly the Moro reflex) and postural reactions can be linked to hearing issues. Whereas many of the reflexes are elicited by stimulation of a specific sensory system – the rooting and sucking reflexes respond to tactile stimuli, the TLR to stimulation of the labyrinthine portion of the vestibular apparatus in the inner ear – the Moro reflex is potentially responsive to multisensory stimuli. A continued relationship can occur in either direction: on the one hand, if the Moro reflex persists, hyperarousal and hypervigilance may render the infant more sensitive to auditory stimuli; on the other, if there has been a history of frequent ear, nose, throat or chest infections in the first years of life, resulting in periods of intermittent conductive hearing loss, the natural defence mechanism for protecting the ear from loud or unwanted sounds (the acoustic stapedius reflex) may be underdeveloped when hearing is restored, and the Moro reflex may continue to be elicited in response to sudden or loud noises or specific frequencies of sound. There can be also an emotional link between these systems if specific sounds are associated with a traumatic event.

Research carried out by Butler Hall (1998) indicated a possible link between audition and the spinal Galant reflex. Continued presence of the ATNR may also influence the development of ear preference. It is believed that the establishment of a leading ear is necessary to develop selective listening (shutting out background noise). Also important for the development of selective listening is the ability to orient to the source of sound. This is because in locating the source of sound it becomes possible to decide if it requires attention or can be ignored. In this context, the retention of primitive reflexes that interfere with orientation could potentially affect aspects of auditory processing. This may be one reason why a reflex integration programme can sometimes improve auditory processing without the need to implement a specific auditory training programme.

Conversely, we also recruit hearing to support spatial awareness. While balance and postural control provide the internal sense of centre in space, and vision provides information about what is happening externally in front of us, hearing informs us about what is happening in the external world beyond and behind the field of vision. By comparing the location and distance of sounds between the two ears, we should be able to locate the source of sounds we cannot see. Sometimes the use of a sound therapy programme alone can improve signs of aberrant reflexes linked to hearing and spatial awareness.

Live music

The value of music for learning has long been recognised, but, with financial cuts and changes in methods of education, music has taken a back seat in the early learning years of many children. Vast improvements have been made in electronic sound equipment. Because it is so inexpensive and easily available, a lot of music is now heard through streaming, where it has been altered by sound engineers who have made subtle changes to the frequency spectrum and beats per minute. Listening to streamed music also removes the vibrational component experienced when listening to a live performance.

Live music, sadly, is today a rare experience for many children. Previous generations of children participated in daily singing led and accompanied by a teacher on the piano; multiplication tables, the alphabet and Latin verbs were learned to tunes. Understanding of what they had learned came later, but the tune and the rhythm aided recall. Most people can still remember the words to all the verses of a song learned in early childhood if someone sings the first few notes of the tune for them. Without the music, they cannot recall the words. In this way, music can act as a key not only for storing information but also for opening a storage unit that has been filled with sequences of information.

The Master of Choristers at an English cathedral said that the reading age of all his choir boys improved by 12 months within six months of their joining the choir. This remained true irrespective of whether they were good or poor readers at the time of joining. It could be said that this was the direct result of the amount of written material they had to sing on a daily basis, but it could also be said that the dual processes of listening, elongating vowel sounds to fit words to music, vocalising, and learning to hear pitch and rhythm enhanced other skills. Audrey Wisbey (1977), in Cambridge, found much the same reading improvement. Moroever, cathedrals and other large old public buildings have acoustics that are rich in the high frequencies and echo and reflect sounds – qualities that are lost in the low-ceiling, carpeted and cushioned buildings of our time.

'Sound is not sound' (Steinbach 1994); sound is vibration, motion and energy. If we hear no sound we perceive danger, for a totally silent world is a dead world. Sound passes through all levels of the brain, affecting not just the ear and the vestibular system but also our bodies through bone conduction. The significance of sound for learning is immeasurable.

Symptoms of auditory problems:

- short attention span
- distractibility
- hypersensitivity to sounds
- misinterpretation of questions
- confusion of similar-sounding words, frequent need to have a word repeated
- inability to follow sequential instructions
- flat and monotonous voice
- hesitant speech
- weak vocabulary
- poor sentence structure
- inability to sing in tune
- confusion or reversal of letters
- poor reading comprehension
- poor reading aloud
- poor spelling
- auditory delay

Vision

Vision is clearly essential for academic learning. The skills of reading, writing, spelling and arithmetic all depend upon the ability to see written symbols. When learning difficulties arise, vision is often the first area to be checked. If the child passes a simple eye test that only assesses distance vision, further investigation into visual problems is seldom pursued. Distance vision is only one component in the complex sense of sight. How we see, the way that we use our eyes and how we perceive the world through sight are the result of a complex series of connections and neural developments that come about in the early formative years and are dependent upon adequate maturation of the central nervous system.

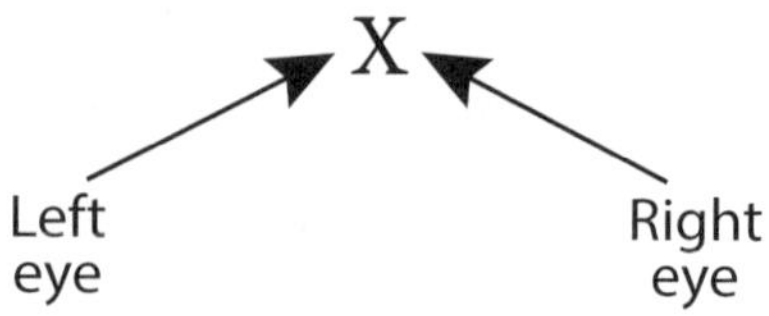

Figure 4.9: Visual convergence.

Each eye sees a different image but the brain must process a fusion of the two. In order to do this, the two eyes must work as a team so that each eye is directed to the same fixation point – for example, on the page – rather like two spotlights highlighting a dancer on the centre of the stage. This is called 'convergence' and must be fully developed for the brain to perceive one clear image (Figure 4.9). Operating as a team, the eyes can then scan along a line of letters and send a clear sequence of images to the brain. Figure 4.10a shows the drawings of one 13-year-old boy, diagnosed with dyslexia, whose eyes had never learned to converge, with the result that he saw a second image or reflection on the page. Figure 4.10b shows the model he had copied from. It is not surprising that he had enormous difficulties with all written material.

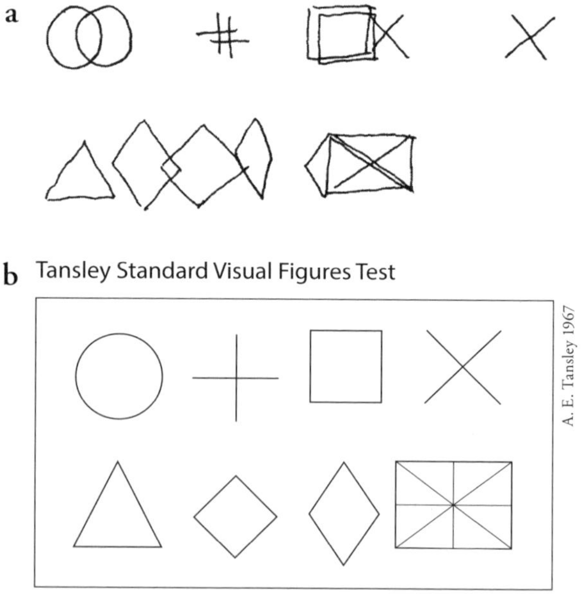

Figure 4.10:

a) Result of poor near point convergence resulting in perception of two images;

b) Tansley standard figures.

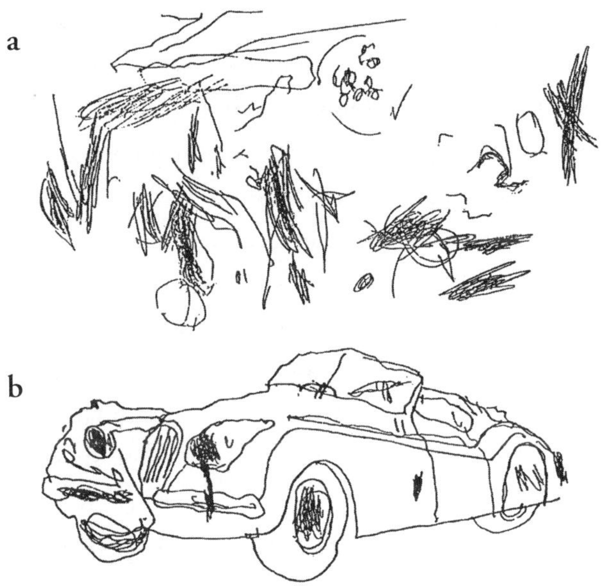

Figure 4.11:

a) First drawing using both eyes;

b) Second drawing using one eye.

Printed by permission of Catharina Johamesson Alvegard, The Institute for Neuro-Physiological Psychology, Gothenberg, Sweden

Figure 4.11a shows a drawing by a boy whose eyes were not working together as a team when he was first assessed. It was his first attempt at copying a picture of a Jaguar sports car –a meaningless jumble of scribbles. Sometime later, the child psychologist who had assessed him asked him to attempt the drawing again, but this time with one eye covered. Figure 4.11b was the result.

When asked why he had drawn the car so differently, the boy's said, 'I thought that everybody else saw flat images like my first drawing and could somehow turn it into the second.' Because the two eyes were not functioning as a team (yoking), the image he was seeing was fragmented and unstable. By removing the confusion of the second image, he was able to make sense of the material in front of him and reproduce it remarkably well. This is not a case for eye patching as a solution to the problem because the two eyes have to learn to work together. Eye patching does not develop yoking ability, but this example demonstrates the devastating effect of a combination of convergence difficulties and lack of yoking ability upon visual functioning.

A second necessity is that the image seen by each eye must be sharp and clearly focused. The focus must be adjusted quickly from one distance or one angle to another. In order to do this, the eyes must converge at one focal distance, then break out of convergence (diverge) to reconverge at the new focal distance. This skill is called 'accommodation'. Difficulties with either convergence or divergence can affect the speed of accommodation. Poor visual accommodation can make the child slower at copying or clumsy when trying to catch a ball.

Furthermore, in order to read easily, it is necessary to be able to scan or track along a line of print smoothly and evenly, so that the brain can receive a flow of sequentially correct information. Tracking is vital for orderly progression from one word to another or finding the way from line to line without loss of place. In addition to the three skills of convergence, accommodation and tracking and the ability to hear the difference between similar sounds, a child also needs to have good directional awareness to distinguish similar but directionally different symbols such as 'p'/'q', 'b'/'d', 'on'/'no', 'left'/'felt', etc.[20]

Directional awareness is in part a vestibular-based skill. Levinson (1984) described the vestibular system as acting like an internal compass that provides a physical sense of 'centre' from which we can automatically judge up from down, left from right, front from back, etc. The development of cerebral dominance at the age of seven to eight years cements this knowledge, but problems with directional awareness may still persist after cerebral dominance has occurred if vestibular functioning is faulty. This may be the child who easily gets lost in new surroundings, has difficulty learning to tell time on an analogue clock, has poor organisational skills and struggles to recognise the difference between similar symbols such as 'b' and 'd', or '2' and '5'.

There is also a theory (Skeffington et al. 1947–50) that concentration on near-point activities when the above or supporting skills are not sufficiently developed may result in a degree of visual near-point stress resulting in compensatory adjustments. Skeffington developed a model to explain why he considered vision to be a function that emerges from four underlying processes: anti-gravity, centring, identification, and speech audition.

> Vision is considered not primarily in terms of optics or accommodation–convergence relationships but rather as an organismic process involved with movement, orientation and localisation in space, language and information processing. (Birnbaum 1994)

The near-point visual stress theory holds that a tendency for convergence to localise closer than accommodation is intrinsic to the near-point visual demands imposed by cultures highly dependent on the use of written language and that these culturally imposed close-work demands 'provoke a biological stress response, characterised in the visual system by a drive for convergence to localise closer than accommodation' (Birnbaum 1994).

This model for understanding the basis of visual function in general ties in with observations from practitioners of the INPP method over many years that – when postural control is well established, primitive reflexes are inhibited and head-righting reflexes present – control of the specific eye movements needed to support reading and writing becomes more efficient. In other words, postural stability and balance, which are contingent upon one another, provide the stable platform for higher centres involved in the control of the various eye movements needed for near-distance work and shifting focus between different distances.

This has implications for times of 'reading readiness'. Rudolf Steiner and Maria Montessori both linked reading readiness to child development – the former to the time of shedding the first milk teeth, normally around six years of age, the latter to the prior development of physical skills – such as learning sounds and letters through singing nursery rhymes and traditional songs to which actions can be added, practical activities like building dens and baking, and touching and recognising materials of various shapes and sizes and tracing and drawing shapes in different media – as well as mental skills based on language development and also social skills learned through the child's inclusion in conversations with family members and peers. While chronological age is used as the primary determinant of time of school entry and year group, developmental age is more individual. Assessment of primitive and postural reflexes at key stages in development is one way in which a child's developmental age in terms of neuromotor skills may be observed.

Reading difficulty is only the tip of the iceberg where visual problems are concerned. Handwriting and spelling will also be profoundly affected, as will coordination, because difficulties with visual adjustment can affect spatial awareness, body image and hand–eye coordination. Many sports and leisure activities will only be performed with great effort, and levels of attainment will tend to be disproportionate to the energy and enthusiasm initially applied to the task. The child can become quickly frustrated and may soon start to avoid activities enjoyed by other children, thereby exacerbating their own sense of isolation.

Since poor visual information can impair the recognition and recall of groups of letters either as units or as a picture (visuo-spatial awareness), spelling can also be affected. Visual imagery or visualisation is necessary for spelling, since it enables the child to form templates or a visual memory for words in the mind's eye. These are then matched against the written word to assess whether the word looks right – that is, is there an element in the word which does not correspond to the remembered visual image of that word? As our hearing deteriorates gradually over the years, we use auditory memory to continue to enunciate words correctly. So, too, do we need a visual memory to be able to spell words accurately.

The effect of aberrant reflex activity upon oculo-motor functioning was discussed in Chapter 1: the ATNR in combination with underdeveloped head-righting reflexes has an adverse effect upon tracking, the TLR upon convergence, the Moro reflex upon the tendency to be stimulus bound and the STNR upon speed of accommodation. Dysfunction in these areas will inevitably result in visual-perceptual difficulties. It is important that an examination be carried out to assess what a child sees and to investigate the ways in which their eyes work together.

Below are two examples of severe visual-perceptual difficulties. Both children were in a mainstream school and struggling to keep up with academic work. They were asked to copy the Tansley Standard Figures and an amended version of the Bender Visual Gestalt Figures (Figure 4.12a) and the Tansley Standard Figures (Figure 4.13a). Despite a history of reading, writing and spelling difficulties, the visual-perceptual and visual-motor integration skills of these children had not previously been investigated. Child A and Child B also had a cluster of aberrant primitive reflexes.

It must be remembered that the eye is only an instrument of vision. To make effective use of the vision that eyes provide, the child must also make use of

Figure 4.12:

a) *Bender visual gestalt figure;*
b) *First drawing attempt by Child A, aged 12 years, with a diagnosis of minimal front brain damage;*
c) *Second drawing by Child A after five months into a reflex stimulation and inhibition programme.*

Bender Visual Gestalt figure

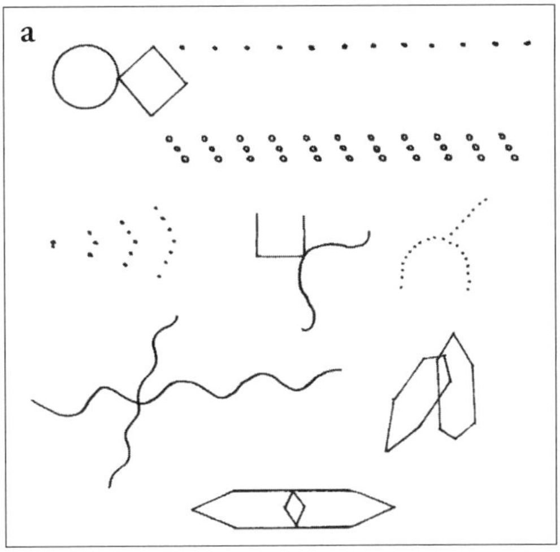

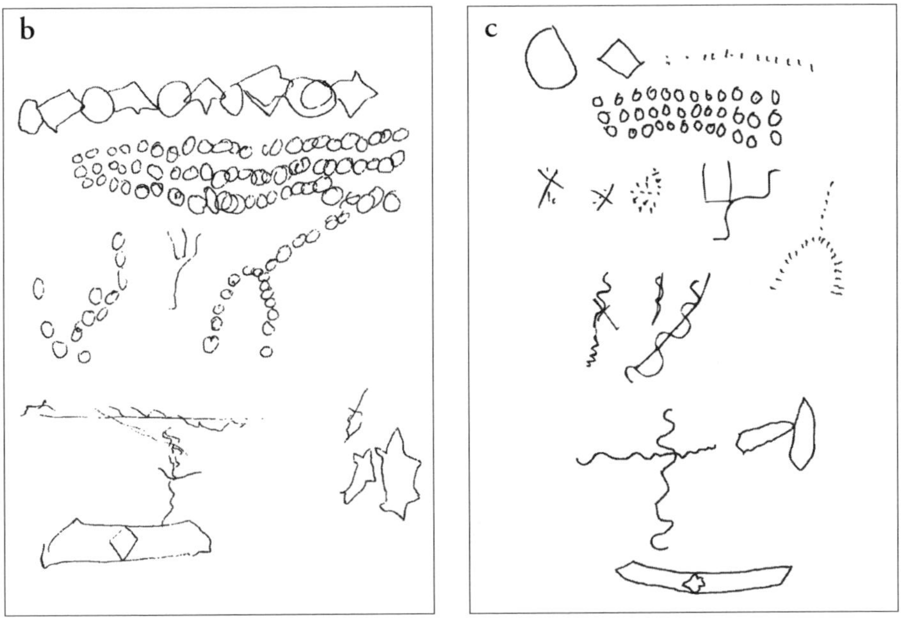

other sensory information. The foundations for these interconnections are laid down during the first year of life, at the time the neural pathways are formed between the eye, the brain and the body. Vision is particularly dependent upon two of these pathways: the vestibular–spinal loop, which provides postural stability, and the VOR (Figure 4.14).

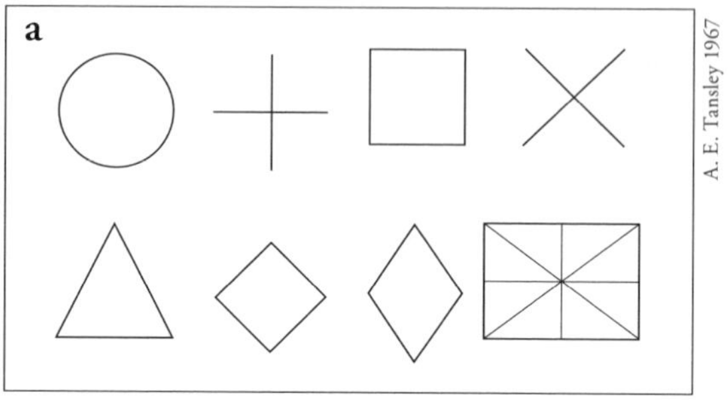

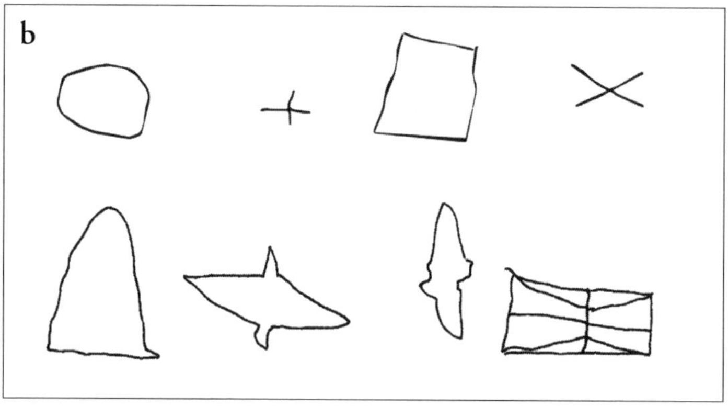

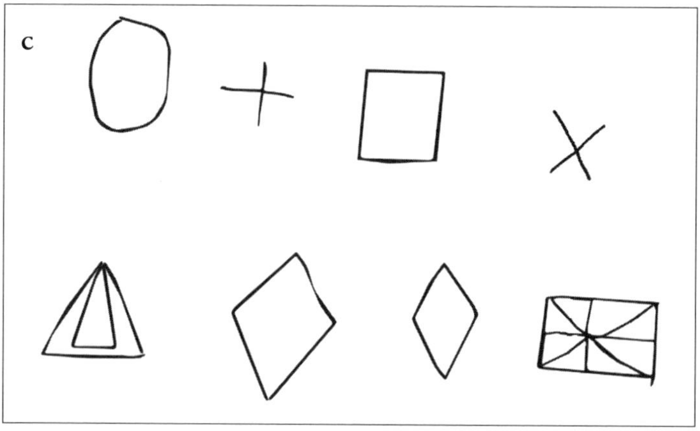

Figure 4.13:

a) Tansley standard figure;

b) First drawing attempt by Child B aged seven years, no diagnosis but underachieving in maths, handwriting and physical education;

c) Second drawing attempt by Child B after three months on a reflex stimulation and inhibition programme.

Interaction between the components of the VOR will determine the efficiency of the visual system in later life, that is, the rapid exchange of information between the vestibular apparatus, the eyes and the level of reflex response to incoming stimuli. Any defect in one of these elements can affect the smooth operation of the whole.

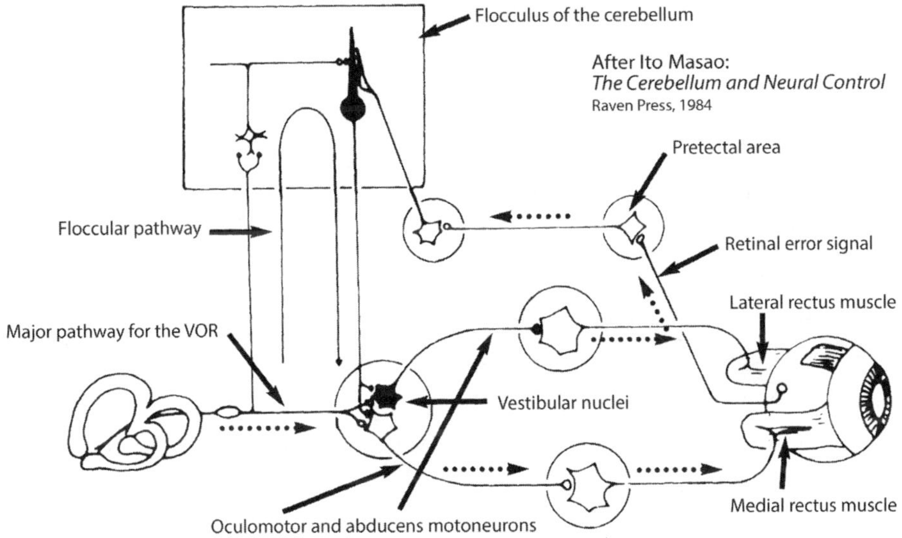

Figure 4.14: Feedback loops involved in the VOR pathway.

Symptoms indicative of visual stress:

- misreading words
- missing or repeating words or lines
- slow reading
- need to use finger or marker as a pointer
- inability to remember what has been read
- poor concentration
- child describes letters that 'move', 'jump' or are poorly focused
- reading at a very close distance
- reading with one eye covered or a sideways posture
- distractibility (stimulus-bound effect)
- poor posture when reading or writing
- head tilted to one side
- poorly spaced work
- handwriting crooked or slopes in different directions, letters poorly balanced

- clumsiness
- difficulty with ball games
- headaches

Proprioception

Closely allied to the other senses and interdependent with them is the compound sense of proprioception. Although it is the result of multisensory information, it also forms an information channel of its own involved in linking interoceptive and exteroceptive experience in terms of body awareness and knowing your place in space.

Proprioception or kinaesthesis enables us to know where the parts of our body are at any time and to make the appropriate postural adjustments. It is an internal sense of physical self which allows us to carry out detailed manoeuvres without conscious awareness and in the absence of other sensory cues.

Proprioceptors are located throughout the body in the joints, tendons, muscles, etc. Their input is processed mostly by the dorsal column and in part by the spino-cervical tract but is also combined with information from the vestibular system to provide internal information about the position of the body and its parts in space. Information derived from proprioceptors also coordinates with information from all other sensory sources to influence body movements and direct adjustments for fine muscle coordination. Needless to say, distorted information coming from any one of these sources can also affect perception that is based on proprioceptors.

Poor proprioceptive awareness is common among children with learning difficulties. Paradoxically, a small number will rely too heavily upon either proprioception or kinaesthesis to perform certain tasks. Proprioception is the awareness of posture, movement and changes in equilibrium and the knowledge of position, weight and resistance of objects in relation to the body; kinaesthesis is the ability to perceive the extent, direction or weight of movement. One example was a seven-year-old boy who was asked to throw a bean bag into a box of sand from a distance of ten feet. The first four attempts missed the target, but on the fifth the bag dropped into the box. Each subsequent throw was successful, until the box was moved one foot closer to him. Theoretically, this should have been easier, but he overshot the target on the next five throws. Thomas had poor depth perception and was relying upon proprioceptive memory to direct the force of his throw. When he had succeeded once he knew the feel of the throw necessary to hit the target. The same feel did not help him once the target was moved.

Many children with poor individual sensory perception will attempt to use proprioception instead of the primary channel for learning that particular skill. It is rather like using a huge net to attempt to catch one individual fish. Learning can only be consistently successful if eyes, ears and balance system are also providing accurate information about changing circumstances. The child who attempts to use proprioception to compensate for weakness in another channel may be the child for whom 'practice makes perfect… sometimes' and who will, at times, produce excellent results but appears to be inconsistent in their performance.

Proprioceptive difficulties can be misinterpreted in terms of causation and diagnosis. Two examples will help to illustrate this point.

The first was a man in his seventies who was receiving chemotherapy for a form of bone cancer. One of the side effects of the medication was the development of chronic peripheral neuropathy. Peripheral neuropathy occurs when there has been damage to peripheral nerves which impairs sensation in the sensory, motor or autonomic nerves involved. In this man's case, sensory nerves in the feet had been badly affected, resulting in numbness to touch and pressure and a reduced sense of position (from the base upwards). When trying to walk up or down steps, he would hesitate, apparently uncertain how to place the first foot and then follow through with the second. To the casual observer, it appeared that he had a major problem with motor planning – of knowing how to direct the motor nerves to execute the sequence of actions required. In fact the issue with motor planning was a secondary result of inadequate proprioceptive signals from the feet to other areas in the brain involved in awareness of position.

The second example is from an experiment in which the functioning of one sensory system is artificially distorted to observe the effect on others. In this experiment the subject is asked to walk across a distance of three or four metres at a slow pace, placing one foot in front of the other, heel touching the toe, while looking straight ahead (tandem walk). The test is performed once going forwards and then once going backwards. Observations are made of balance, accuracy of foot placement (dependent on proprioception) and any extraneous 'overflow' movements involving other parts of the body which may occur but are not normally required to complete the task. A baseline measure of performance is recorded.

The subject is then given a pair of distortion glasses containing mild prisms and asked to repeat the task. In many cases, wearing the distortion glasses results in immediate alteration of posture, impairment of the control of balance, difficulty in knowing how and where to place the feet, and, in some cases, feelings of nausea. If the symptoms were evaluated at face value when the glasses are worn, the subject would appear to have problems with balance, proprioception, motor planning and coordination, but in the experiment the appearance of these symptoms is secondary to the normal relationship between vision, balance and proprioception having been disturbed by the distortion glasses.

Vision also has the ability to override information from other senses. In a similar experiment, one set of distortion glasses make it appear that flat surfaces are concave. When the surface is touched, while the subject is wearing the glasses, the surface also feels as if it was curved. In other words, the visual distortion is powerful enough to overrule perception derived from the haptic sense. These experiments demonstrate that just as important for coherent perception as the functioning of each sensory system is the functional relationship between them.

Vestibular and proprioceptive functioning provide vital internal information about the position of the body and its parts in relation to one another, which is then combined with information about the external environment derived from vision, hearing and touch. If internal systems involved in providing information about position are inadequate, then systems designed to process external information have to work harder to compensate. Signs of compensation in either direction can be observed on a number of tests for soft signs of neurological dysfunction which involve walking both forwards and backwards or carrying out the tests with the eyes open and closed. If performance over a series of tests is consistently better when the task is carried out with the eyes open or when going forwards, it seems that vision is having to work harder to compensate for poor vestibular and/or proprioceptive functioning. If performance is consistently better with the eyes closed or when going backwards, it may be that visual information is not congruent with vestibular and/or proprioceptive function.

Proprioceptive function is also dominant in the formation of the body schema that is represented in drawings of the human figure by children under 13 years of age. Children who have an inadequate sense of where specific parts of their body are either omit them or misrepresent them in terms of scale when drawing the human figure. After they have followed a daily movement programme carried out with the eyes closed, proportions and detail in drawings of the human figure become more age appropriate.

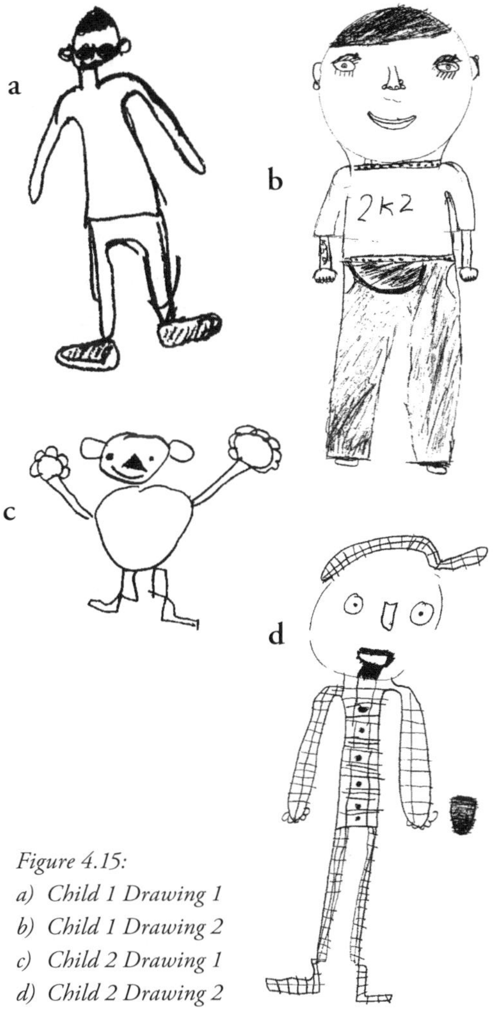

Figure 4.15:
a) Child 1 Drawing 1
b) Child 1 Drawing 2
c) Child 2 Drawing 1
d) Child 2 Drawing 2

Figures 4.15a and 4.15c were drawn by two children before starting a daily developmental movement programme introduced into school (the INPP Developmental Movement Programme for Use in Schools). Figures 4.15b and 4.15d were drawn by the same two children after they had completed the developmental movement programme.

Drawing of the human figure can be assessed using a standardised scoring system to provide one measure of non-verbal cognitive performance. This measure should not be confused with intelligent quotient (IQ), which provides a total score derived from a set of standardised tests and subtests designed to assess a range of abilities. Findings from the 'draw a person' (DAP) test at INPP over many years have revealed that children with NMI consistently omit parts of the body that are not working well for them or represent them disproportionately in their drawings. Figures 4.15a–d provide examples of this. Child 1's first drawing (4.15a) portrays a figure who lacks confidence in space and whose balance is off centre, there is asymmetry in the representation of the body, the hands are omitted and the head is disproportionately small. The second drawing (4.15b) depicts a person who has grown in physical confidence, whose feet are securely and almost symmetrically placed on the ground, and considerable detail has been added, including hands, ears and mouth. The head is still slightly enlarged and no neck links the head to the body, indicating that some problems persist, but the score on one indication of non-verbal cognitive performance has increased from the 14th to the 77th percentile over a period of nine months.

The first drawing (4.15c) of Child 2 (chronological age eight years) was scored as developmentally equivalent to that of a child of five years of age: head, hands and body are disproportionately large, the hands being drawn like paddles; feet and legs lack form, length and symmetry and there is no attempt to add clothing to the drawing. The second drawing (4.15d) shows marked improvement in terms of body awareness and proportions, although the lack of finger differentiation indicates continuing fine motor problems. The score increased from the fourth to the 68th percentile over a period of nine months.

Neither of these children or others in their class had received additional tuition in drawing. They had participated in the INPP Developmental Movement Programme for Use in Schools (Goddard Blythe 1996) – a movement programme carried out for ten minutes per day under teacher supervision – over the course of one academic year. The changes seen across the whole class suggest that there is a relationship between physical awareness and control and aspects of non-verbal cognitive performance, improved proprioceptive awareness being mirrored in improvements in the representation of the human figure.

Symptoms of poor proprioception:

- poor posture
- constant fidgeting or moving
- excessive desire to be held
- may provoke fights to get sensory input
- may have visual problems
- poorly developed knowledge of where different parts of the body are in space
- clumsiness
- poor understanding of personal space – tendency to invade the space of others

Taste and smell

The significance of taste and smell for learning is perhaps largely concentrated in the earliest years of a child's life, when the mouth acts as the primary source of information, exploration, expression and satisfaction. What does it taste like? Is it soft? Can I chew it? How big is it? All early discoveries are made through the mouth.

Much of taste is dependent upon the sense of smell, as we know only too well when we have a bad cold and can only taste the specific tongue tastes of salty, bitter, sweet and sour. Smell is, perhaps, the most evocative of all the senses, instantaneously spanning decades in its ability to remind us of a certain place, person or event. Instead of being routed through the thalamus – like other sensory information – the nerves in the nasal passages send messages directly to the brain's olfactory bulbs, which then spread the impulses to areas of the brain where memories are stored. Thus, a certain perfume will remind us of our mother when we were a small child and she was dressed up to go out for the evening, or the typical sounds and smells of a country will conjure up the memory of stepping off a plane or the restaurants where we ate. Similarly, smell can evoke unpleasant memories: the smell of school can easily become associated with stress, the smell of a hospital with pain. Smell can instantly summon multisensory images. It can also stimulate the production of hormones involved in the control of appetite, temperature, sexuality, and response to fear – in the same region in the brain as is influenced by the Moro reflex: the hypothalamus.

Taste and smell provide important information about an ever-changing environment. In temperate climates it is possible to smell when the season is changing, if rain is approaching for example. Smell thus has the ability to herald change before other sensory systems can. Although the immediate significance of taste and smell to classroom learning is less obvious than that of visual or auditory processing, learning is most effective when we relate to it physically and emotionally in some way. As both taste and smell evoke memories of past experiences, they can enrich a child's ability to link new information to previous experience and commit new information to memory.

Hyper- or hyposensitivity can also occur with taste and smell. Examples of this and the so-called paradoxical behaviour that can result were first described by Carl Delacato (1974) in relation to the autistic child. The child who is hypersensitive to smell may dislike certain environments or be averse to being in close proximity to people whose breath or body odour smell bad and be ultra-fussy about certain foods; as one child asked, 'Have you ever smelled a sprout cooking, then you are expected to put it under your nose and into your mouth – why would anyone do that?' The child who is hyposensitive may also be a fussy eater; this may be the result of nasal congestion and/or enlarged tonsils or adenoids, which can impair the sense of taste to which smell contributes, affecting the bite, chew and swallow pattern and resulting in a child who will only eat a small range of foods that taste bland and are easy to swallow. The child's nutritional status may also be linked to other biochemical factors that enhance or dull the sense of taste; zinc deficiency is one example.

Symptoms of problems with taste or smell (hypersensitive):

- may avoid going to the bathroom and be at risk of wetting their pants because they cannot stand the smell of the cleaning materials used there
- may avoid the school cafeteria because of the lingering smell of stale food
- may avoid school changing rooms

- may avoid other children, especially those who come to school with dirty or smelly clothes
- may misbehave after certain cleaning products have been used
- dislike of close proximity to other people

Symptoms of problems with taste or smell (hyposensitive):

- may eat indiscriminately and be at risk of eating substances labelled 'Keep out of reach of children'

Summary

In some cases, sensory imbalance can be used to produce a rare streak of genius – for example, the accomplished musician who has highly sensitive and highly developed hearing in a specific range; the artist who is able to use slight visual distortion to create an image of the world that is truly unique; the writer who is able to conjure up emotion, experience and imagination to paint pictures with words and give birth to a rich tapestry of characters and events; the actor who can literally feel themself into someone else's persona. These people have been able to gain unique insight from their own brand of sensory experience. They also have the skills that have allowed them to turn this unusual ability to their advantage. This is very different from the child who experiences failure from an early age or lacks the skill with which to profit from their own special window on the world. Our sensory receptors provide us with such an open window, through which we feel, perceive, maintain contact or avoid aspects of the world around us.

Deprivation of even one of the senses will have a profound effect upon the individual, as will any alteration in the transmission of information via one of the sensory channels. Mode, intensity and duration of sensation are also of prime significance, since the type and degree of sensory input will directly influence the level of response that arises. Too little sensation may result in lack of response. Too much can result in overreaction or vastly increased levels of stress as the individual tries to modulate their response. Distortion or blurring of sensation may result in confusion and inappropriate response.

Finally, there needs to be a balance between the different sensory channels so that cross-sensory reference may occur in order to provide the individual with multisensory information about their environment, to which they may then adapt their responses. This is 'sensory integration'.

When assessing a child with learning, language or behavioural difficulties, it is not sufficient to merely identify a hearing problem, a reading problem, a coordination problem, etc. It is necessary to look further and to ask:

- What do they hear?
- How do they see?
- In which specific situations is their balance poor?
- Do they have the mature combination of movements necessary to read, to write and to speak?

If a child does not see, hear or move in the way ideally expected at their age, they may have problems in the physical foundations of learning on which cognitive skills rely.

Chapter 5

Reflex Testing

Tests listed

- Moro reflex standard test
- Palmar reflex
- Asymmetrical tonic neck reflex – Hoff–Schilder test
- Rooting reflex
- Tonic labyrinthine reflex erect test
- Symmetrical tonic neck test
- Landau reflex
- Amphibian reflex prone–supine
- Oculo-head-righting reflexes
- Labyrinthine headrighting reflexes

The following test procedures relating to reflexes discussed in the text should be used for purposes of identification only. They represent only a few selected tests from just one section of a complete diagnostic assessment for signs of NMI. Tests shown as examples in this chapter should not be used in isolation for diagnostic purposes. Reflex stimulation and inhibition training should only be undertaken after a complete assessment and under the supervision of a qualified therapist.

Scoring

Primitive reflexes

0 = no abnormality detected (NAD)

1 = primitive reflex evident (25 per cent)

2 = primitive reflex residually present (50 per cent)

3 = primitive reflex virtually retained (75 per cent)

4 = primitive reflex retained (100 per cent)

Postural reflexes

0 = NAD

1 = postural reflex underdeveloped (25 per cent)

2 = postural reflex underdeveloped (50 per cent)

3 = postural reflex underdeveloped (75 per cent)

4 = postural reflex absent (100 per cent)

In other words, a positive score on any test denotes a degree of dysfunction or immaturity.

The following tests used as part of an INPP assessment are designed for use with children from seven years of age upwards. They are provided as examples only of tests for several reflexes.

Moro reflex

- emergence: 9–32 weeks in utero
- birth: fully present
- inhibited: 2–4 months neonate

It should be noted that the supine test is only one of a series of tests that would be carried out as part of an INPP assessment to detect a Moro reflex.

Figure 5.1: Test position for Moro reflex (supine)

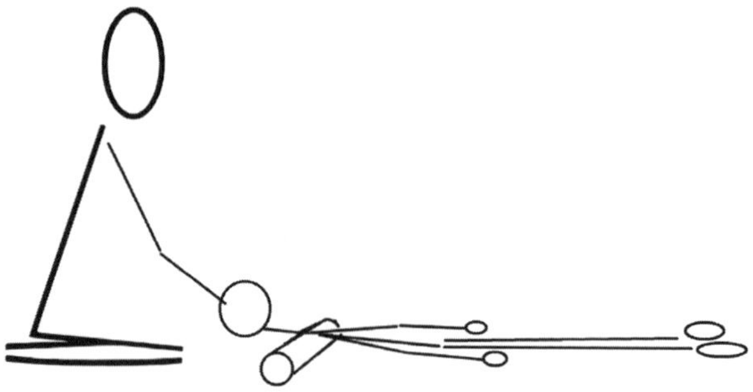

Standard test for vestibular-activated Moro

Test position

Supine, with arms flexed and hands resting on the floor (Figure 5.1). Shoulders should be raised with a small cushion and the child's head supported in the tester's hands and elevated approximately 5cm (2in) above the level of the spine.

Test procedure

After just a few moments, the tester should allow the child's head to drop 5–7cm (2–3in) to just below the level of the spine, but not to reach the floor. Previously the tester will have given the instruction, 'When you feel your head drop you must clasp your hands together across your chest as quickly as you can.'

Observations

Any movement of the arms outwards from the body. Inability to bring the arms across the chest, or delayed action. Disorientation or distress as a result of the test procedure.

Scoring

0. Immediate hand clasp and no adverse reaction.
1. Slight delay in reaction.
2. Delayed reaction; incomplete hand/arm movement or breath-holding.
3. No arm movement, alteration in breathing, and visible dislike of testing procedure.
4. Movement of the arms outwards from the body, leg extension and/or distress.

Also note any reddening of skin or pallor immediately after testing.

Palmar reflex

- emergence: 11 weeks in utero
- birth: present
- inhibited: 2–3 months neonate

Test position

Standing, feet together, with arms bent and palms upturned in a flexed, relaxed position, elbows away from the body (Figure 5.2a).

Test procedure

Gently stroke with a soft brush along the creases of the palm (Figure 5.2b). Repeat twice.

Observations

Any movement of the fingers or thumb inwards towards the stimulus, or extreme sensitivity in the palmar region.

Figure 5.2: Palmar reflex test a) position and b) area

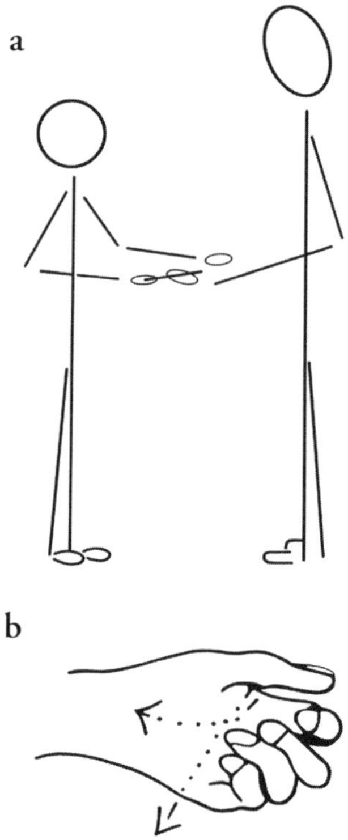

Scoring

0. No response.
1. Slight movement of the fingers or thumb inwards.
2. Definite movement of the thumb or fingers inwards; subject complains touch is ticklish or painful.
3. Movement of the thumb and/or fingers inwards as if to grasp the stimulus; rubbing of the hands immediately after testing.
4. Thumb and fingers close in on stimulation. This may be accompanied by simultaneous movements of the lips.

Asymmetrical tonic neck reflex (Hoff-Schilder test)

It should be noted that this test is only one test from a series of tests for the ATNR which would be used during a full assessment. Suitable for use with children from seven years of age upwards.

Test position

Standing, feet together, with the arms held straight out at shoulder level and height, but with the hands relaxed at the wrists (Figure 5.3).

Test procedure

The tester stands behind the subject and gives the instruction, 'When I tum your head, I want you to keep your arms straight out in front of you, as they are now. This means your arms remain in the same position and only your head moves.' The tester then slowly rotates the subject's head until the chin is parallel with the shoulder. Pause for ten seconds. Return the head to the midline. Pause for ten seconds. Rotate the head to the other side and pause for ten seconds. Repeat the procedure up to four times.

Observations

Any movement of the hand and arm on the side to which the head is turned – that is, do the arms automatically follow the movement of the head?

Figure 5.3: Asymmetrical tonic neck reflex (erect) Hoff-Schilder test

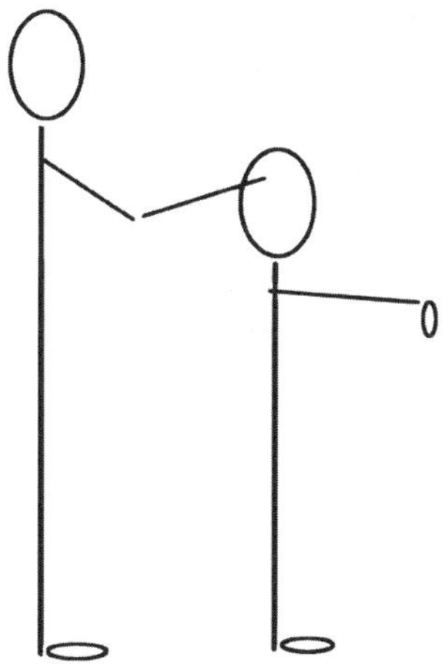

Scoring

0. No response.
1. Slight movement of the arms in the direction the face is pointed.
2. Movement of the arms in the direction of the head to 45°.
3. Arm movement to 60° or flexion of the opposite side.
4. Rotation of the arms to 90° and/or loss of balance as a result of head rotation.

Rooting reflex

- emergence: 24–28 weeks in utero
- birth: present
- inhibited: 3–4 months neonate

Test position

Standing (Figure 5.4).

Figure 5.4: Test position for rooting reflex

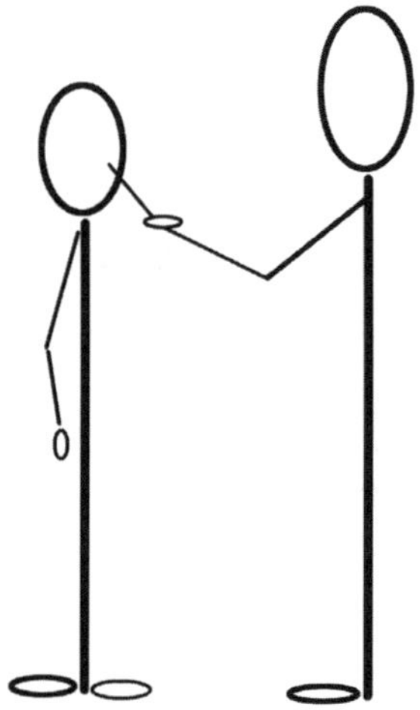

Test procedure

Using a small brush, gently stroke from the outer base of the nose downwards beyond the comer of the mouth. Repeat two or three times on each side.

Observations

Note any movement or twitching of the mouth in response to the stimulus, or withdrawal. Also note any accompanying involuntary movement of the hands.

Scoring

0. No reaction.
1. Slight twitching of the mouth.
2. Definite movement of the mouth and/or dislike of the sensation.
3. Movement and opening of the mouth and/or rubbing of the area stimulated.
4. Movement of the mouth as if to smile; opening of the mouth and turning the head in the direction of the stimulus.

Tonic labyrinthine reflex (erect test)

- emerges: birth
- inhibited: 2–3 months in the prone position; 2–4 months in the supine position, but may still be present in a weakened form up to the age of three years

It should be noted that this test only represents one test in a battery of tests for the TLR.

Test position

Standing with feet together and arms straight at the sides of the body (Figure 5.5).

Test procedure

Slowly tilt the subject's head back into extended position and ask them to close their eyes. (Stand behind to support them in case there is any loss of balance.) After ten seconds ask the subject to slowly move the head forward as if looking at the toes and to maintain that position for a further ten seconds. Repeat the sequence six times.

Observations

Note any loss of balance or alteration of balance as a result of head position, or as a result of head movement from above to below the level of the spine. Also note any compensatory change in muscle tone at the back of the knees as a result of head movement, or any gripping with the toes. Ask the subject for any reactions immediately after testing and note any comments about dizziness or nausea, both of which suggest faulty vestibular functioning and/or the residual presence of the TLR.

Figure 5.5: Test Position for TLR (erect)

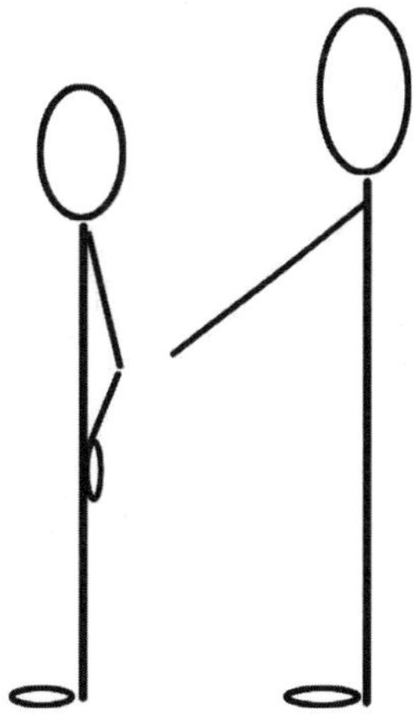

Scoring

0. No response.
1. Slight alteration of balance as a result of head position or movement.
2. Disturbance of balance during the test and/or alteration of muscle tone at the back of the knees.
3. Near loss of balance, alteration of muscle tone and/or disorientation as a result of the testing procedure.
4. Loss of balance and/or massive alteration of muscle tone in attempt to maintain balance. This may be accompanied by dizziness or nausea and, in adults, feelings of panic.

Symmetrical tonic neck reflex

- emerges: 6–8 months of life
- inhibited: 9–11 months

Test position

Four-point kneeling 'table' position.

Test procedure

The subject is instructed to maintain the test position but to slowly move the head to look down 'as if looking between your thighs' (Figure 5.6a). Hold the position for five seconds and then slowly move the head upwards 'as if looking at the ceiling' (Figure 5.6b). Repeat up to six times.

Observations

Any bending of the arms as a result of head flexion, and/or any raising of the feet. Straightening of the arms and flexion of the knees as a result of head extension.

Scoring

0. No response.
1. Tremor in one or both arms or slight hip movement.
2. Movement of the elbow on either side and/or definite movement in the hips or arching of the back.
3. Bending of the arms on head flexion, or moving the bottom back on head extension.
4. Bending of the arms to the floor in response to flexion of the head, or moving the bottom back towards the ankles as a result of extension of the head, the latter resulting in the subject sitting in the 'cat' position.

Figure 5.6:
Test position for assessor and test subject STNR:
a) Flexion; b) Extension

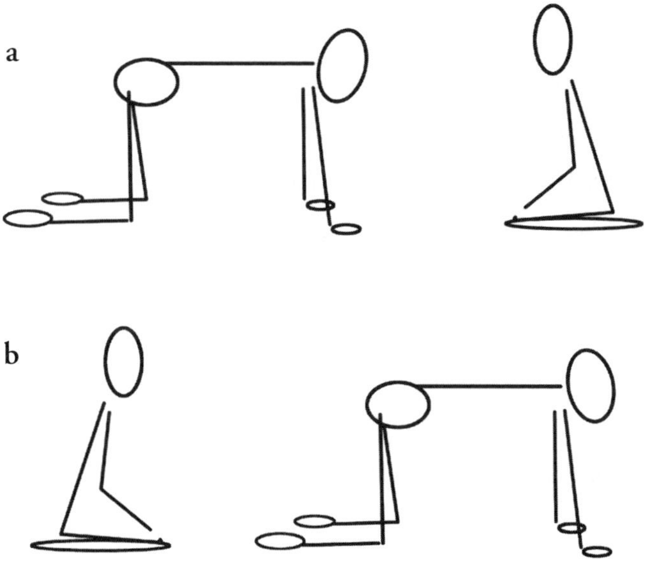

Landau reflex

- emerges: 2–4 months of life
- inhibited: approximately three years of age

Test position

Prone with arms at right angles to the shoulders (Figure 5.7a).

Test procedure

The subject is instructed to lift the upper trunk, arms and hands off the floor, keeping the feet on the floor, and to maintain this elevated position for up to five seconds (Figure 5.7b). This may be repeated twice.

Observations

Involuntary lifting of the feet or lower legs as a result of raising the torso.

Scoring

0. No response.
1. Slight lifting of one or both feet, immediately corrected.
2. Definite lifting of one or both feet.
3. Elevation of both feet away from the floor.
4. Elevation of both feet several inches above the floor and extensor tone throughout the body.

Figure 5.7: Landau reflex test
a) Position 1
b) Position 2

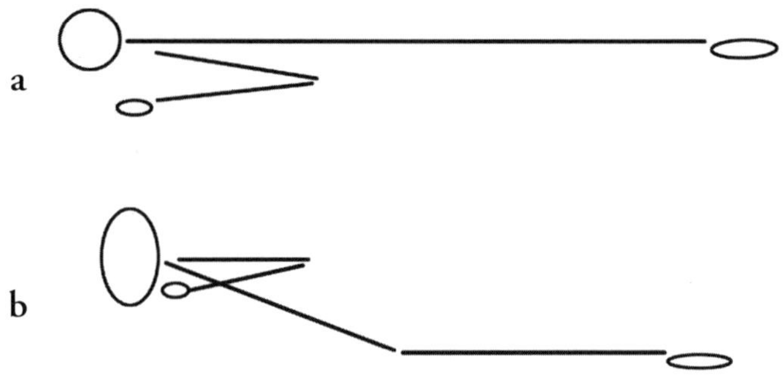

Amphibian reflex

- emergence: 4–6 months neonatal
- postural reflex – should emerge at the developmentally appropriate time and remain active for life (that is, not be inhibited)

Test position

First supine, then prone (Figure 5.8).

Test procedure

Ensure the subject is completely relaxed with the head at the midline. The tester places their hands under the hip and elevates it to an angle of 45°.

Observations

As the hip is elevated, the knee on same side should bend in both supine and prone testing.

Scoring

0. The knee bends on the side of the elevated hip.
1. No visible flexion of the knee, but the leg remains relaxed.
2. The leg remains stiff.
3. The leg is so stiff that it begins to lift.
4. The whole body rolls rigidly

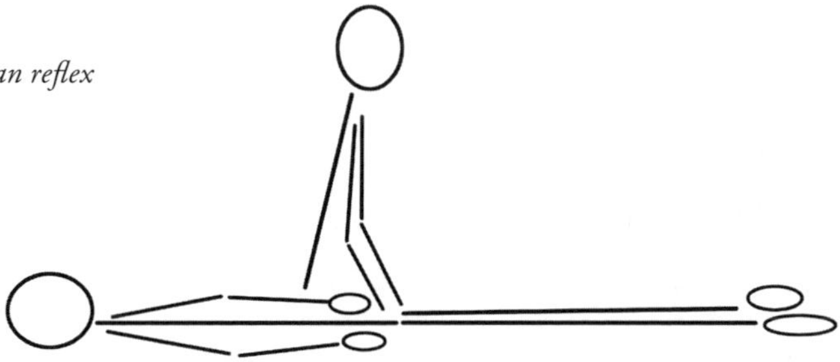

Figure 5.8: Test position for amphibian reflex (prone and supine)

Oculo-head-righting reflex

- emergence: 2–3 months neonatal
- postural – not inhibited

Test position

Subject seated on the floor, legs straight in front, arms resting on thighs (Figure 5.9).

Test procedure

- The subject fixes their eyes on an object at eye level.
- The tester sits behind the subject and slowly tilts the subject to the left in three stages, pausing for two or three seconds at each stage. Pauses are made at 15°, 30° and 45°. Note the position of the subject's head at each degree of tilt.
- Return the subject to the upright sitting position, in the same three stages.
- Repeat the procedure to the right, return to the midline and then repeat the procedure backwards and forwards, ensuring that the subject keeps their eyes fixed on the object at eye level.

Observations

The head should automatically correct itself to the midline (vertical to the ground) as the body position is altered in all four directions. Any flopping of the head or overcompensation in the opposite direction upon return to the midline position suggests an absent or underdeveloped oculo-head-righting reflex. Also note any extension of the leg on the side to which the subject is tilted; this may be an indication of a retained ATNR in the leg.

Scoring

0. Head corrects to the vertical midline position throughout the test.
1. Head slips slightly from the vertical.
2. Head follows the direction of the tilt in line with the body.
3. Head leans below the line of the body.
4. Head drops in the direction of the tilt.

Lack of head-righting forwards/backwards could indicate underlying tonic labyrinthine reflex (TLR).

Figure 5.9:
Test position for oculo-head-righting reflexes

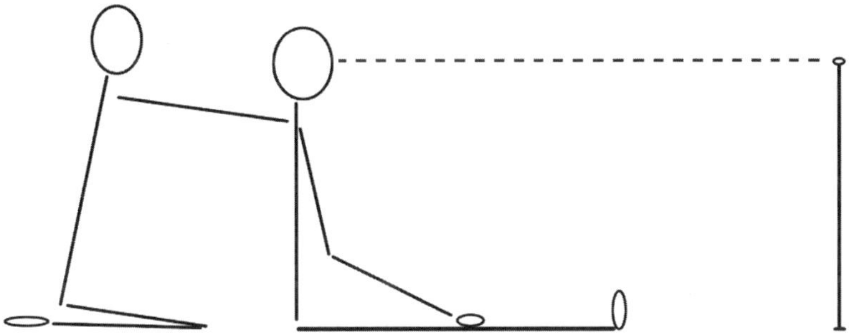

Labyrinthine head-righting reflex

- emergence: 2–3 months neonatal
- postural – not inhibited

Test position

Same as for the oculo-head-righting reflex (Figure 5.9), but the subject is asked to fixate the eyes on an object at eye level and then to close the eyes and imagine looking at the object throughout the testing procedure.

Test procedure

The subject is instructed to fixate the eyes upon an eye-level object and then to close the eyes and visualise the object throughout the testing procedure. Then follow the same testing procedure as for oculo-head-righting reflex.

Observations

Note the position of the head in all four quadrants, but also note where the subject's closed eyes seem to be directed. (Many children can compensate when their eyes are open, but rapidly lose any sense of where they are in space as soon as the eyes are closed.)

Scoring

0. Head corrects to the vertical midline position throughout the testing.
1. Head slips slightly from the vertical.
2. Head follows the direction of the tilt in line with the body.
3. Head slips below the line of the body.
4. Head drops in the direction of the tilt – no righting apparent.

Also note any compensatory turning of the head – this is not the same as automatic righting.

The above tests are presented as examples of test procedures used during an INPP assessment. Assessment carried out by a trained practitioner would include additional tests for many of the reflexes described in Chapters 1 and 2 plus tests for gross muscle coordination and balance, dysdiadochokinesia, cerebellar involvement, laterality (above eight years of age), oculo-motor functioning, visual perception and, if indicated by presenting symptoms and developmental history, audiometric and dichotic listening tests. Remediation would be recommended on the basis of all of the tests listed in the paragraph above.

Chapter 6

What Can Be Done?

Understanding primitive and postural reflexes in the context of remediation

The aim of this book is not to make its readers into therapists, but to give them an understanding of how immaturity in the functioning of the central nervous system can interfere with a child's progress across a range of tasks, and of what developmental intervention may help. Every child's profile is unique; it is in the interpretation of the individual profile of reflexes that the skill and the training of a qualified practitioner are needed.

Assessment of primitive and postural reflexes can be used to:

- identify whether NMI is a factor in presenting problems
- provide indications of the relevant type and developmental level of intervention
- measure/evaluate progress on physical tests carried out at the first screening and during and following an intervention regime

Treatment will depend not only upon the nature and severity of the problem but also on the available resources – physical conditions, special education experts and remedial programmes.

As described in Chapter 5, when performed in a clinical setting each test can yield a possible score of between 0 and 4, a score of 0 indicating no abnormality has been detected on that test (NAD). When assessing primitive reflexes in the older child, a score of 4 indicates that the reflex is fully retained and scores of 1, 2 and 3 indicate the relative strength of the reflex (residual). When assessing postural reflexes, a score of 1–4 indicates that the reflex is underdeveloped (1–3) or absent (4).

Although certain reflexes may be linked to specific problems – the ATNR, for example, often being a factor in specific handwriting problems – it is a cluster of aberrant reflexes in combination with other signs such as difficulties in gross muscle coordination and balance, oculo-motor dysfunction and visual perceptual difficulties – that is, the total score over a number of test and reflexes – that will provide the starting point for recommending types of remedial intervention.

Many years of clinical practice and research derived from the INPP developmental movement programme for schools have shown that if a person exceeds a score of 50 per cent on tests for the ATNR, STNR and TLR combined, then an individual programme supervised by a trained practitioner is recommended. This type of programme is tailored to the individual's profile of reflexes and other issues identified from a detailed assessment carried out by a trained practitioner. Individuals with scores of 25–50 per cent can also benefit from an individualised programme.

If a child exceeds a score of 25 per cent on more than three primitive reflexes, the INPP Developmental Movement Programme for Use in Schools can be used with selected groups or a whole class of children. This programme, developed in 1996, comprises a few key tests from the INPP assessment test battery which can be used by teachers as a primary screening tool to identify children in whom signs of NMI are present and who will be likely to benefit from a general programme of daily exercises. The developmental movement programme is designed to be carried out every day under teacher supervision over the course of one academic year (Goddard Blythe 1996; 2012).

Both the INPP clinical programme and school-based programme have been designed to be used with children from seven years of age and upwards.

Why wait until seven years of age before starting a formal INPP programme?

There are several reasons why the INPP programmes as designed are not generally recommended for use with younger children:

1. The INPP exercises are designed to be performed slowly and precisely. Children under the age of seven years can find this difficult.
2. Balance, postural, motor and visual systems are still learning to function efficiently together. Between six-and-a-half and eight years of age, the developing nervous system goes through a key period of neural pruning and myelination.

Neural pruning is a natural process that occurs at different developmental stages. It involves removing neurons that are no longer used or useful to the brain – rather like clearing out a cupboard of unwanted items to make the space tidier and easier to use. Myelination is the process by which axons acquire myelin – a fatty protective sheath that speeds up impulse propagation along the axons of neurons. In effect, myelination enables signals to pass more efficiently by reducing interference from neighbouring pathways. Although both of these processes are ongoing throughout life, there are key periods in development when the neurological equivalent of a 'spring clean' and 'redecoration' occur.

> Childhood cognitive development is intertwined with brain structural maturation. White matter (myelin) maturation steadily increases throughout childhood. As the formation of the myelin sheath surrounding neuronal axons fastens neural impulse propagation, it is a likely major contributor to processing speed. Indeed increasing processing speed is associated with white matter integrity during middle childhood and adolescence. Similarly white matter microstructure relates to children's cognitive abilities further down the developmental cascades, such as inhibition, spatial working memory, arithmetic skills and reading. (Chevalier et al. 2015).

Major periods of myelination occur in the first two years of life, between six-and-a-half and seven-and-a-half years of age, during the teenage years and again in the early twenties. The period between between six-and-a-half and seven-and-a-half years is of particular significance in the present context because it involves myelination of connections between the vestibular system (balance), cerebellum (fine-tuning of motor output) and the corpus callosum (communication and inhibition of information between the two cerebral hemispheres), which are involved in the integration of balance, posture, eye movements and communication between the two sides of the cortex.

Clinical experience over many years of practice has indicated that, while this dynamic period of development is naturally taking place, the child's system seems to be less responsive to specific reflex integration exercises as used in the INPP clinical and school programmes and so a programme can take significantly longer to achieve the same results if started too soon. For example, a child starting an INPP programme at seven-plus years of age may expect to be on the programme for an average of 12 months; a child starting at six years of age may need 18 months on the same programme to achieve the same results.

3. Compliance can also become an issue with younger children: when they have difficulty carrying out the movements slowly and precisely, there may be resistance to doing the exercises, inconsistency and poorer outcomes. This is not to say that nothing can be done with younger children; rather, the programme used needs to be adjusted to the age of the child. We will return to this later in this chapter.

Intervention

Each category of intervention may involve different levels.

Therapeutic programmes

Movement programmes

Level 1

Individualised reflex stimulation and inhibition programme: If, for example, a child obtains a total score of more than 25 per cent altogether on the tests for primitive reflexes, a specific reflex stimulation/inhibition programme tailored to their individual assessment results is indicated. An individual programme should only be given following an assessment by a practitioner qualified in the management of a reflex programme.

A reflex stimulation/inhibition programme is tailored to the reflex profile of the individual child. Progress should be reviewed at six- to eightweekly intervals and the prescribed exercises adjusted accordingly. Reflex stimulation/inhibition techniques are based upon the theory of replication – that it is possible to replicate specific stages of early development through the repetition of movement patterns naturally made during early development. Reflex stimulation and inhibition movements are grounded on very early primitive movements that an older child would not normally make. In this way the brain is given a second chance to experience input from the developmental stages that were omitted or deficient in the first year of life. These stages should have been fundamental in priming the organism for later learning, and recreating them can help to establish neural connections and reset the neural clock.

As this is taking place some children can regress emotionally for a short period of time. It is therefore important that, even though the programme is carried out at home, it should only be done with careful guidance and qualified supervision.

A specific reflex stimulation/inhibition programme compares with general exercises as a prescription from the pharmacy compares with over-the-counter medication. Playing about with reflexes without training can do more harm than good, which is why this book does not present absolute solutions.

Level 2

INPP Developmental Movement Programme for Use in Schools: A combined score of more than 25 per cent on the tests for primitive reflexes and postural reflexes would also indicate the use of an individualised programme or the INPP Developmental Movement Programme for Use in Schools.

The INPP programme for schools was devised in 1996 with the aim of providing teachers with two short screening tests (for 4–7 years of age and seven-plus years of age) to enable teachers to identify children in class who may be underachieving as a secondary consequence of immature neuromotor skills.

The developmental movement programme itself is designed to be used with children from seven years of age upwards in a classroom setting. Although the screening test will identify children with the greatest need, all children can participate in the daily movements under teacher supervision (the only exceptions being children with underlying physical conditions and children currently involved in other therapeutic interventions; in these cases, advice from the therapists involved should be sought). This programme has been the subject of a number of independent pilot projects carried out in schools (Goddard Blythe 2005) and research commissioned by the Department of Education in Northern Ireland (North Eastern Education and Library Board [NEELB] 2004).

The school programme takes children on a developmental journey that revisits many of the movements that should have been made during the first year of life. Whereas the individual programme personalises exercises according to the findings of an individual child's assessment carried out in a clinical setting, the school programme follows a developmental course that all children can follow in chronological stages over one academic year. The theory behind both programmes is the same – that replication of earlier movement patterns can be used to develop and strengthen pathways that support balance, posture and coordination for the rest of one's life.

Both programmes also rely on three key factors: regularity (every day for the clinical programme; five days per week during term time for the school programme); repetition (repeating the same movements for several weeks before moving on); and duration (following the programme for a sufficient length of time – average of 12 months – to make lasting changes to the pathways involved).

Level 3

Daily movement programmes: Children with scores of less than 25 per cent on either group of reflex tests can benefit greatly from more generalised developmental exercises that can be incorporated into the school day. Many general movement programmes are available. One pilot project carried out at a school in Derbyshire provided an example of the value of daily exercise.

All children in one year group (Year 3) were screened for signs of NMI using the INPP screening test for schools. The year group comprised three classes. One class carried out the INPP developmental movement programme for ten minutes a day every day for one academic year; children in another class participated in daily general movement activities for the same time period each day; and the third class did not receive any additional daily movement activity other than regular physical education (PE) as prescribed by the national curriculum. All children were reassessed for signs of NMI at the end of the school year.

Children who had participated in daily general movement activities had made twice as much progress on neuromotor measures as those who had only followed the national curriculum guidelines for physical education. However, children in the general movement activity group had made half the progress of those in the developmental movement programme group (Micklethwaite 2004). In other words, daily movement activity makes a difference, and if specific movement programmes are not available, encouraging children to be involved in daily physical activity for as little as ten minutes a day can make a difference.

Children under 7 years of age: Although the INPP programmes have been designed primarily for use with children from seven years of age upwards, there is still much that can be done to help younger children develop the physical skills that they will need to support their learning in the classroom. Once again, many excellent movement programmes and activities are available for use with younger children in reception, nursery or home environments.

One of the issues mentioned earlier in relation to the use of the INPP programmes with this younger age group was children finding it difficult to carry out the movements slowly and precisely. One solution is to adapt the movements to make them more suitable for younger children by incorporating them into a play setting. This has been done by means of a series of stories and songs using animal characters that reflect different stages of human beings' evolutionary physical development (Goddard Blythe 2018).

The result of collaboration between me and Michael Lazerev (a doctor who has written a programme of musical education for children from conception to seven years of age), was that the activities suggested in

Movement – Your Child's First Language are designed to be used in pre-school and reception settings. They encourage children to become familiar with the characters in the stories and songs and to act out the movements the stories and songs suggest. Songs and stories are provided on CDs (narrator, singers and accompaniment). Children can carry out movements, designed to follow a developmental sequence, at their own pace. Repetition is encouraged in the use of the stories, songs and accompanying activities. One school in the north of England reported significant improvement not only in children's neuromotor skills at the end of the school year but also in their vocabulary and use of language in written work. The teachers attributed this to the rich use of descriptive words and phrases in the stories and songs the children listened to every day and the songs they had learned to sing by heart.[21]

Duncombe and Preedy (2020) investigated the incidence of motor skills in a group of 108 children using the Movement Assessment Battery for Children (2nd edition, MABC-2). A general physical intervention programme suitable for younger children (Movement for Learning[22]) was introduced into the school day. At the end of the year, children in the intervention group showed significant improvement in measures of motor skills.

The same group of researchers (Preedy et al. 2020) found what appeared to be a significant decline in children's performance on tests for balance, general physical coordination, aiming and catching, and manual dexterity when the results obtained in 2020 using the MABC-2 were compared with the norms last set for this test in 2007.

Among a sample of 120 children aged four to five years from four schools (two state schools and two independent schools) who were assessed in the September they started school, they found evidence of decline in the following skills:

- balance – 6.2 percentile points since 2007
- aiming and catching – 19.7 percentile points since 2007
- manual dexterity – 15.8 percentile points since 2007
- overall physical development – 18.1 percentile points since 2007

Owing to the relatively small size of the sample and a number of other confounding variables, it is not possible to infer causal relationships from these findings, and further large-scale research is needed to identify lifestyle factors that may be influencing aspects of children's physical development in relation to motor skills, but the indication of decline in these areas is concerning.

Level 4

How parents can help: Most parents watch in awe as our children grow from helpless babies to walking, talking and determined individuals. Parents are usually unaware of all the reflexes that play a part in moving from one stage to the next. Growth and development are gradual processes in which reflexes do not simply appear one minute and then disappear the next, but instead gently change from one to another, often coexisting for a short period of time until the next developmental skill is established.

Besides love and discipline, freedom to move and freedom to play are two of the most important gifts that parents can give to their child.[23] If we want to make sure a baby learns to hold their head up, we put them on their tummy, sit in front of them and talk to them. If they do not want to turn over, we hold something bright to their side, so that they are motivated to turn. To help connect their vestibular system to body awareness, we play 'This Is the Way the Ladies Ride' or 'Down in the Deep Blue Sea'. In short, we do all the things that parents have done instinctively with their children for centuries.

'Children learn most when there is joy in learning' (Kiphard 2000). Young children experience movement with joy and will peal with laughter when swung through the air or when they have learned how to roll over. They delight in their own developing mobility and the first shoots of independence that come with it.

A child's learning begins with their own body. Babies are fascinated by their own body parts and will spend any amount of time intrigued by the movement of their fingers and toes before they realise that these moving objects belong to them. A child's earliest exploration of the environment is with the mouth. Through the mouth they learn not only about taste and smell but also about size, shape and texture. The mouth is furnished with millions of neural connections to the brain that, each time they are used, help to map sensory and spatial information in the brain. The child who is free to explore with their mouth is also free to experiment with sounds and with the cooing, babbling and imitation that are the genesis of speech.

Movement and vestibular stimulation are experienced as joy. Through movement, a baby can explore the environment and express their emotions. The word 'emotion' comes from the French *émouvoir*, meaning 'to excite or to move the feelings of'. The word 'joy' is derived from the Latin *gaudere* meaning 'to rejoice'. Posture, muscle tone and facial expression all alter as emotional state changes, and sometimes toddlers will utilise earlier reflexes to express anger or protest.

Have you ever tried to put a toddler into a baby seat when they did not want to go there? If they throw their head back, the body goes rigid as they utilise the TLR in extension. This makes it impossible to bend the body in the middle and helps the child to get their own way. As their anger and frustration increase (decreased cortical control), they will often jerk their head backwards and forwards, strengthening the effect of the reflex and simultaneously working their way into a full-blown tantrum. On the other hand, children roll and tumble, hop, skip and jump for the sheer pleasure of 'being' – of movement in space, release of energy, play with gravity – the simple expression of joie de vivre.

Modern baby equipment has been a godsend for parents, but moulded baby seats, buggies and car seats should never replace parental physical contact or the floor as the baby's first playground. An infant begins to understand changes in mood from the way in which they are handled and carried and from the nature of their carers' movements. These are the seeds of the ability to feel empathy – to feel as another.

Time engaged in free play on the floor helps children to develop head control, essential for the development of good posture. Random and, later, intentional movements of the legs and the arms help them to understand where their body begins and ends in space and also to discover for themselves what they need to do to reach for an object, to roll or to learn to sit and to crawl. All of these activities involving trial and error also involve problem-solving – learning how to assemble previous patterns of movement into new combinations. As a child's physical vocabulary increases, so also do confidence and a sense of body map. In adult life, time spent as a couch potato dulls the mind as well as the body; conversely, in the first six months of life, a clean blanket on the floor provides a playing field in which the infant can start to obtain control over posture and mastery of balance, each stage both reflecting and supporting increased maturity in the central nervous system – an ongoing process – which is realised through a dual process of nature (maturation) and nurture (environmental opportunity and experience). If an adult places a baby in a sitting position, the child does not have the same opportunity or experience of passing through these stages spontaneously and may become afraid of falling because they do not know how to retrieve their balance for themself.

With each new achievement, such as learning to sit, to get on to hands and knees and to stand up, comes a new puzzle – having to cope with a new relationship with gravity. Each stage will need practice and recalibration if automatic balance and coordination are to be acquired. In the first few years of life, the practice of motor skills and play are much the same thing.

Social engagement is also essential. According to Panksepp (1998), rough and tumble play is the direct result of spontaneous neural urges in the brain. Panksepp suggests that it is during play that various neuronal growth factors are recruited. Studies have shown that animals are especially prone to behave in flexible and creative ways. It is thought that games that allow roughhousing help in the development of social skills and enable behavioural change. In short, this type of play affords an opportunity to prime the limbic system, which is the part of the brain largely responsible for emotional affect. This is especially important because it has many connections to the forebrain, which in turn is heavily involved in impulse control and behaviour.

Most parents want to protect their children from the dangers of the outside world, but sometimes this can actually prevent them from developing the very skills they need in order to survive. We learn balance by falling over and then developing strategies to prevent ourselves from falling again. We learn how to tolerate heights by climbing and becoming proficient at it. Most finely honed skills develop out of initial failure and then the desire to overcome the problem. In this sense, early failure is one of life's most important teachers, for it teaches us that we can find new ways to success. Parents who allow their children to test out their environment – within safe boundaries, of course – help them to grow by allowing them the opportunity to learn by experience. Experience is food for brain development.

This early experience also extends to the sounds of speech, of songs and stories, long before a child is ready to read. A study that examined the incidence of Alzheimer's in an elderly population found a connection between early verbal abilities and the continuation of mental agility towards the end of life. The study was carried out among a group of nuns who had had to write a biography of their life before entering the convent. These biographies were examined when the nuns were in their seventies, eighties and in some cases nineties. The ones who had demonstrated an extensive vocabulary at the time of entry into the community still had the most alert mental functioning in old age. In addition to educational background, the factor they had in common was that all had been extensively read to when they were children. One of the researcher's conclusions was a message to parents :'Read to your child, read to your child, and when you have finished, read to your child again' (Snowdon 2001).

Level 5

Awareness in the school: When teachers first meet their pupils, they have not had the opportunity to influence the pupils' previous early development. Assessment of reflexes as an initial screening tool can offer a quick insight into how development has occurred and what special needs may have to be met. A specific programme of exercises to make sure each child will have the necessary benchmarks needed for success in school would be ideal. Although such a programme is not always possible or appropriate for every school, concepts of development can be incorporated into all levels of teaching. Awareness provides the clues to understanding a child's behaviour and is the first step to bringing about change.

Teaching with normal child development in mind: Once the universality and mechanics of normal development are understood, a suitable programme of motor and sensory stimulation can be put together – either for the individual child or for the whole class.

As a general guide, normal development follows a set sequence: Motor development begins in a cephalo-caudal (from head to toe) and proximo-distal (from the centre outwards) pattern. Sensory development begins with the vestibular and tactile systems and is closely followed by proprioceptive, auditory and visual development. None of these systems functions independently. Any attempt at physical remediation should take this normal pattern of development and integration into account.

Figure 6.1 is a simple model of how various systems in early development interact to provide a basis for later learning. At the bottom of the figure are some of the early influences that will affect the child's development. These early ingredients are like the roots of a tree. If the roots are well embedded in fertile soil, the tree has a good footing from which to grow.

Among the roots is the vestibular system, the only one of the sensory systems to be myelinated by the time of birth. After birth, the balance mechanism must learn how to function in cooperation with the other developing sensory systems: touch, vision, hearing, etc. In the early weeks of life, the sensory systems are entrained and integrated through usage, that is, through movement and interaction with the environment. The primitive reflexes provide an instinctive mechanism with which the neonate can respond to sensation through activity. In this context, primitive reflex integration forms the trunk of the tree upon the basis of which the branches (higher brain centres) will later enjoy optimum functioning.

As the primitive reflexes are inhibited in the first six to twelve months of life and are replaced by postural reflexes, so the trunk of the tree which carries neurological connections between the brain and the body grows

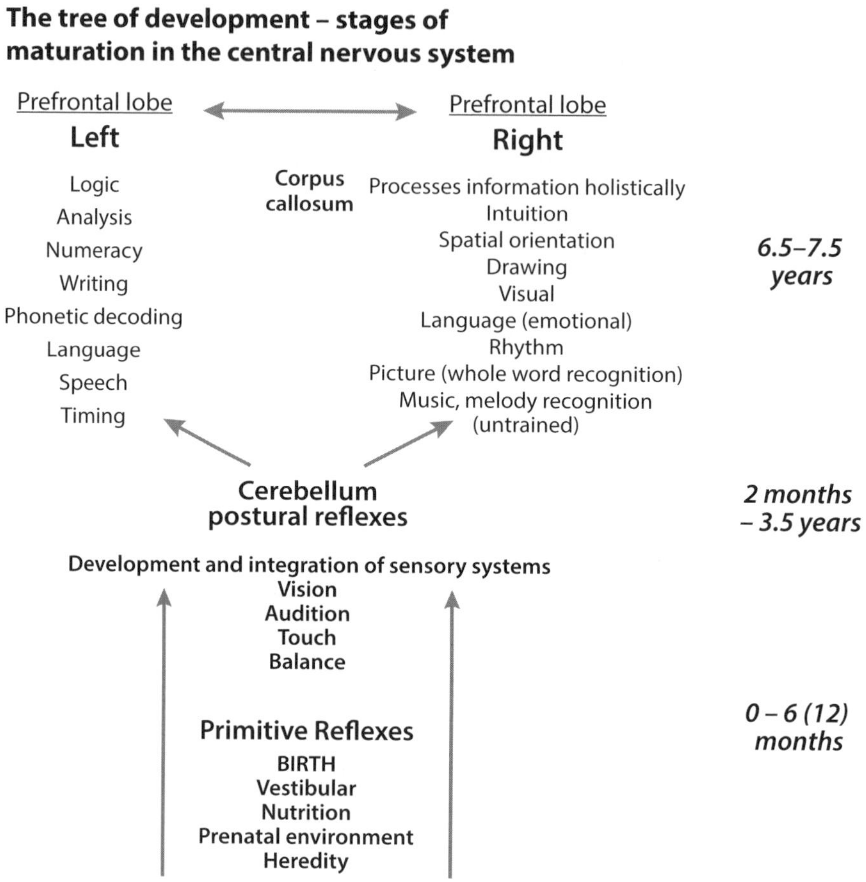

Figure 6.1: Tree of development – stages of maturation in the central nervous system.

stronger. At the same time these changes are taking place, the cerebellum passes through its first major stage of maturation.

Both hemispheres of the cerebral cortex also mature rapidly during the first months and years of life and gain progressively more and more control over the lower centres. Until approximately seven years of age, the right hemisphere is slightly ahead of the left (see Chapter 3), and for certain skills the right hemisphere acts like a training ground for the left. The right hemisphere is particularly good at learning sets and sequences of information through music, rhythm and movement or, put another way, through learning with the body.

A generation ago – and in fact throughout history – it was fairly standard practice to start teaching children younger than seven years old the alphabet and multiplication tables with the aid of music or rhymes. The younger child did not necessarily understand the meaning of what they had learned until later, but the information once learned was filed away, available to be accessed at a later stage when required. Changing trends in educational theory threw out some of these supposedly outdated modes of teaching, asserting that a child needs to understand the meaning of numbers before multiplication tables will be relevant. The result has been that many children do not start learning their tables until seven years of age or above. It is at just this developmental stage that the child should be transferring more direct learning to the left hemisphere, and the left hemisphere does not find it easy to learn batteries of information in this way. Many children above eight years of age struggle to learn their tables even though they may have some understanding of the meaning of multiplication.

Learning by rote or with the body before seven years of age coincides with a time of developmental readiness when the right hemisphere is particularly receptive to stimulation through movement, rhyme, rhythm and song. The cerebellum is also maturing rapidly during these years; the research of Leiner et al. (1986) has shown the cerebellum also to be active during rote learning. It appears that new skills are most easily absorbed if the learning of them coincides with the time of appropriate brain development sometimes referred to as 'the window of opportunity' or the time of neurological readiness.

Children can learn the alphabet to a tune at a younger age and then store that information to be applied at a later stage when the rules of phonetic decoding and spelling are required. Alan Schore (1994) suggests that learning and development are a continuous process of interaction between the two hemispheres, one hemisphere being dominant at one stage of learning and the other hemisphere taking over later on. In this way, both hemispheres are involved in the learning process but eventually one should take precedence over the other for specific tasks. Art, music and physical education are the other face of verbal language. Children who suffer from neurodevelopmental delay (NDD) are often stuck at an earlier phase of development and will benefit from being allowed to retrace some of the earlier stages of learning key skills.

Sensory processing difficulties: Einstein said that all life forms share the characteristic of movement. Of the senses crucial to learning, five share the perception of motion as a common denominator. Where there is motion, there is frequency. Balance, touch, hearing, vision and proprioception are all the result of response to movement at varying frequencies or through a different medium. The vestibular system responds to slow movement (the maximum stimulation for the vestibular system is one degree of arc per second [Guyton 1991]). The sense of touch is felt as a result of movement across the hair cells located in the dermis of the skin, or of pressure applied to the skin. Low-frequency sound is sometimes felt through the tactile system as vibration and only as the frequency of vibrations per second increases does the sense of hearing take over in the perception of sound. Vision is the brain's response to the movement of light waves moving at a higher frequency still. The ability to make sense of movement through the sensory systems is the foundation of learning. The first system in development to answer the call of movement is the vestibular system.

Balance – the beginning of praxis: Balance is not something that happens to us; it is something that we do. It is an adaptive complex behaviour that results from a series of abilities to counter imbalance. Functional balance makes it possible to perform useful actions while maintaining a certain position. This is the foundation for praxis (action). In this way, exercises that improve balance through stimulation of the vestibular system can improve praxis, orientation and behaviour (Schrager 2001).

The most advanced level of movement is the ability to stay totally still. Perfect balance is the action of not moving.[24] Motion helps matter to maintain balance over a narrow base of support. Remember learning how to ride a bicycle? Initially, balance could only be maintained once the bicycle was in motion, and the faster you went, the better your balance seemed to be. The hardest part was learning to start and stop without falling off at low speeds. As control over the centre of balance improved, so less speed was needed to maintain balance.

Children who have difficulty sitting still often have immature control of static balance. They are still at a stage when they need to be on the move to function. In school we require our children to sit still for long periods of time. Those children who fidget and lose concentration after a quarter of an hour often concentrate better for the remainder of the class if they are allowed to get up and move around for a couple of minutes – even in the middle of the lesson. For children with poor balance, movement is food for the brain. Some children will need help to develop new types of movement experience to gain better control and an improved vocabulary of movement. This is where the teacher can help.

Opportunities for vestibular training can be included in the school day and do not necessarily have to be confined to physical education classes. With any exercise regime, the best results are achieved if exercises are practised daily rather than being confined to a 40-minutes class, once a week.

Example of vestibular stimulation:
The vestibular system functions on three planes:

- horizontal head rotation about a vertical (z) axis (yaw)
- head extension and flexion about a horizontal (y) axis (pitch)
- lateral head tilt about a horizontal (x) axis (roll)

Vestibular stimulation can be calming or alerting. Gentle motion such as rocking or the motion of a car may send us to sleep. More vigorous stimulation such as a roller coaster ride has an excitatory effect. Some children are hyper or hypo in their response to stimulation in one of the vestibular planes or to different speeds of stimulation.

Types of stimulation to each one of these planes include:

- horizontal stimulation – spinning in an upright position, lateral head rotation to either side
- rocking – forwards and backwards, forward rolls, swinging
- lateral – rolling along a horizontal surface
- tilting – side to side

The following types of stimulation are naturally a part of activities and games that involve changes of movement in space:

- up and down – jumping, hopping, sliding, see-sawing
- to and fro – running, stopping
- centrifugal force – carousel;
- turning movements of the body such as those used in dance, particularly folk or country dancing
- depth – propulsion of the body above the ground, e.g. scooter board (Kiphard 2000)

These types of movement experiences can be incorporated into a normal school day.

Auditory Training Programmes

The child who has problems in correctly processing auditory information can be helped by sound therapy. An increasing number of methods are currently available, all of which operate upon a common principle that language skills such as speech, reading, writing, spelling and musical expression can only develop if the child has learned to listen. Advanced listening involves both the exclusion of irrelevant sounds and the ability to discriminate and focus on specific sounds. Effective listening is selective in terms of attention and discriminative and in these respects resembles good vision.

The following list is only intended as a guide to help decide which method may be relevant for a particular child:

Dyslexia, reading, spelling and articulation difficulties:

- auditory discrimination training developed by Guy Berard
- Johansen Individualised Auditory Stimulation Therapy (JIAST) developed by Kjeld Johansen
- various levels of listening programme developed by Paul Madaule at the Listening Centre in Toronto

Autism, aphasia, language and general learning difficulties:

- auditory integrative training: the Tomatis method

Listening, language and general learning difficulties; the need to fine-tune musical skills and relieve unexplained anxiety:

- the Tomatis method
- individual centres offering Samonas sound therapy

Johansen's, Steinbach's and Madaule's systems can be used in school and home environments.

Altough the above-mentioned systems of sound therapy help to improve auditory processing through auditory stimulation, the Tomatis system and Madaule's adaptation of the Tomatis method also include exercises that help to train the auditory–vocal feedback loop. This can be important when there is a disconnect between the ear and the voice, which can occur for several reasons. Madaule describes listening as 'a hidden skill behind learning' and voice as the closing link in the loop between the individual and the environment. It is the completion of this loop that enables a person to become self-reliant by connecting linguistically to the outside world.

Auditory processing and learning: The auditory system processes several types of information:

- vibration (with the tactile system)
- sound
- rhythm (with vestibular system)
- timing (with vestibular system)
- orientation in space (whereas vision gives us forward spatial awareness, hearing helps us to be aware of what is happening behind and around us)

Efficient auditory processing is dependent upon:

- adequate hearing in all relevant frequencies, and auditory discrimination
- direct transmission of information to the appropriate area in the brain (laterality)
- speed of transmission (individuals labelled 'dyslexic' often process the sounds of speech more slowly than the norm) (Shaywitz 1996; Merzenich et al. 1996)
- ability to shut out irrelevant sounds

What are some of the stages in early development that a child passes through as they develop auditory-processing skills?

- continuous exposure to the sounds of the mother tongue
- conversational engagement with a sympathetic listener
- language heard without background noise
- vocalisation and action, vocalisation and response
- stage of subvocalisation

As young children start to learn something they very often carry on a personal monologue. This process of vocalisation helps to embed material into memory through the stages of perception, expression, repetition and recognition. The doing stage (vocalisation) helps to pass information to the language centre in the left hemisphere of the cortex. As we mature, we learn to internalise this voice, and later on we may use our inner voice mentally to solve problems.

Signs and symptoms of listening problems

What else other than sound therapy can be done to improve auditory processing?

- regular sounding out as a class
- using song, rhyme and movement to aid memorisation of material (what I know in my body, I know in my head)
- use of song to slow down the sounds of speech

Paula Tallal devised a computer-based training programme (Fast for Word) that artificially slows down the sounds of speech to allow the child time to hear each sound in a word. Setting words to music has a similar effect. Each syllable in a word is given accent, time (spatial dimension) and tonal value, so that a simple sentence such as:

Early one morning, just as the sun was rising...

is sung as

Ear-ly one mor-or-ning, just as the sun was ri-i-sing...

This elongates the time span of individual sounds and syllables in the enunciation of sounds, which in turn helps the child to register and articulate individual sounds in each word. Children with spelling problems often spell exactly as they hear, so that a word like 'remember' may be written as 'rembr' when the middle syllable in the word has not been registered.

To create an external feedback loop to improve the ear–voice connection, Madaule suggests cupping the right hand in front of the mouth and speaking into it. This creates an external resonance chamber that transmits vibrations back to the right ear through bone conduction and encourages more efficient right-eared listening.

Music as a primary teacher

Music can be used to help develop listening acuity, language skills and timing. Music is language without words. In common with other languages, it imposes order, structure, rhythm, timing and sound frequency discrimination upon random sound. It gives meaning to sound. In terms of both evolution and development, music can be understood at the most primitive levels, for music is processed at all levels in the brain.

Music is one of life's earliest natural teachers. Before birth, the foetus reacts to music with changes in motor activity; infants respond to music and can imitate simple rhythms before they develop speech. The early cooing of the baby has melody, intonation and cadence. Even in the absence of musical training, these non-verbal elements of pre-speech are perceived primarily by the right side of the brain, the side of the brain responsible for melody recognition, language comprehension, picture recognition, spatial orientation and rhythm. Although reading does not become proficient until the two sides of the brain are working together, these are the very skills that the young child needs when starting to learn to read. Nursery rhymes, songs and movement to music can all be used in the first five to seven years of life to develop other skills in preparation for literacy.

Just as language varies from one region of the world to another, so music carries within it the colour and flavour of the region in which it has grown. Hence, although there are common elements in the folk tunes of the world, there are also language characteristics that are unique to the area of origin. In this sense, the native language and music of an area share a common accent.

Musical activities give a child a second chance to learn accurate codification and tonal quality of language. This is true even for children who may have suffered intermittent hearing loss in the early years, a time generally considered to be essential for tuning into the sounds of language that are so important for later verbal and literacy skills.

Rhythm and the perception of pitch begin with the body; the former is a vestibular function and the latter involves frequency perception within the body as well as the brain. Emile Jacques Dalcroze, a professor of harmony at the Conservatoire of Geneva in the 1890s, noticed that many of his music students were unable to appreciate the chords that they had to write. It was as if they could not hear inside their heads what they had written with their hands. This is similar to the reading and spelling difficulties experienced by children who are unable to match the phonetic features of a word to the visual symbol. Dalcroze concluded that his students had not had sufficient physical experience of chords (singing different parts – treble, alto, tenor and bass – for example) at the beginning of their studies when brain and body were learning to hear and discriminate the individual elements that make up chords (Bachman 1991).

He developed a series of physical exercises put to music that were designed to develop the inner hearing and musicality of students through the use of the body as a musical instrument. This provided the basis for the Dalcroze approach that can be taught to music teachers for use in schools today. By harnessing a child's natural movements such as walking, running, hopping, skipping, rocking, bending and stretching, the fundamentals of rhythm, rhythmic patterns and phrasing can be taught.[25] These are also important elements of language.

One masterclass in the Dalcroze method for professional musicians involved playing an instrument or singing while standing on a giant trampoline. The effect was to unify the body and instrument in such a way as to significantly improve tone, dynamics and musical expression. In other words, instead of the instrument being an external extension of the body, with residual tension held in the body, the body and instrument moved together to play as one.

In the monastic schools of the Middle Ages, music formed an integral

Type of brainwave	Frequency Hz	Associated state	Implications
Beta	13–22	Alert waking state	May be inconsistent in ADD and ADHD
Alpha	8–12	Relaxed consciousness	Daydreaming
Theta	4–7	Deep meditation; when drifting off to sleep	Optimum creativity; reduced environmental vigilance
Delta	0.5–3.5	Deepest phase of sleep; unconsciousness	

Table 6.1: Brainwaves and associated states

part of education: 'To medieval thinkers, arithmetic, the science of number, was fundamental. Music was the expression of number in time, giving pitch, duration, rhythm, stress and accent to the words. Language regulated by number was song. Number structuring space was geometry' (Le Mée 1994).

In this sense, music can also supply the architecture for many aspects of learning. Certain sound frequencies have the ability to alter brainwave states. There are four major brainwave states that take us through our cycles of waking and sleeping, relaxation and arousal, lethargy and creativity (Table 6.1).

Different combinations of sound and rhythm can both mimic and induce the frequencies that are active in different brainwave states. Music and sound therapy can help to attune the brain to a frame of mind that we would like to induce. Many of us subconsciously use this process in the music we select at different times in the day and in different emotional states.

> Baroque music such as Vivaldi, Bach and Handel has a strong intellectual component and is related to the head, although the rhythm affects our active principle and the timbre and sonority of our emotions. Mozart's music seems to provide food for all three principles whilst some rock and roll music that makes the pelvis gyrate hardly moves above the belt. (Le Mée 1994)

A teacher accidentally utilised this effect when she started to play Mozart as background music during her high school science classes. She observed that the general noise level of a normally disruptive class dropped and concentration and behaviour improved. To back up her observations, she also had the children's blood pressure measured both before and after the class in which the Mozart had been played. The blood pressure of the students was consistently lower after the classes in which background classical music had been present. This is not to suggest that classical music should be played as a backdrop to every class. Some children will find it as distracting as others find it helpful, but classical music can be used to improve concentration and enhance creativity under certain conditions (Savan 1999).

Music lessons can also be used to teach simple exercises that involve listening and vocalisation. Play two notes and then teach the children to hear which one is higher using movements up and down an imaginary staircase. Help them to judge the interval between two notes. Do two notes played together clash or harmonise? What is the difference in interval between sounds that blend and sounds that clash? Even if the child cannot sing in tune, encourage them to sing each note, record it and then modify their singing after listening to the sound of their own voice. Encourage the singing of simple rhymes and sequences to tunes, such as the days of the week, months of the year, multiplication tables, the alphabet and tongue twisters.

An entire system of general teaching is now available based upon the concept of the 'self voice'. The system ARROW – an acronym for Aural–Reading–Respond–Oral–Written – requires the child to read a section of text into a recording device. They have to listen to the sound of their own voice, then to playback and then use their own voice to dictate. They also write down the relevant information. Significant improvements in reading and spelling age have been reported after only a few weeks of use (Lane 2012).

For many children, a tune can act as a code to a memory-filing system, that is, help in both the laying down and the retrieval of information into and from memory storage. These are only a few preliminary ideas upon which more sophisticated exercises can be based.

It is also important to remember here that inadequate exposure to vocabulary as a result either of intermittent hearing deficit or of lack of stimulation can result in the emergence of auditory processing difficulties later on. If we were to visit a foreign country whose language were new to us, we would not suddenly develop an auditory problem. Inability to understand or express what we want to say would owe to lack of exposure to the association of objects and symbols with specific sounds as well as to the vocabulary, grammar, tones, cadences and nuances of speech. Conversation and extensive reading aloud can help a child who has suffered a language deficit for social or environmental reasons.

Visual processing

The range of problems a child may experience with visual processing was outlined in Chapter 4. Symptoms observable in the classroom may include:

- loss of place following a line of print
- need to finger-point to maintain visual fixation
- frequent mistakes when copying
- flat, monotonous voice when reading aloud
- poor reading comprehension
- inability to draw accurately
- misalignment of columns in arithmetic
- difficulty catching a ball

Many visual problems will need professional investigation and may involve a visit to:

- an optician to check visual acuity
- an orthoptist who may be able to recommend special glasses or eye exercises
- a developmental or behavioural optometrist

Eyesight should always be checked before any other exercises are attempted, even if a profile of abnormal reflexes is known to be present.

If eyesight is found to be normal, but there is a cluster of abnormal reflexes, a reflex stimulation/inhibition programme can make a profound difference to both oculo-motor and visual-perceptual skills. A vision therapist working in

Reflexes	School problem	Remediation approach
Moro reflex	Overreactive, hypersensitive, stimulus bound, difficulty with ball games.	Professionally supervised reflex stimulation and inhibition programme. Sensory: vestibular training; tactile stimulation; sound therapy.
Palmar reflex test: Light stimulation of the palm of the hand	Poor manual dexterity, immature pencil grip. Speech and hand movements may be connected.	Clasping and unclasping of the hand around an object (e.g. stress ball or various textures). Independent thumb and finger movements progressing to thumb and finger opposition movements. Finger exercises with hands separately and then making different movements with hands together.
Asymmetrical tonic neck reflex test: Supine – slow lateral head rotation. Erect – Hoff–Schilder test.	Handwriting. Expression of ideas or knowledge in written form. Possible eye-tracking issues. Difficulty crossing the midline. Ambilaterality or cross-laterality.	Slow exercises that begin with homolateral movements of the limbs in response to lateral head rotation in the same direction when lying on the back: • progress to extension of one side of the body in the opposite direction to head rotation • independent cross-pattern movement of the arms and legs with head at the midline Both of the above should be performed in slow motion while lying on the back. Train eye-tracking movements by asking the child to slowly move the thumb of the dominant hand from side to side at visual reading distance from the face, keeping the head still while focusing on the thumb. First, ask the child to do this six times with the eyes closed, imagining they are following the thumb, then repeat with the eyes open. Slowly move the thumb back and forth from near point visual distance to arm's length while focusing on the thumb. Extend the distance of focus to a point on the wall (far distance) and then back to the thumb at arm's length and near point.
Rooting and Suck reflexes	Poor articulation. Prolonged sucking of thumb, finger or comforter. Poor mouth control when eating; dribbling. Oversensitive to being touched on the face. Possible need for orthodontic treatment later. Swallowing movements too near the front of the mouth, which may lead to development of a high palate and narrow jaw.	Reflex inhibition programme.

Reflexes	School problem	Remediation approach
Spinal Galant reflex	Inability to sit still or remain silent. Poor concentration. Continued bedwetting above the age of five years.	Reflex inhibition programme if other retained reflexes are present. If it is the only primitive reflex detected, exercises carried out lying on the back, such as cycling movements in the air, can inhibit the reaction. Sound therapy may also be indicated in some cases.
Tonic labyrinthine reflex test: Movement of the head through the horizontal plane (flexion and extension).	Poor balance. Rigid or floppy muscle tone. Oculo-motor dysfunction, e.g. convergence and accommodation inadequacy. Visual-perceptual difficulties. Spatial difficulties.	Reflex inhibition programme under the supervision of trained practitioner or therapist. • Vestibular stimulation such as gentle rotation, rolling or rocking movements, initially carried out with the eyes closed • Extension and flexion exercises performed on the floor in supine or prone with the eyes closed If TLR or Moro reflexes are present to a score of 50 per cent, or in combination, then an individually supervised reflex inhibition programme is recommended.
Symmetrical tonic neck reflex Test: Head extension and flexion in the quadruped position	Sitting posture; tendency to slump on work surface when writing or eating. Poor hand–eye coordination. Possible delay in adjusting focus between varying visual distances. Clumsy.	Creeping on hands and knees . Provision of a sloping or tilted surface for writing and drawing.

Table 6.2:
General remediation suggestions for residual or underdeveloped reflexes (score >25 per cent).

the Netherlands found that he achieved the greatest success if he delayed using vision therapy until a child had had at least six months on a reflex stimulation/ inhibition programme. In many cases, vision therapy was not required after the reflexes had matured. In those cases where residual oculo-motor problems remained, the time needed on a vision therapy programme was halved.[26]

Until other methods of therapy have succeeded in improving the child's vision, teachers can help to reduce the effect of some visual problems in a number of ways. To help children who have tracking problems to maintain visual fixation on the correct line, allow them to use a ruler under the line. A rectangular 'window' cut into a small piece of cardboard will allow them to concentrate on a few words at a time. This can also help the child who is visually stimulus bound and cannot cope with a lot of visual information presented at one time. If they are reading from a screen, increase the size of the font and margins to decrease the amount of text on one page.

Creating a better learning environment with NMI in mind

The class teacher is usually too busy with the daily curriculum to focus individual attention on the child with immature neuromotor skills. Signs of some retained reflexes, however, are not only easy to spot but, with the awareness gained from reading the material in Chapters 2 and 3, almost impossible to miss. A range of skill levels are always seen in any classroom. The following methods will make it easier to adjust teaching methods to the needs of each child. Tables 6.2 and 6.3 have suggestions that may be used by all teachers, but the following strategies outlined by Jane Field (1992) may also help to accommodate in the classroom the child with NMI and/or auditory-processing difficulties.

Moro reflex: Given that a child with a retained Moro will overreact to almost all stimuli, the most important accommodation a teacher can make for such a child is to create the classroom as non-threatening an environment as possible. This can be done by keeping noise levels to a minimum – both the teacher's own and that of the children. General movement during teaching should be reduced as much as possible, so that the child's eyes are more able to attend selectively to what is of immediate concern to them. Careful planning can seat certain children in positions where much of the general bustle of the classroom is outside their field of vision.

All children hate to be singled out – to be different – unless that difference increases the status among their peers. The child with a Moro reflex already feels at variance with others and has difficulty fitting into a group. As a result, their self-esteem is usually low or, at best, fragile. A teacher who is aware of such a trait and understands the underlying reason can do much to build confidence without making the child feel conspicuous.

Asymmetrical tonic neck reflex: The child who still has an ATNR needs extra space to write in order to accommodate the effect of the reflex. This is the child

Reflexes	School problem	Remediation approach
Head-righting reflexes Test: Tilting of the body while seated focusing on a fixed point ahead.	Oculo-motor dysfunctions. visual-perceptual problems. Gravitational insecurity, possibly influencing spatial awareness. Motion sickness	Vestibular training, e.g. slow rotation (eyes closed), rolling and tilting, progressing to eyes open as balance and head-righting improve; use of scooter board, wobble board, first lying, then sitting, then standing; use of swing, see-saw, playground equipment involving rotation; trampoline.
Landau reflex	Imbalance between flexor and extensor muscle tone.	Prone – lifting torso off the ground while keeping feet on the ground.
Amphibian and segmental rolling reflexes	Lack of segmental or differentiated movement through the body.	Rolling from prone to supine and vice versa. Initiating movement from one portion of the body and following through sequentially with other sections.
Equilibrium reactions		These will only develop fully if the Moro and tonic labyrinthine reflexes are inhibited; absence of equilibrium reactions may be symptomatic of other retained primitive reflexes.

Table 6.3: General remediation suggestions or strategies for underdeveloped postural reflexes

who may rotate the page as much as 90° to allow for the fact that every time they turn their head to write, their arm wants to stretch. They often push the paper to the far side of the working surface, particularly when writing near the bottom of the page. Seating a right- and left-handed child together at a table will cause enormous problems for this child. If the child also has retained a Moro reflex, then the distractions of group teaching may make concentration impossible for them. Simple changes such as arranging the classroom so that there at least some individual desks or placing tables in rows facing the teacher will help to minimise distraction and allow each child maximum personal space.

Difficulty with the physical act of writing will prevent the child from expressing ideas in written form even though it is easy for them to do so orally. Ideas can be reinforced by allowing a period of discussion which can then be condensed into key words or phrases as an outline for an essay or a short piece of creative writing. Similarly, the child can be taught to underline salient points. When they are given a paragraph that is intended to test their comprehension or that is part of an exam question, this practice will enable them to identify the main points for discussion.

Use of a laptop computer can aid spelling, grammar and content, since the finger control required for keyboard skills is different from that required for handwriting. Posture and movement at the keyboard do not trigger the ATNR and so the computer frees the child from the physical constraints of the ATNR. Spellchecks can help to reinforce correct spelling and thereby develop better visual memory of how words should look. Not all children, however, can master the visual-motor integration skills needed for fast and accurate typing (some children with dyspraxia find this particularly difficult) and in these cases a computer will only be of limited assistance.

Where improvement in handwriting is essential, some of a child's homework may be done on a computer and then the correct version copied by hand into the exercise book. This, in effect, separates out the two processes of cognitively processing information and physically writing it down.

Symmetrical tonic neck reflex: This is the child whose posture will be affected by any movement of their head forwards or backwards. This will be particularly noticeable when the child sits at a desk, since inclining the head forward to focus on work will cause the arms to bend and the head to fall nearer and nearer to the working surface. The effect of this can be minimised by altering the angle of the work surface so that the head can be maintained in a more upright posture. The old-fashioned sloping desks were ideal for this, but a triangular structure that can be placed on top of the table will have the same effect. The effects of STNR will usually diminish quickly if a motor-training programme is provided.

Spinal Galant: The effect of the retained spinal Galant is that it creates an 'ants in the pants' child. There are other reasons why a child can't stay in their seat, yet some teachers have found it possible to cease constant complaints and reminders to keep children still. The main offenders in the classroom are given flat, plastic pillows filled with water. Such simple devices give them enough wriggle room so that they can stay in their seats, and peace and quiet will be restored.

Sometimes even after reflex abnormalities have been corrected a child continues to have problems with integration of the two sides of the body. Independent use of the left and right hands, use of opposite hand and foot, etc. may be difficult. These movement disabilities reflect the inability of the two sides of the brain to cooperate in facilitation, inhibition and transmission of information back and forth across the corpus callosum. Efficient communication between the two cerebral hemispheres in both directions is necessary for all academic learning, particularly for solving problems that require a sequence of procedures. (Solving one simple multiplication problem involves at least nine interactions between the two sides of the brain.)

Sheila Dobie and colleagues at the INPP in Scotland developed a series of exercises that help to train different parts of the body to operate with each other in any number of combinations and sequences. As a child's movement vocabulary increases, basic movement patterns become automatic. Not only does the child's motor competency improve, but corresponding cognitive abilities also show greater flexibility and improved performance.

Simple changes in the classroom

- Seat a child at the front of the class rather than leaving them to daydream or be overlooked or distracted at the back. This can help to focus their attention and enable the teacher to notice whether the child has understood what is being taught or the task in hand.
- Give clear instructions, speaking slowly and enunciating each word. Some children with dyslexia process the sounds of speech more slowly and will miss part of the information while others with attentional problems may zone out if too much information is given at once. Short sentences and stopping to ask the child (or other children) to repeat what they have to do, before an activity commences, can embed information in short-term memory and also reveal whether any part of an instruction has been misunderstood.
- Ensure written instructions are clear – that writing or print is large enough for the whole class to see – and do not stand in front of the board.
- Where possible, provide concrete examples of what is being discussed. For example, if a child is struggling with a basic concept in maths, introduce physical materials to demonstrate what the concept means.

The last point above was illustrated for me when one of my children was struggling to understand fractions, decimals and percentages. As soon as the subject was brought up, a glazed expression would appear and the shutters would come down to block any further abstract explanation. A resourceful learning support teacher put 100 toy Roman soldiers on the table and asked the child to count them. The teacher then asked him to divide them into two equal halves and count how many soldiers were in each half. He then asked the boy if he understood what the word 'centurion' meant and asked him to write down as many words as he could think of starting with 'cent': 'centurion', 'century', 'centimetre', 'centipede'. He then explained that 'cent' means 100 and that a centurion was one soldier in charge of a group of 100 other soldiers. 'So,' he said, 'you now have two groups of 50 soldiers, one group out of the two is one half – or 50 out of 100 – which is equivalent to 50 per cent. This means the same if written as a decimal (out of ten) and is shown as 0.5.'

The teacher then used the soldiers in different groupings and combinations to revisit basic arithmetic concepts such as counting out three groups of six and then explaining with verbal language that 3 × 6 = 18. Equally, if 18 soldiers were divided into three groups, each group would comprise six soldiers. In this way, the child started to understand not only that multiplication and division are opposite processes, but also to apply the known methods (multiplication tables for example) he needed to employ to solve new problems. Much of the mental blank that had previously existed had been bridged by working with concrete examples of mathematical concepts.

Tables 6.2 and 6.3 have many further suggestions for those who are in a position to do more than is usually possible in the classroom.

When a child is experiencing difficulties, it is often tempting to try to provide the maximum stimulation and support. A study by Kavale and Mattson (1983) suggests that if too many types of intervention are made at the same time the results are less than chance. In other words, there is no significant improvement.

The brain can only take in a certain amount of new information at one time and often needs time to absorb and integrate new information. It is therefore advisable to start with only one method of intervention and allow time to assess progress before building anything further into the programme. If the child's behaviour starts to deteriorate shortly after something new has been added, this may be a sign that they are overloaded and the amount of stimulation needs to be decreased. More is not necessarily better.

Although the above are general suggestions for parents or teachers who have the time to dedicate to carrying out daily exercises with a child, if a cluster of abnormal reflexes are present the child ideally needs a structured programme based on the findings of assessment.

Nature and nurture – a complex picture

The presence of a primitive or lack of a postural reflex at key stages in development can be seen as evidence of subcortical interference in the control of neuromuscular functions. Voluntary control of movements directly reflects the degree of cortical control in the individual: the cortex represents purposive behaviour whereas subcortical control tends to be limited and stereotyped.

Subcortical systems may remain overly involved for a variety of reasons: pathology, metabolic imbalance, injury or lack of use at any early stage in development. Retained primitive reflexes are not the primary cause of the presenting difficulties, but rather a symptom or signpost of immaturity in the functioning of the central nervous system. Damage or disease affecting higher centres can release primitive reflexes (as in cerebral palsy, multiple sclerosis or Alzheimer's disease, for example), or retention of primitive reflexes may in itself interfere with the establishment of consistent cortical control. Assessment and analysis of primitive and postural reflexes can therefore be used as a valuable tool to assess the level of functioning under specific conditions, and the developmental level, type and intensity of remediation required by the individual. The ability to pinpoint the arrested stage in development can also help to determine the teaching methods and strategies from which a child is likely to benefit most, as well as bring understanding of aspects of behaviour and emotional regulation.

The reflexes provide only the substrata for later learning. By the time a child has reached the age of eight years, other systems, learning styles and compensations will also have become involved, which may be accompanied by dysfunction in how the brain processes and integrates auditory information, visual information, vestibular functioning, etc. These differences in sensory integration and process can affect perception and influence emotional response to different environments.

It is therefore important to unravel which area presents the greatest stumbling block for the individual and to devise a personalised programme. For, although the symptoms of dysfunction may be similar for many, the developmental route through which the individual has travelled to accommodate their problems is as individual as they are. This is why a battery of tests that examine a cluster of reflexes and more than just one area of functioning can be invaluable in assessing the needs of the individual.

Complicating the search for answers, other factors may have contributed along the way. Poor nutrition is just one. Allergies, food intolerances, a surfeit of junk food, or dietary restrictions – increasingly features of affluent societies – can result in a profile of vitamin, mineral and trace element depletion which increases craving for one food group at the expense of another. Paradoxically, vitamin, mineral and trace element deficiencies can also be linked to obesity, which constitutes a new form of malnutrition. Nutritional status influences the availability of neurotransmitters, the body's chemical messengers. These are the molecules used by the nervous system to transmit messages between neurons or from neurons to muscles. They influence a neuron in one of three ways: excitatory, inhibitory or modulatory.

Allergies, social deprivation, neglect or abuse, genetics, biochemical influences and psychological factors may all play a role. Human beings do not grow and develop in the tidy context of departments and professional disciplines, but are the product of genes, environment and experience in a constantly changing world.

Social and environmental factors may also be behind an apparent increase in signs of NMI in children in societies ever more driven by economics and technological advances, since sedentary lifestyles provide less opportunity for movement and engagement in real physical time and space. Gadgets of convenience such as infant bucket seats (some with built-in entertainment), bouncers, walkers and electronic devices and games replace the experience of movement, social engagement with another human being, and learning by physical trial and error.

Overuse of baby equipment in infancy can result in reduced 'tummy time' in the first nine months of life. Tummy time, when a child is awake, is important to support the development of head-righting reflexes and neck and shoulder strength and to afford physical space, freedom of movement, and opportunity to learn how to crawl. Social engagement is important for the development of non-verbal and verbal language. Conversation involves listening, waiting and reflecting based on what the other person has said. Trial and error learning is important for problem-solving and learning how to do something. These physical experiences also act as cognitive building blocks that support cognitive learning.

Use of electronic media

The last 25 years have seen a transformation in the media through which children in technological societies learn and in how they spend their leisure time. Although electronic media provide benefits in terms of access to information and the speed and organisation of output and entertainment, if overused they can have harmful effects, including various influences on the child or adolescent's developing brain. The impact of these media is twofold:

- what it prevents a child from doing
- what it does

What screen time prevents

Physical activity

When children are using electronic media they are not engaging in large physical movements, physical interaction with another human being, or free, spontaneous and self-generated creative play.

Sensory experience of content

The limited interaction with and integration of multisensory experiences with images viewed on screen does not produce the same physical and biochemical changes as occur in response to sensory experiences in the real world.

Figures 6.2 and 6.3 show children playing in a field of lavender, exploring the feel of the flowers with their fingers and releasing the aroma by brushing against the plants. The combination of colours constantly changing in the light, touch, smell and the chemical effect of scent on the brain will become associated with the scent of lavender for life. The screen image of a lavender field (Figure 6.4) will only conjure up those physical changes if the feel and scent of fresh lavender are already known.

Figure 6.2:
Children playing in lavender field.

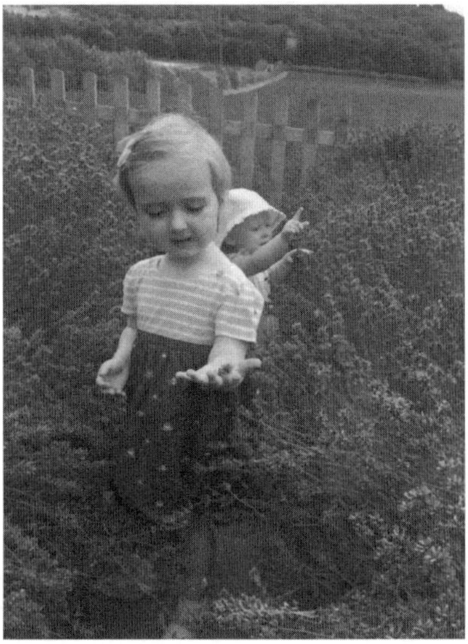

A similar dulling of sensory and emotional involvement may also develop when someone is exposed to images of violence. The revulsion that naturally occurs when one is an unwilling witness to violent scenes does not necessarily have the same impact or intensity when the violence is viewed remotely and there is a physical buffer between reality and its consequences. This can result in a person becoming detached from the real effects of violence, inured to the suffering of others and less empathically responsive.

Figure 6.3:
Children walking through lavender field.

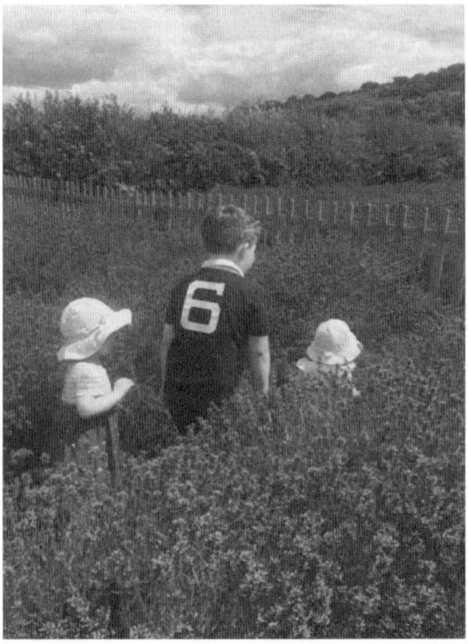

Social skills

Unlike an adult's brain, a child's brain is still developing. As a result, it is more malleable. Too much time in front of a screen not interacting with other people can lead to trouble with social interaction. There may be a lack of opportunity or practice in picking up on non-verbal cues. Facial expressions, postural changes, speed

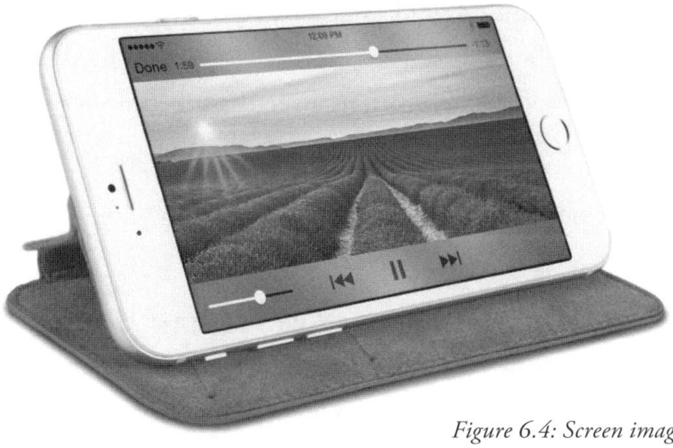

Figure 6.4: Screen image of lavender field.

and quality of movements, tone of voice, and eye contact all provide important insights into the feelings and intentions of others and how to respond to them. Even the sense of smell can provide subliminal messages about a person's state of arousal. If indulged at the expense of real interpersonal relationships, excessive screen time could lead to social and relationship problems later in life. Sympathy or 'common feeling' begins with the ability to feel as another.

Screen time, if not used for social interaction, may reduce the amount of time spent in conversation. Conversation is key to language development through the exchange of thoughts and ideas and through listening to each other. Conversation is not just about the exchange of information; it's about sharing thoughts, expressing feelings, understanding, interpretation and seeing situations in new ways. Conversation connects us, forms bonds, enables us to articulate feelings and anxieties that may have become locked in the self, as well as providing a melting pot for the generation of new ideas. Conversation is the alchemy through which the raw materials of random thoughts and observations can be turned into creative gold. It can challenge our accepted view of the world, introducing us to new ideas and perspectives, and motivate the flagging will.

Sleep

Sleep is essential for physical growth (growth hormone is secreted during sleep), development, learning, memory, emotions, behaviour and overall mental health. Electronic devices emit blue light from their screens. When exposed to this blue light before bedtime, a child's body may interpret it as daylight and the brain may signal the body to stay awake after the screen has been turned off. Long-term exposure to blue light can result in disturbed sleep patterns and imbalances in a child's biological clock.

What screen time does

Attention

Prolonged screen activity has greater impact on brainwave states in children, reducing their vigilance to external stimuli and increasing their propensity for passive attention. When children are exposed to technology frequently or for long periods of time, their brain may adopt an internet approach to thinking – quickly scanning and processing multiple sources of information and making rapid shifts of visual attention. Although this type of processing is useful for scanning novel environments, it is not good for developing listening skills, retaining information in short-term memory or developing the specific eye movements needed for reading. This type of processing has many features in common with aspects of ADD.

Thinking styles

Computer programs are pre-set, often developed by a particular type of 'digital thinking' mind, and therefore lead the child to explore or follow a designated programme as opposed to responding in innovative creative ways. If a child spends long periods of time engaged in activity through a single medium, the developing brain starts to think in a similar way – expecting to be provided with binary options or solutions to problems or challenges.

A study carried out in Japan in 2022 indicated that boys who watch screens at the age of one are more likely to show signs of autism at the age of three. Among boys, longer screen time at one year of age was significantly associated with autism spectrum disorder at three years of age (Kushima et al. 2022). The reason was uncertain, since it is possible that children with autistic tendencies seek out and demand more screen time, but screen time also affects the brainwave state of children differently from adults and this may play a part in children's difficulty in shifting attention away from screen activity. Difficulty in shifting attention between different sensory modalities is also a feature of ASD.

Mood regulation

Excessive screen time has been linked to issues with attention, frustration, aggression and other behaviour. Children who have more than two hours a day of screen time are more likely to have angry outbursts or be irritable when asked to stop using their devices, or when they are not using them. The latter finding is thought to be related to the potentially addictive properties of screen time, including the ways screen time affects brainwave states and may increase the neurotransmitter dopamine, which is linked to the sense of reward.

Brainwaves

More than 50 years ago, Krugman (1971) discovered that TV screen time dampens the activity of the critical left brain within 30 seconds of starting to view. Brainwave activity switches from an alert waking state, associated with increased beta activity, to a predominance of alpha waves, indicating an unfocused, dreamlike state in which adults and children alike are more receptive to images and feelings. 'Both advertisers and politicians intuitively know how powerful the TV/Brain effect is!' (Large 2006).

The brain constantly generates electrical activity in both sleeping and waking states. This can be recorded using an electroencephalograph (EEG) machine. German psychiatrist Hans Berger (1873–1941) was the first to record brainwaves from the scalp and discover that there was a change in activity when subjects became drowsy or fell asleep. Other scientists subsequently confirmed Berger's observations. The technology for detecting and analysing brainwaves states has advanced considerably. The two fundamental aspects of brain activity measured using the EEG are the frequency and amplitude of the waves. The specific frequencies of different bands of brainwave and the associated mental states in relation to arousal are listed in Table 6.1.

Exposure to screens has been shown to reduce attention span in children. Increased slow-wave (theta band) and decreased fast-wave (beta and gamma bands) generated from EEG, as well as an increased theta/beta ratio, have been observed in children with ADHD. Results support a negative relationship between screen exposure and attention-related patterns from the EEG in typically developing pre-school children (Zivan et al. 2019).

In a study carried out to investigate associations between screen-based media use and brain white matter integrity in pre-school children researchers, reported:

> In this cross-sectional study of 47 healthy prekindergarten children, screen use greater than that recommended by the American Academy of Pediatrics guidelines [Table 6.4] was associated with lower measures of microstructural organisation and myelination of brain white matter tracts that support language and emergent literacy skills and corresponding cognitive assessments.
>
> These findings suggest a need for further study into the association between screen-based media use and the developing brain, particularly during early childhood. (Hutton et al. 2020)

Research carried out at the Australian National University in Canberra found that television viewing reduced the quantity of the highest-frequency brainwaves involved in alert attention and decision-making and caused an increase in theta activity. Whereas alpha activity is associated with relaxed waking states, theta is associated with drowsiness and a generalised dampening of the brain's ability to send or receive information, associated with reduced vigilance and states of passive inattention. Merrelyn Emery, one of the researchers in the Australian study, concluded that abundant constant theta activity, which approaches a drowsy or hypnogogic pattern when one is watching television, affects the way that knowledge is processed and acquired. 'We can confidently predict that as theta activity increases during viewing, there will be at the ontogenetic level, a corresponding increase only in 'knowing of' and not 'knowing' (Emery 1987). Theta activity is also associated with a different kind of perception. 'An increase in theta represents a breakdown between person and environment in the sense that environmental vigilance is neglected' (ibid.).

This type of second-hand knowledge derived from passive observation rather than experience is not integrated in the same way as information learned from direct experience, which roots knowledge into the self. Krugman (2000) described such knowledge derived from passive observation as involving 'recognition without recall, exposure without perception'.

Addictive properties

Researchers have discovered not only that screen time is habit forming, but that dopamine, strongly connected with addiction, is implicated. Screen use releases dopamine in the brain, which can negatively affect impulse control. Studies have shown that screen time affects the frontal cortex of the brain, in a way similar to the effect of cocaine. Like drugs, screen time sets off a pleasure/reward cycle that can have a negative impact.[27]

Dopamine is a neurotransmitter involved in pleasure and reward systems in the brain as well as the inhibition of involuntary movement when one is at rest. It is one of three neurotransmitters collectively known as 'monoamines', of which the other two are norepinepherine (noradrenaline) and serotonin. Norephinepherine is a key chemical in mediating the physical changes involved in arousal and is important in the regulation of hunger and alertness. Serotonin is important in the regulation of sleep, particularly the onset of sleep. Dopamine plays many roles in the body and is involved in reward, motivation, memory, attention and body movements. Low levels may negatively affect mood, motivation and memory. All of the monoamines are closely linked to mood states and, when poorly regulated, to emotional disorders.

In *Healing ADD: The Breakthrough Program that Allows You to See and Heal the 7 Types of ADD*, Amen (2013) says that children with ADHD are particularly susceptible to the addictive properties of electronic games. In a study published in *Nature*,[28] researchers carried out PET scans on subjects playing action video games and discovered that the basal ganglia, where dopamine is produced, were more active when the subjects were playing the game than when they were at rest. Amen (2001) goes on to say that 'both cocaine and Ritalin™ (a stimulant drug used to treat the symptoms of ADHD) work in this part of the brain as well'. One of the properties of Ritalin™ is to make more dopamine available to the brain.

> Video games bring pleasure and focus by increasing dopamine release. The problem with them is that the more dopamine is released, the less neurotransmitter is available later to do schoolwork, homework, chores and so

on. While the brainwave theory partly explains the dulling effect of television on the brain, the neurochemical theory explains some of its addictive properties with the let down or withdrawal symptoms that follow. (Amen 2001)

Visual skills

Overuse of computers and computer games may also affect the developing visual skills of young children. Whereas concentration on near-point activities too soon (such as early reading before the necessary supporting postural and visual skills are in place) may be associated with visual near-point stress (Skeffington 1943), possibly leading to the development of non-hereditary short sight, computer use requires intensive periods of focus at extended near distance – a focusing distance just beyond the ideal reading distance – with a tendency to develop convergence and focusing problems at reading distance. A significant number of children assessed at the INPP in recent years appear to have difficulty with near-point (reading distance) convergence and can benefit from a small, temporary plus prescription, easing near-point stress at reading distance until reflex status has matured and accommodative and convergent skills have become more flexible. This symptom has become increasingly evident in the last decade or so. Whether it is related to increased use of screen time is not yet known.

Although many hand-held computer games help to train accommodation between field vision and central vision, they do not train the eye-tracking skills needed for reading. Children become good at rapid shifts of visual attention within their field of vision, but hand-held computer games do not develop the smooth sequential eye movements needed to follow a line of print without the eyes jumping further along the line or to the line above or the line below. Children become good at rapidly decoding individual symbols, shapes or pictures on a screen, but are not as good at following a series of symbols from left to right and decoding them in an accurate sequence. This is important for spelling.

Prolonged screen time can also result in symptoms of digital eye strain which may include burning, itchy or tired eyes. As well as affecting sleep, blue light is damaging to the retinal cells and can speed up macular degeneration. Depending on the type of device in habitual use – for example, hand-held devices tend to be used at near distance whereas laptops involve extended near distance – this can also lead to the development of myopia or near-sightedness in children.

Posture

Being hunched over a smartphone or tablet for long periods of time can affect posture and the developing spine (Figure 6.5). This can lead to harmful physical effects that can last for the rest of one's life, such as back pain and headaches.

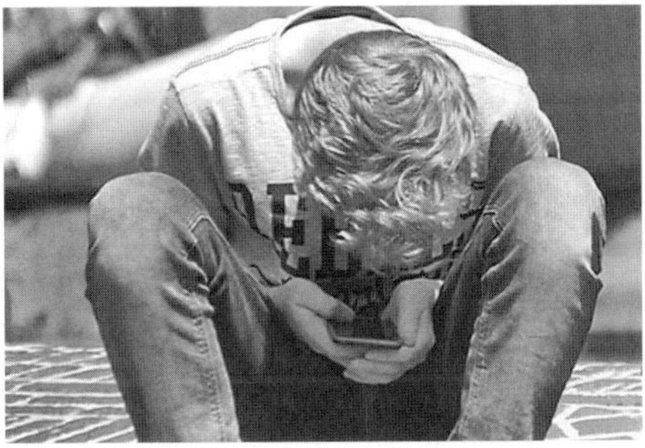

Figure 6.5: Sitting posture of teenager using a mobile electronic device.

Weight

As mentioned above, screen time is a sedentary activity. This, coupled with eating high-calorie junk foods and reduced physical exercise, can lead to childhood obesity and poor muscle tone. When children and adults have meals or snacks while watching and sitting in front of a screen, they have less conscious control over what or how much they eat.

Fast foods are exactly what they say they are: instantly available, eaten fast, often on the hoof, and they generally have high fat, sugar and refined carbohydrate content. When food is eaten at speed, the satiety centre in the brain does not have time to recognise signals sent from the gut that the body has had enough and to respond by switching off the hunger signals before more food is eaten (Goddard Blythe 2001).

The gut–brain axis normally controls appetite and satiety via neuronal and hormonal signals when entry of nutrients into the small intestine stimulates the release of peptides, which act as negative feedback signals to reduce meal size and terminate feeding, but it takes at least 20 minutes for this feedback to be recognised in the brain. Fast food can overtake this system. Satiety also occurs in relation to the ratio of nutrients to calories, protein and fibre content and the insulin response.

In this context, children who have a habit of eating during screen time are at increased risk of becoming overweight. The combination of increased weight and less physical activity can affect the development of muscle tone, making the taking of regular exercise more difficult and less appealing.

In balance

Although mindful (and regulated) use of digital devices can support well-being, conditions imposed on societies by the COVID-19 pandemic in 2020 resulted in a significant increase in the use of screen time for children and adults. Pandya and Lodha carried out a review of screen use in an attempt to understand virtual social connectedness, excessive use of digital technology and their consequences and to suggest strategies to maintain healthy use of digital technology. They reported:

> … excessive screen time to be associated with a range of negative mental health outcomes such as psychological problems, low emotional stability, and greater risk for depression or anxiety (Allen et al., 2019; Aziz Rahman et al., 2020; Ministry of Human Resource Development, 2020).
>
> Negative consequences often result when digital use is impulsive, compulsive, unregulated or addictive (Kuss and Lopez-Fernandez, 2016). (Pandya and Lodha 2021)

How much is too much?

Electronic media are not all bad. During the COVID-19 pandemic, they enabled communities in isolation to remain connected, families to see one another online, essential items to be delivered, businesses to survive and technological advances to be made. Before the pandemic, they provided a source of education and entertainment and access to images and knowledge and data way beyond the scope of individual physical proximity and will continue to do so; but, as with medication, the difference between benefit and harm or the emergence of side effects is dose dependent, which raises the question: how do we ensure that children's exposure to screen time is age appropriate? Table 6.4 presents the recommendations of the American Academy of Pediatrics.[29]

Age	Recommended screen time/use
18 months and younger	Avoid use of screen media other than video-chatting.
18–24 months	Choose high-quality programming and watch it with their children to help them to understand what they are seeing.
2–5 years	Limit screen use to an hour per day of high-quality programmes.
6–12 years	Place consistent limits on the time spent using media and the types of media and make sure media do not take the place of adequate sleep, physical activity and other activities essential to health.
12 years and older	Designate media-free times together (parents too should adhere to this), such as mealtimes, walks and driving as well as having media-free zones at home such, as bedrooms.

Table 6.4: Screen time recommendations for children (American Academy of Paediatrics 2022)

Summary

Irrespective of culture, every child's experience of growing up is unique. Children growing up within the same family do not share equal proportions of their parents' time, attention or affection. Siblings in the same family home will often describe the parenting they received and their memories of childhood very differently from each other. Even identical twins who share the same genetic make-up will have occupied different positions in the womb, birth experiences, feeding and parental involvement. These are just a few examples of how nurture works alongside nature to fashion the neurological and emotional connections that make each one of us who we are.

Whether there really is an increase in the number of children in mainstream schools with signs of immature neuromotor skills, or whether such problems have become more evident simply because studies have examined them, has not been conclusively established. The reasons for these problems are multi-factorial. Irrespective of the reasons, immature neuromotor skills can impact on children's ability to achieve to their full potential in the classroom and have been shown to be linked to emotional insecurity in later life.

No matter what the cause, a neurodevelopmental approach to understanding and resolving signs of specific learning difficulties, underachievement or behavioural/emotional problems will enable the teacher, therapist or clinician to take the lid off the symptoms to see what lies beneath. Primitive and postural reflexes reveal information about maturity in the inner functioning of the central nervous system, providing a window through which we can view the developmental level of the child. They prompt us to look again at the observation posed by Tansley over 50 years ago:

> For far too long teachers have concentrated upon the psychological problems of the child, or the socio-economic environment, instead of asking the question, does the child have the equipment which he needs to succeed at the educational level asked of him and the methods imposed on him. (Tansley 1967)

This question, which first led Peter Blythe into the search for a physical basis for learning disabilities and emotional problems that did not respond to therapies available at the time, remains as relevant today and to future generations as it did more than half a century ago. If the physical foundations upon which learning and emotional resilience are built are made strong, then teaching can be effective and the child can start to grow. In our modern world, there is little leeway for academic failure, and if it seems to exist we must continue to ask the question 'WHY?'

Chapter 7

A Short History of Reflexes and the INPP Method

> All truth passes through three stages: First, it is ridiculed. Second, it is violently opposed. Third, it is accepted as self-evident. (Arthur Schopenhauer)

The word 'reflex' is a derivative of the word 'reflection', which etymologically means to 'bend it back'. The earliest use of 'reflex' in this context can be traced back to Thomas Willis (1621–75), who was one of the first medical physiologists in the 17th century to place his faith in clinical and laboratory observation as opposed to the theory of the 'humours' and the philosophies of the Graeco-Roman tradition. Willis (1670 cited in Finger 2000) used the terms 'motus reflexus' and 'reflexion' to describe how impulses or 'spirits' in the nerves to the central nervous system could be 'reflected' back to the muscles. The automatic action generated by the process was similar to the action of light bouncing off a mirror. It was also Willis who gave us modern medical terms such as 'neurology', 'lobe' and 'hemisphere'

Roger Whytt (1751) carried out experiments on animals and attempted to list the functional relationship between reflexes and protective behaviours. He was intrigued by the continued motor activity of animals following decapitation – a well-known, but not understood phenomenon. This is woven into the 17th-century English children's rhyme, 'King Charles walked and talked for five minutes after his head was cut off!' The term 'reflex' reappeared in the 18th century when Georg Prochaska of Vienna described 'the reflexion of sensorial into motor impressions… which takes place in the common sensory centre and which may take place with consciousness or without' (cited in Shepherd 1994).

In 1820, Charles Bell and Françoise Magendie recognised that 'between the brain and the muscle there is a circle of nerves; one conveys the influence of the brain to the muscle, another gives the sense of condition of the muscle to the brain'. The action may vary in intensity according to the stimulus or internal state, but the basic pattern remains the same. These and other scientists were thus able to show that it is the brain and not the individual body part that 'feels' sensation, but they were unable to explain how different regions in the brain and the body communicated this information.

It was the Spanish histologist Santiago Ramon y Cajal (1843–1926) who pieced together a vital missing link when he proposed the neuron theory and the law of dynamic polarisation. Cajal traced the nerves from the sensory organs such as the eyes to the brain and found that the sensory nerves project inwards from peripheral dendrites and axons towards the brain. The motor nerves operate in reverse; the dendrites of the motor nerves are in the brain and spinal cord with axons projecting outwards towards the muscles. However, the question remained, how do impulses pass from one neuron to another? The neuron theory stated that every nerve cell branches and each branch meets at a junction. Sherrington was later to name these junctions 'synapses', although the question of how impulses passed across these gaps remained unanswered until 1914, when Henry Hallett Dale isolated a compound called acetylcholine found in the ergot fungus. Dale found that when this substance was applied to a nerve ending it produced a response in the muscle. A further series of experiments by Dale together with the work of Loewi suggested that acetylcholine was secreted by motor nerves in response to electrical stimulation and that acetylcholine was the chemical agent by which nerves worked on muscles. It was the first neurotransmitter to be identified.

Charles Sherrington (1857–1952) carried out a series of animal experiments in which he separated and identified nerves leading to and from the spinal cord and the brainstem. He then divided the brainstem and spinal cord from higher regions in the brain and undertook further experiments to see what happened to such 'brainless' creatures when the central nervous system acted without the executive control of higher regions in the brain. Through this process he was able to establish the existence of the reflex arc – the path along which sensory signals are gathered together and passed through the central nervous system, which reacts by turning specific groups of muscles on and off. He also realised that reflexes do not act in isolation; rather they act together in a coordinated system (of systems). The detailed findings of this work were published in *The Integrative Action of the Nervous System* (1906).

Therefore, it was through the work of many of scientists over many years that the beginnings of our modern understanding of reflexes and of the central nervous system was born. Subsequently, reflexes have been chronicled by many authors for diagnostic, functional and developmental purposes.

It is now recognised that certain reflex reactions provide outward signs of levels of functioning within the central nervous system. They can be used as tools to assess damage, disease and dysfunction in the central nervous system. The cardinal feature of a reflex is that the basic pattern of response remains unchanged and, once initiated, the action cannot be modified. This final observation provides the reason why there is such a profound impact upon the functioning and adaptability of the individual, who is the servant rather than the executive master of their reflexes.

The model for assessment and remediation of reflexes in the context of learning and emotional problems outlined in the previous chapters started its journey to its present form from several sources. No history can ever paint a true picture of the past, because ideas are born not from a neat sequence of events but rather from knowledge and multiple influences collected over a long period of time. 'The real history is the story of the struggle – the searchings, successes and failures as well as the personal interactions of everyone in the field.'[30]

History of the development of the INPP method

In order to understand a method, it is not enough simply to learn the procedures and techniques of the system; it is essential to know its history: how it evolved; the ideas that underlie it and contributed to its development; the people who built it and the problems they were attempting to solve; the discussions, debates and even conflicts that arose along the way. The method that emerges is but a crystallisation of this history. It can be taught and replicated, but to understand how it works, to solve problems, to recognise when it is being misapplied or misused, it is necessary to know its history and the thinking that led to where it is today.

Peter Blythe, founder of the INPP method, said that the origins of the method began in 1969 shortly after he was appointed as a senior lecturer in applied psychology at a college of education in Lancashire. He was informed that he was expected to deliver a lecture on reading difficulties to a group of students and teaching faculty – a subject on which, as a former psychotherapist, he freely admitted he knew nothing. In preparing for the event, he scoured a local bookshop, where he came across a small book, *Reading and Remedial Reading* by AE Tansley (1967). In his haste to find content and a rationale for his forthcoming lecture, the message he extracted from the book was never to assume that, because a child looks normal, they have the neurological organisation or equipment in place to meet the demands of the classroom. This concept – that rather than looking to treat the presenting problem, a practitioner should investigate the underlying mechanisms – was the beginning of the journey that led to the INPP method today.

Blythe always referred to himself in jest as a 'reductionist' and this was certainly true of his later summary and simplification of the genesis of the method down to just one event in the 1960s. Many moments of inspiration occur when new facts or challenges converge upon a mind that is searching and prepared. Blythe's practical need to understand reading difficulties had followed many years of working in private practice as a psychotherapist and consultant hypnotist. He had noticed that a number of adult patients suffering from what were described as 'neuroses' at the time were either unable to enter hypnosis or were recidivists, unable to benefit in the long term from the therapies of choice despite a desire to get better and often having a good intellectual understanding of their problems.

Blythe had come to realise that many of these patients were unable to cede control sufficiently to enter hypnosis and/or held tension in particular parts of the body, which he named the 'locus of control'. He discovered that if, instead of trying to teach them to relax, patients were encouraged to increase the intensity of tension in the body, they would eventually lose cortical control. As tension and feelings became stronger than the cortex's capacity to contain them, the patient would spontaneously abreact and emotional memories that had not been available to consciousness would come flooding to the surface.

The technique of locating and building up areas of physical tension in the body later became known as 'psycho-muscular release therapy' (PMRT). Blythe used this technique extensively in his own practice in the United Kingdom and taught it to practitioners of psychotherapy in Sweden in the 1970s. It mirrored some of Wilhelm Reich's theory that an inherent part of emotional conflict for which there is no immediate solution can be a tendency to armour the body, somatising the stress and making the body a physical container for emotions. Blythe wrote:

> The first glimmer of light came to me when I read the work of the late Dr Wilhelm Reich and learned that he had faced a similar dilemma. He discovered that people developed a 'character armour' to protect themselves, or, put more simply, Reich came to the conclusion that we mirrored our neuroses in our bodies and there is a definite body language which the psychotherapist and psychoanalyst has to understand.
>
> The man who holds back what he would really like to say to other people learns to physically control himself by keeping his mouth tightly shut, his teeth and jaws clenched, and before long he forgets what he wanted to say as it is firmly buried behind the 'character armour' of his mouth and jaws.
>
> The person who is frightened of recognising his or her own body feelings in certain situations will tighten up the muscles in the solar plexus, the abdomen, and soon find themselves holding their bodies in an upright, permanently tensed position. (Blythe 1974)

Although PMRT was effective in unlocking residual tension held in the body, it did not answer the question 'why'? Why are some individuals more sensitive and prone to stress? Why are they unable to regulate their emotions to relieve their stress? Why are they more sensitive to life events than others? Why do they remain stuck in self-destructive behaviour despite a strong motivation to be well? These were questions that remained in the back of Blythe's mind and to which psychodynamic theories of the time did not have satisfactory answers.

In his new teaching post, Blythe was comfortable with aspects of teaching the college curriculum based on theories of personality disorder and he introduced his trainee teacher students to various controversial projective tests including

Karen Machover's (1942) 'personality projection through the drawing of the a human figure', the Rorschach (1964) plates and their interpretation, and other projective tests developed by Berkowitz and Rothman (1960) for use in the classroom. Blythe duly delivered his lecture to faculty and students, in which he summarised the main message he had gleaned from Tansley's book.

Tansley (1967) had mentioned three main areas identified as commonly present in children with reading difficulties:

- immature or aberrant patterns of motor development
- visual–motor integration (VMI) or hand–eye coordination difficulties
- cross-laterality or ambiguity of laterality

One of Blythe's mature students, David McGlown, was equally captivated by Tansley's theme and, together, Blythe and McGlown set about devising an informal test battery to examine a child's physical, emotional and perceptual functioning.

Physical assessment was influenced by Delacato's neuropsychological approach to reading difficulties and included observations of how a child crawled and crept together with tests for lateral preference.

Emotional functioning was investigated by assessing children's drawings in response to 'the thing I hate most', 'the thing that makes me happy', etc. in addition to 'draw a person', 'draw a family', 'draw a good person' and 'draw a bad person'. The child was asked to explain why the person they had drawn was good or bad. Children were also asked to write short pieces on 'the kind of person I would like to be' and 'the sort of person I am' and responses to suggested 'headlines'.

Perceptual functioning was determined by asking children to copy geometric shapes developed by Tansley (1967), Daniels and Diack (1962) and Bender (1946), which provided indications of difficulties with visual discrimination (recognising similarities and differences between shapes and forms), VMI (hand–eye coordination) and spatial awareness.

As part of his normal teaching practice, McGlown cooperated with a local headmaster who allowed him to use this informal test battery with a number of children in his school who were presenting with diverse learning difficulties. The results enabled Blythe and McGlown to isolate three specific areas of functioning that appeared to play a significant part in specific learning difficulties:

- aberrant patterns of motor development (children who had failed to go through the developmental stages of crawling on the stomach and creeping on hands and knees); it was noticed that these children were either unable to crawl or showed deviant patterns of creeping several years later
- evidence of cross-laterality or marked ambiguity of laterality
- definite visual-perceptual problems including difficulty with VMI

When all three criteria existed, Blythe and McGlown (1980) called the syndrome 'organic brain dysfunction' (OBD).

The term 'organic brain dysfunction' was chosen to try to alert teachers and educationists to the fact that children with average or above average intelligence who were failing in the classroom might have a cluster of small physical dysfunctions that prevented them from performing and demonstrating their intelligence, that is, that the brain and various parts of the body failed to work together automatically.

Besides identifying key signs of physical dysfunction, Blythe and McGlown also developed a physical remediation programme to try to correct underlying faults. Based on their knowledge at the time, it relied heavily on the methods used in the United States by Carl Delacato and Glen Doman in rehabilitation programmes for individuals who had suffered brain injury. Although the Delacato–Doman methods were modified and reduced to make them more suitable for children with specific learning difficulties, Blythe (1990a) commented that, on reflection, they were crude, taking up to 40 minutes a day and using exercises intended to train or impose developmentally later patterns upon earlier ones.

McGlown graduated after writing up their findings in his academic dissertation (1971), and the two pioneers parted. Blythe returned to private practice, concentrating on adults suffering from stress-related emotional problems, while McGlown went on to pursue a career in teaching. Now aware of the role of underlying physical factors in specific learning difficulties, Blythe realised that many of the adults he was seeing suffering from neuroses resistant to therapies of choice, and from stress-related problems, shared many of the same dysfunctions as children identified with specific learning difficulties.

His observations in relation to stress were published as a book entitled *Stress Disease: The Growing Plague* (Blythe 1973). Thanks to its popularity, he had the opportunity to examine a significant number of stress-prone individuals for possible signs of OBD. He was also invited to lecture to a group of Swedish doctors, dentists and psychologists who were following a three-year postgraduate course in hypnosis and psychosomatic medicine.

My part in their programme was to teach them the new techniques I had developed to make hypnosis more scientific, less time consuming and more effective, and, more importantly, to teach them the methods I had devised to treat those patients who had failed to respond to or benefit fully from hypnosis. This particular methodology I called 'psycho-muscular release therapy', known in Sweden simply as 'release therapy' (Blythe 1990b).

Meanwhile, McGlown was becoming increasingly frustrated by professional constraints within mainstream education. These meant that as a teacher he recognised children who were failing, but he was not allowed to investigate the underlying mechanisms or do anything about them. In 1975, he joined Blythe in private practice and they decided on the name 'the Institute for Neuro-Physiological Psychology' to cover the areas they would specialise in. Neuro because the underlying connections were neurological; physiological because the processes involved were functional, physical and biological; and psychology because these systems affected emotional and cognitive functioning.

The aims of the INPP were:

- to research the effects of central nervous system dysfunction (OBD) on children with specific learning difficulties and adults suffering from neuroses who failed to respond to treatment
- to develop reliable and replicable methods of assessing signs of OBD
- to develop appropriate central nervous system remedial and rehabilitation programmes

In the early years of the INPP, much of the diagnostic assessment focused on observation of patterns of motor development, laterality and visual perception, but by 1977 Blythe had become aware of the role of one primitive reflex – the ATNR – in development, and its influence if it remained active beyond the first six months of life. Tests for the ATNR were introduced into the diagnostic assessment but it was not until later the same year that Blythe came to realise the significance of primitive and postural reflexes generally.

On yet another trip to Sweden to lecture, I was staying with Bengt-Goran Fasth and his wife Marie-Louise at their home in Molndal, Gothenburg, when I noticed on one of his bookshelves a book entitled *Pictorial Manual of Neurological Tests* (Van Allen and Rodnitzky 1981). In it were various tests for primitive reflexes that should only be present in the first few months of life, after which they should be inhibited – controlled – by a higher part of the brain. Following their inhibition, the brain should release further reflexes – the postural reflexes – to help the individual to cope with gravity and develop good coordination.

This became yet another major milestone along the way. From then onwards we could examine the central nervous system for dysfunction with accuracy, rather than checking for possible soft signs, such as crawling and creeping. We were also able to measure the degree of dysfunction present.

We were then able to devise new test procedures to ascertain if the primitive reflexes were still present or the postural reflexes were absent. We were able to recreate new reflex-inhibition movements to inhibit primitive reflexes still present, and thereby give higher parts of the brain the opportunity to release the appropriate postural reflexes. These new procedures were subsequently written up in *The Clinician's Handbook for the Detection and Remediation of Organic Brain Dysfunction* (Blythe and McGlown 1990).

As the theory aroused curiosity and the remedial programmes started to produce results, interest in the methods increased among a range of other professions. In recognition of the dangers inherent in people copying and applying aspects of the methods without sufficient knowledge, a decision was made to offer training in the techniques that had been developed.

One of the first people to train was a child psychologist from Gothenburg who had attended Blythe's postgraduate lectures to students in Ulricehamn, Sweden and had started to incorporate some of the ideas into the child guidance clinic where she practised. Catharina Johannesson (later Johannesson-Alvegård) trained with Blythe and from 1975 they held training courses for hundreds of teachers, educational psychologists, speech therapists, physiotherapists and school doctors in Sweden. In 1977, she founded the Swedish INPP and became responsible for the provision of training in Sweden.

In parallel with the INPP in Chester, one of the Swedish institute's aims was to carry out research based on the method. The most notable of these early research projects was undertaken by two teachers specialising in special education and published as the *Dala Clinic Final Report* (Bernhardsson and Davidson 1982). The remediation methods developed by Blythe and McGlown were used with a small group of learning-disabled children for whom nothing else had helped to close the educational gap. Those children who completed the programme all made significant educational gains. Other studies included a master's dissertation by Christer Telléus in which he discovered that, as early as 1947, Arnold Gesell (sometimes referred to as the grandfather of child development) and Louise Bates Ames had linked retention of the ATNR to the development of handedness.

Publications in English included *Agoraphobia – An Organic Basis?*, which investigated signs of OBD in a group of adult agoraphobes and panic victims, including a patient's description of her journey through and treatment of agoraphobia (Hurst Vose 1981); a shortened version of a presentation on minimal brain dysfunction (MBD) and OBD made at a symposium on minimal brain dysfunction in Boden, Sweden; and *The Developmental Check List and Evolution of Primitive and Postural Reflexes* (McGlown and Blythe 1980). Determined to provide an academic trail of supporting literature and clinical findings for others to follow, Blythe and McGlown published a book, *An Organic Basis for Neuroses and Educational Difficulties* (1979), in which they described the rationale, research and tools of assessment and remediation that they had developed to date.

From the outset, it had been agreed that the INPP would not work with individuals of any age who were brain injured. These patients would be referred to other organisations already specialising in providing intensive rehabilitation programmes for brain injury. This was to change later, since McGlown had both a personal and growing professional interest in brain injury, initially based on the successful treatment of one child, which led to an influx of enquiries from other parents of brain-injured children. It was decided that a new division of the INPP would be set up under the directorship of McGlown, to be called ' the Centre for Brain Injury, Rehabilitation and Development' (BIRD).

By 1982, BIRD was registered as a national charity and slowly the work being done with children with specific learning difficulties and adults with secondary neuroses began to diverge from the programmes used with brain-injured patients. The INPP premises was not well adapted to patients with physical disabilities; when BIRD relocated to more suitable premises in 1983, the partnership between McGlown and Blythe was dissolved.

From this junction the methods used for the treatment of the two groups separated. Whereas BIRD continued to practise patterns of motor development such as crawling and creeping as major elements of the remediation programme, Blythe realised that there are many other motor patterns, which precede crawling and creeping in development, that naturally play a part in the integration of primitive and postural reflexes at corresponding stages of development. Crawling and creeping are products of early reflexes becoming inhibited and postural reflexes developing. Although crawling and creeping remained important elements of the INPP programme, they were no longer used as the primary mechanisms of inhibition and integration.

Following the parting of ways, the INPP confined its reflex-inhibition programme to trying to replicate the stereotyped movements that all normal human infants make at specific times to facilitate neurodevelopment, in order to inhibit the primitive reflexes and encourage emergence of the postural reflexes (Goddard 1990). This refinement of the methods used to integrate early reflexes meant that a programme that had formerly taken 40 minutes a day was reduced to ten minutes a day.

By the late 1980s, it had also become clear that the original definition of OBD and terminology were no longer accurately descriptive of the INPP method. In 1987, the INPP accepted the medical terminology 'neurological dysfunction' to describe adults who had a cluster of aberrant reflexes and 'neurodevelopmental delay' when referring to children who had a cluster of reflexes underlying specific learning difficulties.

Professionals who had trained with INPP and passed the qualifying examinations became Associates of the INPP. As part of their associate membership, they attended regular update training days. Associates made a number of contributions to the theory and practice of the method.

Associate contributions

Some of the most significant of these contributions were in relation to understanding the effects of the Moro reflex if retained and, later, one of its functions in infancy. As described in Chapters 1 and 2, the Moro reflex is a reaction to a sudden unexpected stimulus and is particularly sensitive to vestibular stimulation in the first weeks of life.

The Moro reflex acts as an infant's primitive fight or flight response and is replaced by an adult startle or Strauss reflex from about four months of age. Sean Cottrell (1987) – an INPP Associate – had observed that the testing methods being used at the time only seemed to detect the Moro reflex in 3–4 per cent of the cases he assessed, despite the symptoms of many patients suggesting that the reflex was uninhibited. The testing method for the Moro reflex was the same procedure used by paediatricians with newborn babies and by clinicians assessing older children suffering from brain injury. In those groups muscle tone is usually underdeveloped and the reflex is easily elicited when tested in the supine position. It was Cottrell's belief that these tests were not sensitive enough to detect traces of the Moro reflex in older children and adults who had developed muscle tone and postural control.

Cottrell (1987a) presented his findings in a paper entitled 'The Moro revisited', which described the physical and psychological effect of the Moro reflex when it remained. In response to this paper, three other Associates – Roger Benett, John Rowston and Steve Clark – developed a new and more sensitive test carried out in the erect position to elicit the Moro reflex if it was still present in older children and adults. The test was checked to ascertain its validity and reliability and was subsequently incorporated into the INPP assessment protocol for children and adults.

Benett was also intrigued by the effect an uninhibited Moro reflex had upon a person's personality structure and described his observations of the relationship between the Moro reflex and personality traits in a paper entitled 'The hidden Moro' (1988).

These detailed observations of the Moro reflex under different testing conditions and its association with specific symptoms and personality traits led to an alteration in how the reflex was treated. Blythe and McGlown had originally constructed an exercise to try to inhibit the Moro reflex using a position and movements that were either opposite to the reflex response or contained it. This seemed to be effective for a while, but often the reflex would re-emerge later, indicating that it had indeed been restrained by the exercise but not integrated into higher patterns of response or behaviour.

It was at this time, 1988, that the remedial programme was changing from exercises that involved practising patterns of motor development to using the reflexes themselves as instruments for integration. Blythe's gradual realisation that the normal developmental stereotyped movements made by infants at about the same time have a natural inhibitory and integrative function led him to observe normal infant movement patterns and to develop exercises based upon them.

In 1988, I joined the INPP and took part in one of the continuing professional development (CPD) days for Associates. I heard the ongoing discussions about the Moro reflex, and Blythe's assertion that if a reflex reappears that is normally present in early development and apparently inhibited early in the remedial programme, it must be because an earlier reflex is still active. In regard to the Moro reflex, this presented a conundrum, because at that time the Moro reflex was said to be the earliest of the primitive reflexes to emerge. If this was the case, what earlier reflex or pattern could undermine long-term inhibition of the Moro reflex?

At an earlier meeting, Ernest Keeling had introduced colleagues to a small book written by a Norwegian professor, Birger Kaada (1986), that describes the FPR and Kaada's theory that this reflex may act as a trigger mechanism in SIDS. On reading this book a few months later, I suggested that there might be a maturational relationship between the fear paralysis and Moro reflexes, the former acting as the earliest and most primitive of the startle reactions and later being modified as the Moro and then adult reflexes emerge. This was only ever mooted as a hypothesis, but, if correct, it suggested that the Moro reflex has a function in overriding the more primitive 'withdrawal' reaction that is a characteristic of the FPR. If this were the case, then simply attempting to inhibit or contain the Moro reflex would not be sufficient. In some cases it would be necessary to stimulate the Moro reflex in order to inhibit it.

At the same time, I realised that the FPR may act as an underlying mechanism in the presentation of selective mutism – the inability to speak under specific conditions. A series of papers followed: 'The fear paralysis response and its interaction with the primitive reflexes' (1989); 'The continued presence of the fear paralysis reflex in its effect upon subsequent central nervous system development' (1989); 'Elective mutism – the unchosen silence' (1991); 'The developmental basis for learning difficulties and language disorders' (1990). The last-mentioned was an attempt to summarise changes that had been made to the methods originally developed by Blythe and McGlown and to define the INPP method as it had become by 1990.

I wrote:

> The work of The Institute for Neuro-Physiological (INPP) in Chester is concentrated upon the detection, and then the correction of aberrant reflexes. At a full Neuro-Developmental assessment, tests are carried out for the presence of both primitive and postural reflexes, together with tests for cerebellar functioning, dysdiadochokinesia, balance, gross and fine muscle coordination, oculo-motor functioning, visual perception and visual-motor integration ability. Thus both the effect and potential cause are screened for. At the end of the examination, an index of dysfunction can be evaluated on the basis of the scores in each section. It is then possible to decide from which

stage of development an individual programme of remediation should be constructed. It is also possible during treatment to look back, and to measure a correlation between reflex inhibition and improvement in different areas of functioning.

Blythe (1980) asserted that, 'the innate mechanistic processes involved in the inhibition, modification and transformation of the basic reflexes are observable, and more importantly replicable at any age, to assist in the rehabilitation of neurological impairment'. The theory of replication is the basis for all the reflex-inhibition techniques used by INPP, i.e. that it is possible to give the brain a second chance to register the inhibitory movement patterns which should have been made at the appropriate stage in development, or, to recapitulate a stage of development which may have been omitted, or incompletely worked through, for one reason or another during intrauterine life or infancy.

The remediation of aberrant reflexes is based on the primary concept of replication, together with three concomitant theories:

1. Every reflex has a purpose and will not be fully suppressed unless it has successfully completed the job it was designed to do.
2. All human babies make certain stereotyped movements during the first year of life (Thelan 1979). These movements contain within them the natural antidote to the appropriate reflex at that stage in development, thus facilitating inhibition of a primitive reflex, on the one hand, and the subsequent release of a postural reflex, on the other, together with continued CNS [central nervous system] development.
3. There is a sequence and pattern to reflex inhibition. Starting with the emergence of each reflex, then seeing it strengthen and reach its peak, and finally undergoing inhibition; its inhibition coinciding with the strengthening of the next reflex in the chain and the latter assisting the inhibition of the former. E.g. the ATNR may play a part in inhibiting the Moro reflex with the Landau and Symmetrical Tonic Neck (STNR) reflexes aiding inhibition of the TLR. In this way, nature seems to have ordained that she should close the door on one reflex by opening the door on the next.

> Each developmental stage is like a building block, carefully placed in the right position so that the structure as a whole will be solid when it is complete. A misplaced block at the foundation or near the bottom of the building will affect all the floors that are built on top of it, so that the earlier the malfunction, the greater are the possible effects on the expression of subsequent development. In constructing a remediation programme, the earliest detected aberrant reflex will form the starting point for replication.
>
> On average, a child is on a programme for approximately one year, about the same period of time that it takes a baby to make the transition from helpless neonate to walking. As the aberrant reflexes are modified and corrected, so many of the presenting symptoms also undergo transformation.
>
> To summarise, it is suggested that the primitive reflexes present the earliest developmental markers from which it is possible to chart specific areas of dysfunction. They also provide the trunk of the tree from which the branches of motor development, perception and cognition will grow and if there is cluster of aberrant reflexes, the cortex will be required to work harder to compensate for the dysfunction.
>
> It is further suggested that if the aberrant reflexes are detected and the appropriate reflex inhibition movements are replicated on a daily basis, higher parts of the brain and associated pathways will have a second chance to inhibit the aberrant reflexes and permit the emergence of the postural reflexes. When this occurs the cortex is freed to concentrate upon the intellectual tasks which are its specialty. (Goddard 1990)

In 1989, Jane Field cooperated with Blythe to produce a new, shortened version of the original clinician's handbook, intended to provide instruction for students of the method in the testing of those reflexes included in INPP diagnostic assessment.

Another Associate, Patricia Faulkner, investigated the incidence of abnormal reflexes in a group of 18 children of high intelligence (IQ of 140+) who presented with handwriting difficulties. Her working hypothesis was 'that children with high intelligence who experience difficulties with the mechanics of writing have a degree of CNS dysfunction' (Faulkner 1988a; see also Faulkner 1988b).

Central nervous system dysfunction was defined at the time as comprising:

- aberrant primitive reflexes
- cross-laterality of ambiguity of laterality
- visual-perceptual difficulties

In order to explore her hypothesis, Faulkner gave her subjects (aged eight to twelve years) standardised educational tests in verbal reasoning, reading, comprehension and writing. All were tested for the presence or absence of a number of primitive reflexes thought to be connected with learning difficulties, namely: ATNR, STNR, spinal Galant reflex and head-righting reflex. Tests were also administered to check the functioning of the vestibular system, oculo-motor functioning and visual-perceptual performance.

The results obtained support the hypothesis that children with high intelligence who have difficulties with writing have a degree of central nervous system dysfunction. All showed the presence of aberrant primitive reflexes, cross-laterality and visual-perceptual difficulties.

In 1994, Gwen Wilkinson undertook a replica of a study that had been carried out by Barbara Rider in the United States in 1972. Rider had compared the reflex responses of a group of normal second-grade children with a group of learning-disabled children. She had found that the incidence of abnormal reflexes in the learning-disabled group was significantly higher than in children in the group with no learning disabilities. Wide range achievement tests (WRAT) were also applied to both groups; the results showed that children with normal reflex status all scored higher on WRAT tests. Wilkinson not only confirmed a link between abnormal primitive reflexes and lower educational performance but also that it was possible to identify children who were underachieving, simply by looking at the reflex profile. In analysing the results, she noticed that the common denominator in terms of reflexes among the groups performing below expectations on achievement measures was the presence of the TLR, which was evident in all learning-disabled and underachieving subjects. She also identified a possible relationship between a residual Moro reflex and problems with maths.

The INPP in Germany

Between October 1993 and 1994, a group of postgraduate students studying education at the University of Hamburg trained with Peter Blythe in Chester. This project had been initiated by Thake Hansen-Lauff and supported by her husband W. Lauff, both of whom had attended the Fifth European Conference of Neuro-Developmental Delay held in Chester in March 1993. As educationalists they felt that the work of INPP Chester could be an extremely valuable and important enrichment of the praxis and theory of education in Germany. The group of postgraduate students who attended the course in Chester had been prepared beforehand by Thake Hansen-Lauff.

In 1995, Hansen-Lauff was appointed by the INPP to act as the Institute's representative in Germany. This role gave her permission to start training courses there. The first two training courses took place at the University of Hamburg, still with the participation of Peter Blythe. Thereafter and until 2020, most of the courses took place in Laboe, then the seat of INPP Germany.

Between 1996 and 2018, Hansen-Lauff trained around 400 professionals. In 2021, around 280 active practitioners were listed as INPP International Licentiates complying with the specified standards and quality management of INPP International. Since 2016, in order to meet the still growing interest in the INPP method, three further co-trainers have offered INPP training courses in five different locations in Germany.

Programmes for auditory-processing difficulties

In 1987, Peter Blythe organised the first international conference on neuro-developmental delay in children with specific learning difficulties. Among the presenters were Harold Levinson, one of the first clinicians to recognise and research the role of the vestibular–cerebellar system in the presentation of dyslexia and phobic states; Harry Wachs, a developmental optometrist working with vision therapy; and Damian Downing, who specialised in the assessment and treatment of nutritional factors in a range of disorders. These three areas seemed to represent the major links to other systems involved in the presentation of the same difficulties that the INPP was treating. The only missing element at the first conference was auditory processing.

In subsequent years, the INPP was introduced to: the Tomatis method, a number of Associates attending a training workshop weekend; AIT, introduced by Svea Gold by way of Annabel Stehli's book *The Sound of a Miracle* (1992), which tells the story of Stehli's family's quest to find help for her daughter who had a range of problems linked to ASD; Samonas sound therapy, developed by Ingo Steinbach; Paul Madaule's programmes delivered through the Listening Centre in Canada; and Alex Doman's Listening Program. All had value in identifying and treating problems associated with auditory-processing difficulty or auditory hypersensitivity, but the method that seemed to fit best with the population the INPP mainly worked with, and with Blythe's original aim of being able to evaluate and thus carry out evidence-based research on whatever methods were employed, entered INPP's ken in 1993.

Kjeld Johansen, a former Danish schoolteacher who had attended one of Catherina Johannesson-Alevgård's training sessions in Sweden, contacted Blythe and asked if they could meet when he was en route to Canada to meet with Alfred Tomatis's protégé Paul Madaule. During his college years, Johansen had worked with people using an auditory stimulation method developed in California by the Danish-American researcher Christian A. Volf (1894–1967). Later as a teacher, Johansen noticed that several pupils with written language problems who were categorised as dyslexics actually suffered from problems with basic auditory sensing and perception of certain frequency ranges and at the same time often had problems with ear preference and some kind of cross-laterality. On the basis of ideas from Volf, Tomatis, Orton and many others and on his own work, Johansen has developed over the years a system of assessing auditory perception using a combination of pure tone audiometry and tests for binaural and dichotic listening. In cooperation with the composer Bent-Peder Holbech, he produced music to train auditory perception using frequency specific stimulation – the method known as Johansen Individualised Auditory Stimulation Therapy. JIAST is used to support students suffering from learning and/or behavioural problems.

A modest man, more interested in making a difference to individuals than promoting his own methods, Johansen (1993) introduced Blythe and me to the concept of using frequency-specific music to improve auditory discrimination, lateral preference and auditory processing. Blythe was immediately interested by the laterality element, and I, coming from a family background steeped in classical music, was keen to find out more about the influence of music beyond that of musical training. At our request, Johansen returned to Chester in October 1994 to train us in his method.

The method appealed to us both for two different reasons. Firstly, it involved detailed assessment using accepted measures of pure tone audiometry and binaural and dichotic listening, thereby providing a clear clinical baseline from which to make a clinical judgement about which music to select for therapy and the evaluation of change during and following intervention. Secondly, it was also a gentle system of training, which could be carried out at home and reviewed at six-weekly intervals over the course of one year. This fitted neatly alongside the structure of the INPP programme, as well as being a system that seemed to carry minimal risk of overloading a patient.

The concept of overload

The risks of overload had long been recognised. Overload occurs when a patient is overstimulated by remedial programmes that require the system to adapt more rapidly than it is ready to do. It is similar to the concept of overdose in the use pharmaceutical agents – something known but often overlooked in psychiatric treatment. If a patient is given the wrong medication or a dose that is beyond their tolerance level, it can have the paradoxical effect of leading to an increase in the very symptoms that it is intended to treat.

In a paper written in 1975 Arnold M. Ludwig wrote:

> Higher brain centres are continually at work to filter, modify, regulate and control sensory input and determine the meaning attributed to it. The resultant interaction between central and peripheral processes tends to produce types of cognitive–perceptual styles which not only shape the personalities of individuals but also influence their views of the world.

He continued:

> The interaction between man and his environment can be noted in countless trivial and profound ways both in the normal and psychopathological behaviour, as man seeks out the environments that either soothe or arouse the senses. Hyperactive children and manic patients tend to display a type of stimulus hunger, while depressed patients seem predisposed to shut out stimuli. With chronic schizophrenics, some seem impervious to most forms of sensory and social stimulation while others frantically tend to seek outside or even self-administrated forms of stimulation. (Ludwig 1975)

In the early 1980s, when the INPP remedial programme was moving from training patterns of motor development or using exercises devised to inhibit reflexes towards the selection of natural infant movements, it was noticed that the latter seemed to be more potent and that a smaller 'dose' yielded more immediate and lasting results. However, with increased potency the risk of overload also increased. From paying careful attention to the experience of families and adult patients between reviews, it quickly became apparent that only a small number of exercises was needed to achieve beneficial results without inducing overload.

Signs of overload may include increased incidence of bedwetting in children who suffered from nocturnal enuresis, bad dreams, behavioural issues at home or school and tantrums. Adults, more able to identify and articulate their experiences, described increased sensitivity to everything around them combined with an inability to protect themselves before feelings became too strong. This hypersensitivity could be to sensory stimuli, emotional events or a combination of the two. Crucially, sensory overload, which can occur as a result of hypersensitivity in one or several sensory modalities, or be heightened by emotional stress or the adaptations required by remedial intervention, can induce intense emotional reactions and vice versa. Underlying hypersensitivity can be exacerbated by increased emotional excitation and emotional stress can reduce thresholds of arousal, resulting in the two conditions mutually reinforcing each other. Adults also described dreaming about and remembering events from much earlier in their lives which they had not thought about for many years or had not been able to recall consciously. These reactions seemed to be similar to the more explosive spontaneous abreactions induced by PMRT in the 1970s.

The question was: why? What was it about these exercises that seemed to have an emotional/psychological impact as well as fulfilling their primary purpose of integrating primitive and postural reflexes? The precise answer and the mechanisms involved are still not known, but it has been suggested that hypersensitivity may arise as a result of a number of adaptations required by the system.

One theory is that emotional memories have physical correlates and that repetition of earlier movement patterns not used for many years can trigger suppressed memories; that the body has a memory and that the body's vocabulary of movement is linked to preverbal expression of feeling or affect. When these movements are re-enacted on a regular basis, they may act as a key to open and release buried emotional memories held within the body.

Another is that alterations in how the body and nervous system respond require adaptation at a psychological as well as a physical level. This involves changing habits and compensatory behaviours that have developed over time. While new systems are developing to replace established but less efficient ones, there can be a short 'no man's land' period when the old systems are diminishing in usefulness and the new ones are not yet sufficiently established or familiar to feel comfortable or secure. It can feel rather like being asked to use new technology without any training. For a short period of time, the effect can be one of increased disorientation, insecurity and arousal.

Observation over time started to paint a profile of individuals who seemed to be more susceptible to overload on a programme and reactive to different combinations of exercises. The common denominators among this group were definite vestibular disturbances with or without evidence of a residual Moro reflex. It was found that this group responded to the programme better if given only one or two exercises aimed specifically at improving vestibular function and/or integrating the Moro reflex. These individuals also seemed to be more sensitive to more than one type of programme being applied at a time. For example, if sound therapy was applied at the same time as vestibular work was being done in the early stages of the programme, signs of overload were more likely to appear.

For this reason JIAST was selected as the preferred method of sound therapy to be used alongside the INPP programme. As a general guideline, if vestibular dysfunction were evident on the INPP assessment, the vestibular dysfunction would be addressed first and sound therapy introduced a little later in the programme. It should be stressed that this is not an absolute rule for practice. The approach will vary according to the presenting problems, needs, age and profile of the patient. Other methods of sound therapy are sometimes recommended either before or after completing an INPP programme. During training, INPP practitioners are taught how to tease some of these factors out of the developmental history and auditory screening questionnaires used at the initial consultation and make recommendations based on an individual's profile of needs.

Developments in the United Kingdom

Meanwhile in the United Kingdom – as more patients were seen, both at the INPP in Chester and by Associates in their own practices – observations, experiences and ideas were shared, discussed and tested. Some were discarded and others were incorporated to become part of accepted practice. There was also increasing concern that people who had heard about the method were attempting to use aspects of it without adequate knowledge or training and thus the method at risk of falling into disrepute, since misinformation exchanged during informal conversations and meetings was fast becoming a series of memes passed between different professional groups.

Literature

In response to this growing problem and to a request from Björn Gustafson, a psychologist working in Sweden, for a pamphlet on the significance of primitive and postural reflexes in the presentation of specific learning difficulties for readers in Sweden, I wrote my first book *Ett Fönster in i barnets huvud* (Goddard 1996). In this I described key reflexes and their specific effects upon different areas of functioning. A few months later, on hearing of its forthcoming publication, Svea Gold, publisher and author of *If Kids Just Came With Instruction Sheets*

(1998), suggested that the book be extended and published in English. The first edition of *A Teacher's Window Into The Child's Mind* was published by Fern Ridge Press in 1996. The book was later updated as *Reflexes Learning and Behavior* (Goddard 2002) and published in many languages.

The next step was to examine critically the reliability of some of the clinical tools Blythe and McGlown had developed, to set an accepted standard for other professions.

In 1998, I analysed parental responses to the INPP screening questionnaire. The questionnaire was used as an initial screening tool to decide whether a child should be recommended to proceed to an INPP assessment. It comprised 26 criteria covering aspects of developmental history from family history to the present day. If a child scored more than seven 'yes' answers to questions concerning potential causes or markers of developmental problems, it was highly probable that detailed assessment would reveal signs of neurodevelopmental delay that were likely to respond to intervention using the INPP method. The questionnaire had been in use for 20 years but had not been reviewed for validity and reliability.

I compared the questionnaire responses from the parents of 72 children who had contacted the INPP, because their child was underachieving in reading, writing or spelling, with responses from parents of 72 children across the same age range in a local primary school who had no history or presenting symptoms of underachievement in reading, writing or spelling. The results were submitted for independent statistical analysis both to check the reliability of the score of seven 'yes' answers and to analyse whether specific factors carried a high weighting in terms of risk. The statistician's report read:

> The results of the Student *t*-test suggest that the INPP Developmental Screening Questionnaire does discriminate between children with specific learning difficulties and those without specific learning difficulties on the basis of a cluster of factors in early development, a score of 7 or more differentiating the two groups.

This simple screening device could be of use to teachers, educational psychologists, occupational therapists and other professionals in the initial assessment stages of a child's needs, to determine whether neurological/

developmental factors lay beneath a child's presenting difficulties. Children who have neurodevelopmental delay, as defined by the continued presence of a cluster of aberrant reflexes, respond to a physical sensory programme of remediation, and this should be taken into account in any recommendations that are made to address their specific learning difficulties (Goddard Blythe and Hyland 1998).

Meanwhile the number of people being trained in the United Kingdom and Germany was slowly growing. Not all of those who trained wished to become or remain Associates of the INPP; some went to pursue independent research or to practise the method outside the constraints of associate membership. Some of them are worthy of mention not only for their findings but also to understand the origin of other programmes that have grown up.

In 2000, Martin McPhillips, a former Associate of the INPP, together with his colleagues, published the findings of a randomised double-blind controlled trial that had investigated the efficacy of replicating primary reflex movements on specific reading difficulties in children.

> We assessed the efficacy of an intervention program based on replicating the movements generated by the primary-reflex system during foetal and neonatal life. A randomised, individually matched, double-blind, placebo-controlled design was used and children (aged 8–11 years) with persistent primary reflexes and a poor standard of reading were enrolled into one of three treatment groups: experimental (children were given a specific movement sequence); placebo-control (children were given non-specific movements); and control (no movements).
>
> From an initial sample of 98 children, 60 children, 20 in each group were matched on age, sex, verbal intelligence quotient (IQ), reading ability, and persistent asymmetrical tonic neck reflex. For asymmetrical tonic neck-reflex levels there was a significant (group by time) interaction ($p<0.001$). The experimental group showed a significant decrease in the level of persistent reflex over the course of the study (mean change –1.8 [95 per cent CI –2.4 to –1.2], $p<0.001$), whereas the changes in the placebo-control and control groups were not significant (–0.2 [–0.9 to 0.6] and –0.4 [–0.9 to 0.2]). (McPhillips et al. 2000)

Following publication, McPhillips set up Primary Movement as an independent non-profit-making charity.

Blythe was initially elated that an independent academic study had confirmed that the theory and underlying methodology he and McGlown had created, and many colleagues had helped to develop, had been proven to be sound, but he was later crestfallen to discover that the research carried only a minimal acknowledgement of the original source of the theory and some of the tests and exercises used in the study.

Later the same year, Blythe succumbed to a critical illness and, fearing that he might not live, in 2001 he appointed me as director of INPP.

In 2001, I was invited to present a paper at the Fifth International British Dyslexia Association Conference in York. Recognising that the classical view of dyslexia, which at the time chiefly focused on specialist teaching, was very different from the INPP's view that underlying physical factors could contribute to the presentation of dyslexic symptoms, I decided to analyse the clinical findings of a group of children, previously diagnosed with dyslexia, who had been assessed at the INPP for evidence of neurological dysfunction. The rationale behind this study was to demonstrate that oculo-motor and visual-perceptual problems, often features of dyslexia, did not exist in isolation and could be part of a more general picture of NMI.

A series of standardised neurological tests for abnormal reflexes were carried out on a sample of 54 children who had previously received an independent diagnosis of dyslexia, to see if neurological dysfunction was a significant factor underlying their dyslexic symptoms. Additional tests were carried out to assess oculo-motor functioning, visual-perceptual performance and cerebellar involvement including dysdiadochokinesia to see if other areas related to motor development were also significant factors in the sample.

> Abnormal primitive and postural reflexes were found to be a universal underlying factor in this sample. A high percentage of the sample also demonstrated difficulties with oculo-motor functioning, visual-perceptual skills and dysdiadochokinesia, suggesting a positive relationship between abnormal reflex activity and immature postural, motor and visual functioning. (Goddard Blythe 2001)

Following the presentation, there was valid criticism that the study had not included a control group. Acknowledging this, I asserted that the aim of the study was to demonstrate that neurological dysfunction indicated by the presence of aberrant reflexes was present in some children diagnosed with dyslexia and that, though aberrant reflexes might not be the primary cause of the dyslexic symptoms, if these reflexes were corrected some of the symptoms associated with dyslexia might diminish. In other words, dyslexia should not be treated simply as a problem of cognitive processing; underlying mechanisms should also form part of the assessment and treatment of symptoms associated with dyslexia.

As awareness and interest in other interventions complementary to the INPP method increased, it was recognised that the terminology used to describe the INPP approach needed to be more precise. 'Neurodevelopmental delay' – the term used at the time – tended to suggest a wider range of symptoms than simply immature neuromotor skills and was increasingly being used more generally to describe children with neurological and/or intellectual impairment. Although the INPP approach also screens for indications of other factors such as auditory-processing difficulties and nutritional and skeletal problems, the INPP method is based on the assessment and remediation of neuromotor skills. The term 'neuromotor immaturity' is therefore a more accurate description of the specific problems the method sets out remediate. The term 'neuromotor immaturity' is used in the medical context to describe generalised or specific immaturity in neuromotor functioning. The INPP uses this term to describe the presence of a cluster of aberrant reflexes that provide evidence of immaturity in the functioning of the central nervous system.

Assessing and addressing neuromotor readiness for learning in the classroom

Several Associates in different parts of the world had attempted to adapt the clinical programme and integrate it into a school setting in an informal way (Johannesson-Alvegård 1990; Lloyd 1994/1995). In 1995, the first group of students from Germany returned to Chester to attend their first CPD days. The feedback from Germany was that, although there was definite interest in the method in educational circles, the prime demand was for something teachers could do at the cutting edge of education. About the same time, I was asked to give lectures to several schools in the Chester and North Wales area, which wanted not only information about physical bases for underachievement in the classroom, but also something practical that teachers could do. In answer to this gap, I started to put together a shortened test battery based on the much longer INPP clinical assessment, and a general developmental movement programme designed to be used daily with a whole class of children in school under teacher supervision over the course of one academic year.

The idea behind the screening test and developmental movement programme was that teachers could be instructed in a one-day training course how to administer the shortened test battery – to be used not as a diagnostic tool but as a screening device to identify children in class who might be at risk of underachieving as a result of immature physical skills. The developmental movement programme could then be introduced as a class-based activity for all children, although the programme would be aimed primarily at helping those with immature physical skills. Teachers would not select individual exercises (as practitioners do, according to the results of the individual clinical assessment), but would follow a sequence of developmental movements over the course of one academic year.

This project was initially produced by the INPP as a restricted publication (Goddard Blythe 1996) and was soon translated into German. Interest in the one-day training courses offered in Chester and as in-service training for schools in the United Kingdom and Germany grew rapidly. Teachers started to introduce the screening test and intervention programme into schools. Many carried out small pilot projects investigating:

- incidence of immature neuromotor skills in mainstream primary schools
- improvement on measures of neuromotor skills before and after completing the school programme using the screening test as the pre- and post-intervention measuring tool
- a link between immature motor skills, educational performance and behaviour
- improvements in motor skills and performance on educational measures such as reading, writing and spelling

Over the years a wealth of empirical evidence has been amassed from small-scale projects in schools that have shared their results in individual reports. These have consistently shown:

- the presence of residual primitive reflexes in school-aged children (NEELB 2004)
- improvement in primitive reflex status, balance and coordination in children who took part in the programme (ibid.)
- improvement in some academic assessments in children who took part in the programme (Goddard Blythe 2005)
- improvement in behaviour in children who had been referred to behavioural support services before the implementation of the programme (Marlee 2008)
- general teacher observation of improvement in playground behaviour, concentration and deportment (Silvester 2006)

Many of these projects were written up as independent reports by the schools involved for their local authority or funding body, but this was not sufficient to answer the challenge from academics that the programme had not been formally and independently evaluated using control or comparison groups.

In 2003, after providing a one-day training course to a group of teachers in Northern Ireland, I was contacted by the adviser for English and literacy in County Antrim to be told that the Department of Education Northern Ireland had approved funding to carry out a formal research project to investigate the impact of residual reflexes on children's literacy progress and to address the correlation between a movement programme and progress in reading and writing.

> The study involved seven schools who were invited to participate as they had no contaminating factors, i.e. not involved other literacy initiatives such as the Early Years Enriched Curriculum pilot nor the Reading Recovery program. The schools had two P2 [Primary 2] and P5 [Primary 5] classes, one P5 class who acted as the control group. The experimental group of P5 pupils received the daily program of exercises from September 2003 to June 2004. The second tier of the research explored the correlation between those children who had

> retained reflexes and their literacy progress at the end of Year 2. The school proved to be performing at, or indeed above, the Northern Ireland average in literacy as evidenced by the end of key stage assessment. We recognise that this may have impacted upon the study. (NEELB 2004)

The INPP's only involvement in the project was the provision of training to teachers who would be carrying out the assessments and supervising the movement programme and independent evaluation of scores that teachers were applying to screening tests at the first assessments to ensure inter-test reliability from the outset. Thereafter, the actual testing of children, implementation of the programme and collection of data were carried out by teachers, data were submitted for independent statistical analysis, and the findings were reported by an independent body commissioned by the North-Eastern Education and Library Board (NEELB). The executive summary of the project reported:

> Measures of retained reflexes, balance, educational ability and concentration/coordination were made in a controlled study of P5 children in seven Northern Ireland primary schools at the start (September 2003) and end (June 2004) of the school year. In each school one P5 class undertook the exercises and the other did not. Two P2 classes in each school also participated in the research. None of the P2 classes undertook the exercises, and the extent to which the presence of retained reflexes at the start of the school year can predict educational progress at the end of the year was assessed. A total of 672 P2 and P5 children participated in the research. The following conclusions were drawn:
>
> - 35 per cent of P5 children and 48 per cent of P2 children showed elevated levels of retained reflexes at the first assessment.
> - 15 per cent (49) P5 children had a reading age below their chronological age. Of these, 28 also had elevated levels of retained reflexes.
> - Elevated levels of retained reflexes are correlated with poor educational achievement at baseline.
> - Children who undertook the exercise program showed a statistically significant greater decrease in retained reflexes than children who did not undertake the exercises.

- Children who undertook the exercise program showed a highly significant improvement in balance and coordination, and a small but statistically significant increase in a measure of cognitive development over children who did not undertake the exercises. No difference was found in reading, handwriting or spelling in children who were already achieving at or near their chronological age, but for children with high levels of retained reflexes and a reading age below their chronological age, those who undertook the exercise program made greater progress.
- Retained reflexes are correlated with poor cognitive development, poor balance and teacher assessment of poor concentration/coordination in P2 children. Neurological scores and teacher assessment at baseline predicted poorer reading and literacy scores at the end of the study. (NEELB 2004)

Critics maintained that the report had not been published in a peer-reviewed journal. I therefore wrote a summary of the findings from the Northern Ireland study and some of the independent reports from other small-scale studies that had been carried out in schools and submitted the report for peer review. It was published in 2005 in the peer-reviewed professional journal *Child Care in Practice.*

If representative of the general school population at the time, these findings suggested that nearly half of children entering the school system in Northern Ireland at four or five years of age (P2) were not ready in terms of the physical skills needed to support learning in the classroom, and that there was a correlation between less mature motor skills and lower educational performance, and yet the findings were greeted with polite disinterest.

Results from the older group (P5) who participated in the intervention programme invited criticism that the results did not show conclusively a link between improvement in neuromotor skills and school performance. I acknowledged that further large-scale independent research needed to be carried out but pointed out that the Northern Ireland study had included children of all abilities – including those with a reading age already at or above age expectations – and that these latter children would not be expected to make significant further gains. The number of children in the sample who met the criteria for which the programme had been designed – more than 25 per cent signs of immaturity in neuromotor skills and performing below age expectations on educational measures at the outset – was not large enough to yield statistically significant results, but the intervention group did show greater gains than the comparison group.

Academics are rightly sceptical, advising caution in relation to any claims that an intervention improves any skills other than those trained by the exercises in the programme, but such scepticism has made it difficult to access pathways to ongoing and future research. The aim of the programme is to strengthen the physical foundations for learning, not only balance and coordination, but also oculo-motor functioning and visual perception. Individually and collectively, these abilities support more than just reading and writing. They affect how a child interacts with their environment, the child's body language and their ability to interpret the body language of others correctly and to respond appropriately. These abilities can affect self-awareness, self-control, and levels of arousal and anxiety and self-confidence. Teachers in schools where the programme has been used report improved attention, perseverance, playground behaviour (fewer fights and more controlled use of personal space) and self-esteem. In one area, children who had been referred to Behavioural Support Services were removed from the waiting list one term after starting the programme without any specific behavioural work having been done (Marlee 2008).

It should also be stressed that the introduction of a developmental movement programme into schools is not intended to replace normal teaching or remedial teaching in any way. Children with NMI will continue to need educational support to make up the deficits that developed while they were unable to keep up earlier on. The screening test is simply intended to help teachers identify children who may be at risk of underachieving as a result of NMI and to give them an opportunity to improve neuromotor skills by using the developmental movement programme. The Northern Ireland study revealed that NMI measures of children who took part in the programme improved significantly more than those who did not.

Meanwhile, training and the spreading of general awareness had all continued. I was invited by Hawthorn Press to write a book for parents and general readership. In 2004, *The Well Balanced Child* was published, followed a few years later by *What Babies and Children Really Need* (2008), *The Genius of Natural Childhood* (2011) and *Movement – Your Child's First Language* (2018). I was also approached by Wiley (later Wiley-Blackwell) and invited to submit a proposal for a book intended for a more academic readership. *Attention Balance and Coordination. The ABC of Learning Success* was published in 2009, followed a few years later by formal publication of the school programme – *Assessing neuromotor readiness for learning: The INPP screening test and school intervention programme* (Goddard Blythe 2012) – and then a screening test for clinicians and health practitioners (*Neuromotor immaturity in children and adults: The INPP screening test for clinicians and health practitioners* [Goddard Blythe 2014]).

Neurodevelopmental delay in adults and adolescents

Although in Chester the demand for children to be seen overtook enquiries relating to adults, in the United States Lawrence Beuret, who had trained in Chester in 1985, started to specialise in the assessment and treatment of adolescents and young adults. In 2002, he prepared a paper for the INPP conference in Chester on his findings.

At a previous conference he had summarised common reactions observed during assessment of this group, which included, vertigo, sensations of falling, and headache. These symptoms varied widely from almost no extraneous reactions in the early-identified learning-disabled patient to:

> … irritatingly voluminous and distracting in the panic-agoraphobic patient. This variation, as later emerged, depended on whether reflex presence or absence was accompanied by vestibular–proprioceptive dysfunction/mismatch. In effect, vestibular malfunction and its relationship to proprioceptive function served to amplify the underlying primitive and postural reflex abnormalities. (Beuret 1992)

He later went on to discuss how NDD is far more elusive in this older population of adolescents and young adults than in children presenting with specific learning difficulties or underachievement, being characterised less by the presence of a cluster of primitive reflexes than by a combination of underdeveloped postural reflexes, vestibular anomalies and highly developed compensatory behaviours, which have served to mask or distort a uniform symptomatic picture. Consequently, this group is often assumed to be working to potential, and symptoms only start to surface when the system is required to make life adjustments or is overloaded.

The most severely debilitating circumstance results when three factors coexist: persistent primitive reflexes, absent or markedly underdeveloped postural reflexes, and vestibular–proprioceptive mismatch. 'These patients present with multiple system involvement, cognitive and processing impairment, immunological disorders, psychological symptoms and exquisite sensitivity to stress' (Beuret 1992). Beuret identified a particular profile among these patients:

> Early academic success followed by a gradual decline, partially compensated for by increased study time. Temporal headaches and fatigue accompanied extended reading, compensated for by increasingly frequent breaks. Oculo-motor symptoms – unreported frequent skipping of rereading of lines of print, occasional doubling or 'moving' of letters or words. Early printing and writing success followed by reversion to printing to lessen hand fatigue. Early reading for pleasure which stopped in grade 5. A family history of motion sickness being exaggerated by reading.
>
> The clustering of these initial changes around grade 5 (age 10) closely correlates with the beginning of escalation of academic demands – critical reading comprehension, inferring and synthesizing from reading material, more creative writing, increased volume of homework. Stopping or reducing reading for pleasure is one of the consistent signs of this disorder.
>
> Possessing of a superior IQ made it possible for this student to perform well enough through high school to be admitted to college (university). The 'tipping point' appeared connected to going to university away from home. (Beuret 2009)

To determine whether NDD was a key factor, Beuret used the Holmes–Rahe Social Readjustment Rating Scale, which scores a series of life events. A score of less than 150 across all criteria indicates a relatively low amount of life change and susceptibility to stress-induced health breakdown; 150–300 points implies a

50 per cent chance of major health breakdown in the next two years; a score of more than 300 points raises the odds of major health breakdown to 80 per cent. The difference in presentation of health problems across the scores will depend on resilience. Beuret's theory was that the compensations required by NDD would reduce resilience to stressful life events and that the transition to university, which involves multiple adaptations, including the development of new study techniques, leaving home and forming new social relationships, could catalyse the development of symptoms previously masked by a stable environment.

Some years later he added the Minnesota Multiphasic Personality Inventory (MMPI-2) to the tests he used in assessing patients before starting and after completion of the INPP clinical programme. The MMPI-2 is the most widely used and researched clinical assessment tool employed by mental health professionals. Although Beuret's findings were not published, empirical evidence derived from case studies suggested that young adults with significant levels of NMI scored highly on measures of mental health problems (depression, anxiety), personality characteristics and general personality traits such as anger, somatisation, hypochondriasis and poor ego strength when first assessed. After they had completed the INPP programme some of these scores were diminished. These clinical findings were in line with Blythe's theory and observations from treating adults presenting with agoraphobia and panic disorder – that NMI predisposes an individual to experience high levels of arousal with associated hypersensitivity to environmental stimuli and tendency to somatise affect.

In 2009, Curtis Cripe, a psychologist specialising in neurofeedback, presented his clinical findings of changes on EEG analysis of patients who had followed the INPP programme. The EEG is a test used to find problems relating to electrical activity of the brain. Electrical activity in the brain appears in an EEG as a pattern of waves. Different levels of consciousness, like sleeping and waking, have specific normal ranges of frequencies of waves per second. For example, the wave patterns move faster when one is awake than when one is asleep, are faster in an alert waking state than in relaxed contemplation and are slowest in deep sleep. An EEG is used to investigate whether the wave frequencies or patterns are normal but the brain wave activity also reflects levels of arousal in different situations. Cripe noticed that patients who presented with a Moro reflex at the first assessment showed increased levels of arousal, which diminished as the Moro reflex was inhibited and symptoms of anxiety receded after use of the INPP programme.

Neuromotor immaturity and ADD/ADHD

In 2004, a postgraduate student in Australia undertook a shortened training with Blythe to equip her to test for certain reflexes in the course of her master's thesis, which investigated the incidence of retained primitive reflexes in children diagnosed with ADHD. The results of her research concluded thus:

> The present research studied the symptomatologic overlap of AD/HD behaviours and retention of four primitive reflexes (Moro, Tonic Labyrinthine Reflex [TLR], Asymmetrical Tonic Neck Reflex [ATNR], Symmetrical Tonic Neck Reflex [STNR]) in 109 boys aged 7–10 years. Of these, 54 were diagnosed with AD/HD, 34 manifested sub-syndromal coordination, learning, emotional and/or behavioural symptoms of AD/HD, and 21 had no (or near to no) symptoms of AD/HD. Measures of AD/HD symptomatology and of the boys' academic performance were also obtained using the Conners' rating scale and the WRAT-3, respectively. Results indicated that, in general, boys diagnosed with AD/HD had significantly higher levels of reflex retention than non-diagnosed boys. Results also indicated both direct and indirect relationships between retention of the Moro, ATNR, STNR and TLR reflexes with AD/HD symptomatology and mathematics achievement. The pattern of relationships between these variables was also consistent with the notion of the Moro acting as a gateway for the inhibition of the other three reflexes. (Taylor et al. 2004)

Subsequently a group of independent researchers investigated the presence of primitive reflexes in a group of 80 children aged eight to eleven years diagnosed with ADHD. Their findings showed that ADHD symptoms and balance deficits are strongly and specifically associated with persistent ATNR in girls and STNR in boys when compared with a control group. They concluded, 'These results provide first evidence in medical literature that ADHD in girls and boys is specifically related to distinguished neurological developmental mechanisms related to disinhibition of primitive reflexes' (Petr et al. 2021).

Use of the term 'disinihibition' is interesting, since it assumes that primitive reflexes had been inhibited at an earlier stage in development. The author's view is that, unless these reflexes were assessed during the first year of life and found to be inhibited, it is possible that full inhibition had never taken place.

Neuromotor immaturity and school performance

In 2011, I was invited to present findings from the INPP school programme in two school districts in the United Kingdom at a conference organised by the Academy of Special Education in Warsaw. Two independent projects had been undertaken with 64 children in schools in Northumberland and children in Berkshire to investigate whether:

- retention of three primitive reflexes (as indicators of NMI) was present in children in mainstream primary schools
- there was a link between immature motor skills and lower performance in reading, writing, spelling, maths and drawing, and
- retained primitive reflexes responded to a developmental movement programme (the INPP programme for schools)

Eighty-eight point five per cent of children aged seven to eight years and 40 per cent of children aged four to six years in Northumberland had residual (>25 per cent) primitive reflexes. Higher scores on tests for retained primitive reflexes correlated with lower performance on the DAP test. Children in the INPP group enjoyed a significantly greater decrease in abnormal reflexes than children who participated in a daily general movement programme.

Six out of six children who followed the INPP programme in Berkshire showed significant decrease in abnormal reflexes and improvements on the Salford Sentence Reading Test compared with six children who did not take part in the INPP programme (Goddard Blythe 2011b).

Meanwhile, others were carrying our similar projects in schools in the Midlands (Griffin 2013), London (Harte 2015) and Jewish kindergartens in New York City.[31] All showed similar trends: that the incidence of NMI among children in mainstream school settings is significant; that there is a correlation between higher levels of NMI and lower performance on standard educational measures (standard attainment tests [SATS] were used by schools in the Midlands). Despite this growing body of evidence to suggest that motor skills matter in school, resistance persists among educational authorities and politicians to considering, or commissioning further independent research into, the possible role of reflex integration movement programmes in supporting children's performance.

Indeed, rather than investigating further whether there is a link between the two, there is a tendency to sweep empirical findings under the academic carpet whenever they point to unwelcome trends. In 2017, Preedy and Duncombe released the results of a project they had conducted using the MABC-2 test battery, alongside some of the tests from Assessing neuromotor readiness for learning (Goddard Blythe 2012), with 120 children aged four to five years across four schools (two state schools and two independent schools) (Preedy et al. 2017).

In 2007, when the MABC-2 was produced and the data normalised, the mean would have been 50 (based on a normal distribution) (Sugden and Henderson 2007). The data obtained from this sample of children showed a decline from this in all areas tested:

- balance: 43.8 (n = 116), indicating a 6.2 percentile point decline since 2007
- aiming/catching: 30.3 (n = 119), indicating a 19.7 percentile point decline since 2007
- manual dexterity: 34.2 (n = 118), indicating a 15.8 percentile point decline since 2007
- overall physical development: 31.9 (n = 115), indicating an 18.1 percentile point decline since 2007

When these findings were presented at a conference, one reaction was that the norms on this test need to be revised. Although this may be true in terms of how the figures appear on a distribution scale, simply resetting the norms would obscure the fact that in this sample there appears to have been a significant decline in children's physical abilities over a ten-year period.

Further large-scale comparative research is needed to establish whether there is a corresponding link between decline in children's physical skills and lower levels of academic achievement.

Further studies, in Norway, investigated the efficacy of the INPP clinical programme in remediating signs of NMI and, in Poland, investigated the incidence of NMI.

Norway

This study, carried out by two INPP practitioners between 2004 and 2011 (Berg and Fitzgerald 2013), involved 87 children (66 boys and 21 girls) and investigated the effects of the INPP clinical programme on children's motor skills using the MABC-2 as an independent measure of children's motor skills before and after use of the INPP clinical programme. The mean pre-test age was nine years.

All participants tested positive for ATNR, STNR, TLR and Moro at the outset. The average training period during which the participants carried out prescribed exercises once a day, every day, under parental supervision, was 9.6 months. Follow-up reviews were carried out every seven to eight weeks.

Results showed a significant improvement of reflex status upon completion of training ($t = 17.99$, $df = 86$, $p < 0.001$). After training aimed at inhibiting primitive reflexes, motor skills were also significantly improved ($t = 15.09$, $df = 86$, $p < 0.001$).

The researchers concluded that the results indicated that primitive reflexes can be inhibited using the INPP method and that improvement in reflex status is reflected in a significant improvement in motor skills using the MABC-2 as an independent measure of change. They also advised caution in interpreting the results, owing to weaknesses in the validity of the study.

Poland

A series of independent studies have been carried out in Poland using the screening test *Assessing neuromotor readiness for school* (Goddard Blythe 2012). The first investigated the persistence of primitive reflexes and associated motor problems in healthy pre-school children. In a sample of 131 children aged four to seven years of age the TLR was found to be the most common non-integrated primitive reflex, one that the researchers (Madejewska et al. 2016) thought might have been linked to other imbalances identified during the study. Girls in the group showed significantly higher results in tests of neuromotoric efficiency i.e. neuromotoric skills commensurate with age expectations. Madejewska et al. (2016) concluded that it would be helpful 'to examine children for their neurological maturity and apply early stimulation for children with developmental delays'.

A second study (Gieysztor et al. 2017) involved 135 children divided into two groups:

- four to six years of age
- seven to nine years of age

Results showed that reflexes are spontaneously integrated as children get older and this process is more complete in school-age than in pre-school children but that some non-integrated reflexes persist. The authors concluded:

> Introduction of screening tests and treatment of reflex integration at the stage of pre-school and early childhood may be a part of the prevention of developmental disorders. Conducting wider populations studies showing the presence and impact of persistent primitive reflexes in various spheres of life of healthy children, would help to define age standards for the reflex integration. (Gieysztor et al. 2017)

The third study investigated the degree of primitive reflex integration as a diagnostic tool to assess the psychomotor development of healthy pre-school and early school-age children (one of the purposes of the INPP screening test):

> The primary purpose of this study is to present the activity of three tonic reflexes in a sample of 112 Polish children aged four to six in relation to their motor skills. The children were examined for the presence of the asymmetric tonic neck reflex (ATNR), symmetric tonic neck reflex (STNR), and tonic labyrinthine reflex (TLR). Motor performance was

> examined with the MOT [Motoriktest für Vier- bis Sechsjährige Kinder] 4–6. Statistical analysis shows an inverse correlation between the score in the test of reflexes and motor efficiency (MOT 4–6) at $p < 0.05$ (–0.33). Children with increased reflex activity presented a lower level of motor efficiency. The multiple regression model showed that with the older age of the child and the decrease in the level of reflex activity, the motor skills of children improve. Thus, there is a need for early screening of primitive reflexes in children. Properly selected exercises and therapeutic activities aimed at integrating APRs [aberrant primitive reflexes] in children with developmental difficulties can improve their motor skills, perceptual abilities, and emotional behavior. (Pecuch et al. 2021)

As the author of the screening test they were using, I would question whether use of the tests would prevent developmental disorders, since the presence of NMI is already an indicator of immaturity in the functioning of the central nervous system, but the identification of NMI before or at the time of school entry could enable teachers and therapists to introduce effective movement programmes to reduce the incidence and effects of early NMI on later development and performance.

Other research examined whether there is a difference in primitive reflex integration in musically versus generally educated primary school children. In a sample of 45 children aged six to seven years, the status of the ATNR, TLR and STNR was examined in 22 musically trained children and compared with the reflex status of the 23 non-musicians. Musically educated children had a significantly better level of primitive reflex integration than the comparison group, leading the authors to conclude that 'Musical training can be a stimulus influencing primitive reflex integration (PRI). Musical training may influence the maturation of the CNS measured by PRI. Musical training may be part of the reflex integration therapy in children' (Gieysztor et al. 2019).

Matuszkiewicz and Gałkowski (2021) investigated whether there was a relationship between developmental language disorder (DLD) and motor deficits, including the persistence of primitive reflexes:

> Developmental language disorder (DLD) is a developmental disorder where children fail to acquire language in the absence of a clear cause. Many studies have reported general motor deficits in children with DLD, but no studies have uncovered a cure. The purpose of our study is to better understand the underlying motor deficits in DLD, starting from uninhibited primary reflexes – which are the most basic stage of motor development. Knowledge of this motor–language relationship should lead to earlier and more targeted interventions in young children with DLD. Method: Children with DLD (n = 75, age range: 4–10 years) and 99 age-matched typically developing (TD) children completed a nonword repetition test to assess DLD and six other tests to assess primitive reflexes. Results: Children with DLD demonstrated higher levels of persistent primitive reflexes compared to typically developing children.

Although this study demonstrated a link between DLD and immature neuromotor skills, it did not investigate whether aspects of DLD respond to motor intervention programmes designed to inhibit primitive reflexes.

This group of studies, while confirming a link between residual primitive reflexes, lower performance in motor skills and DLD have not examined the efficacy of physical intervention programmes. There is a pressing need for further independent research to investigate and confirm whether:

- reflex integration programmes are effective in reducing the incidence of residual primitive reflexes in school-aged children (the study carried out in Northern Ireland in 2004 showed a significant decrease in abnormal reflexes in the experimental group relative to the control group)
- reflex integration is associated with improvement in motor skills
- reflex integration is linked to improvement in standard measures of academic attainment
- reflex integration is linked to improvement in measures of behaviour

Although the above topics have been the subject of earlier pilot projects, larger-scale independent research is needed to verify trends identified by these earlier projects (Micklethwaite 2004; Goddard Blythe 2005; Marlee 2008).

Neuromotor immaturity and oculo-motor dysfunction

A link between specific aberrant reflexes and impaired oculo-motor functioning has long been recognised and discussed (Goddard 1995). In 2004, Wibke Bein-Wierzibinski, one of the group of postgraduate students from the University of Hamburg who had trained in Chester in 1994, presented the results of a study she had carried out investigating the relationship between retained primitive reflexes and immature eye movements.

Using an infrared computerised eye-tracking machine alongside INPP tests for reflexes before and after intervention, she not only confirmed a relationship between a retained ATNR and impaired horizontal eye-tracking movements, but also discovered one between retention of the STNR and impaired vertical eye-tracking movements, with potential impact on tasks such as aligning columns correctly in maths and perception of height and depth.

More recently, Andrich et al. (2018) examined the relationship between visual skills deficits (VSD) and retained primitive reflexes in children. In a sample of 135 children aged 6–14 years they found significant relationships between VSD and three of five primitive reflexes (TLR, ATNR and STNR):

> Scores taken from the Draw-a-Person Test and Motor Speed and Precision Test also suggest relationships with primitive reflex retention and VDS. Logical Regression analysis suggested that the Tonic Labyrinthine Reflex is a potential predictor of VSD.

The authors conclude that children with VSD may be at risk of developing issues with attention, depression and anxiety as a result of an inability to match performance to expectations.

Memes and diversions

As the work of INPP has spread through a combination of literature, training and word of mouth, there has been a tendency for people to short-cut access to the method without training from the source. This has resulted in the spread of various memes among different groups – a meme being a unit by which cultural ideas, symbols or practices can be transmitted from one mind to another through writing, speech, gestures, ritual, etc., which can also mutate, altering the fundamental characteristics of the original information.

Such mutation has occurred with respect to the INPP method. It was in answer to concerns about misunderstanding and possible misrepresentation of the method in a number of circles that Blythe and Goddard Blythe wrote an article, 'Correcting clinical facts' (2012), in which they itemised a number of tests and erroneous interpretations of tests which had unintentionally crept into the professional practice of other groups.

Along the way there have been many others who have been enthused by the concept that use of the body reflects maturity in the functioning of the central nervous system and that physical exercises can be used to assist the body to train the brain, but who wanted to explore and develop it in other ways. Some acknowledge the source – like Harold Blomberg, who developed Rhythmic Movement and acknowledges that his programme is based on rhythmic exercises he learnt in 1985 from a Swedish body therapist, Kerstin Linde, who had attended INPP training in Sweden – and others do not.

As memes pass from one generation of students to another, using different methods, some of which may be based on the theory and/or practice of the INPP method, subsequent generations often do not know the origin of the theory and practices they are using. Many of these offshoot methods have introduced more exercises over a shorter period of time, or have mixed and matched several interventions or different levels of intervention at the same time. Although these approaches may be successful with resilient children, or children in whom the identified level immaturity arose later in development (full integrated primitive reflexes but immature postural reflexes, for example), there is a greater risk of overloading the sensitive child, producing initially successful results, which tail off several months after the programme ends, or acting as a sticking plaster that improves the surface symptoms but fails to address or integrate all of the underlying mechanisms. Some methods rely on tests for primitive and postural reflexes which are not recognised as valid tests by the medical profession.

Blythe and the INPP have been adamant that the testing procedures used to assess patients in clinical practice and in screening for signs of NMI in other settings must be recognised and replicable by other professions.

Differences between the INPP programmes and other motor-training programmes

Motor-training programmes have been around for many years (Kephart 1960; Frostig 1970; Cratty 1973; Lefroy 1990; Kiphard 2000). Many start at the crawling and creeping stages of development. The difference between reflex stimulation and inhibition programmes and more general motor-training programmes is that the former use the reflexes as indicators of stages when development may have been temporarily arrested or omitted. The child who has retained early reflexes proceeds to the next developmental skill apparently without ill effect. Subtle gaps, however, remain in the wiring of the central nervous system which are linked to a bypassed stage of development.

A reflex stimulation and inhibition programme aims to give the brain a second chance to experience the movements that should have been made in the early months of development. It thereby creates a bridge across the gaps and facilitates more efficient transmission and execution of messages passing between the brain and the body. Whereas many other methods of intervention work from the cortex down towards the brainstem, reflex stimulation/inhibition programmes start primarily from the spinal cord and brainstem and work up towards the cortex to access improved cortical control by providing more efficient pathways. Just as the brain directs the body in carrying out coordinated actions, so also can the body, through repetitive practice of movements, help to improve the functioning of the brain.

New directions

'Correcting clinical facts' (Blythe and Goddard Blythe 2012) was to be the last publication of Blythe's life. Following a long and difficult illness, he died on 18 August 2013. For me, his death was the loss not only of my husband and closest friend but also of my mentor and professional partner. I have often said that the developments we accomplished together at the INPP over 26 years were 'not the ideas borne of individuals, but the sparks that flew between'. Following Blythe's death, I saw my future role as being to prepare the method to pass on to future generations.

To this end, between 2013 and 2018 much was done in establishing a code of practice for practitioners. In the late 1990s, the concept of Associates of the INPP was abandoned; it was later replaced by one of Licentiates of the INPP. Licentiates are practitioners who have qualified through INPP training in the United Kingdom or licensed training in other countries. Licentiate membership is voluntary and involves agreeing to a code of ethical practice, attending two supervision (CPD) days biannually and being responsible for one's own professional liability insurance. In return, practitioners can use the INPP logo and will be listed on the INPP national websites as qualified and approved practitioners. Membership is renewed annually.

The aim of licentiateship was to ensure a basic standard of practice so that the public could be assured that the version of the INPP method they received would be consistent with training and standards set by the INPP. These aims were intended not to stifle development of the method but to ensure that new findings would be evaluated before being incorporated into future practice and training.

Content, presentation and delivery of training have been standardised in all countries in which national principals have been licensed to provide training in the INPP method. This, together with setting a minimum entry qualification for students to be admitted to the four-module practitioner training course, led to the INPP practitioner course being accepted in 2018 by the Department of Medicine, Faculty of Science at a university in the United Kingdom as equivalent to 60 postgraduate credit points (50 per cent of a master's degree). External accreditation is an optional extra for students who have completed the INPP practitioner course, since many students already hold a postgraduate qualification.

Postscript: International development

In 2022, training in the INPP method was available in 12 countries under the direction of national principals of the INPP. Principals of the INPP are responsible for the provision of training in the INPP method in a defined territory, provision of CPD days, and administration of matters concerning

Licentiates practising in their territory. Principals meet at least once a year and, increasingly, decisions about training and practice are made collectively.

Cultural and historical differences are reflected in professional uptake of the method and specialisation. In the German-speaking countries, for example, the method has been embraced and accepted more easily than in many other countries. Thake Hansen-Lauff, INPP Principal for Germany since 1996, suggests that:

> One reason for this may be that from the beginning we – as educationalists – considered education as the main theoretical (and practical) frame of reference for INPP. For us the INPP-concept was a revelation because it made it possible to compliment education with the neuro-physiological dimension. Therefore education was the broad umbrella under which other disciplines could become subsumed.
>
> We also avoided use of the term 'therapy'. Instead we took 'Entwicklungsförderung' (approximately translated as developmental support), which was also helpful in the idea and method becoming accepted in educational settings.
>
> Also important might be the German health care system. Unlike in England and also – as far as I know in Scandinavia – people in Germany do not expect to have free access to all therapies through a national health care system. Parents are used (and many are willing) to pay privately for extra services for their children.
>
> In all professions (teachers, doctors, therapists of all sorts) people are expected to be conscientious in continued education. In the German-speaking countries, professionals seek out training in the INPP method without a need for INPP to advertise training. It also helped that soon after we completed our own training we started to translate many of your papers and later books into German so that the concept did not only spread by oral transmission but through published literature. I also believe that the extensive support and supervision of course graduates that trainers in the German-speaking countries undertake might have played a role.[32]

In other European countries 'ergotherapy' is an accepted concept. Ergotherapy (from ancient Greek ἔργον = 'work', and θεραπεία = 'service' or 'treatment') is a form of therapy that deals with the execution of concrete activities and their effects on humans and our environment. Impairments are treated through the targeted use of individually meaningful activities. Areas of ergotherapy may be applied to paediatrics, neurology, orthopaedics, traumatology, rheumatology, geriatrics and psychiatry and therefore encompass a number of professional disciplines, such as OT, physiotherapy, SALT and psychology. This broader concept of interdisciplinary application may have made it possible for the INPP method to be included under the umbrella of ergotherapy in these countries.

In contrast, in the United Kingdom, funding and provision of services in the National Health Service (NHS) are restricted by the National Institute for Care and Excellence (NICE), which recommends whether interventions are safe, effective and cost effective for use in the NHS. INPP practice is not currently recommended for use in the NHS by NICE, meaning that practitioners can only operate in private practice. Furthermore, because the INPP trains professionals from a range of disciplines (education and psychology as well as professions allied to medicine), the method does not fit neatly under the medical umbrella or referral system. Teachers in the UK, with the exception of physical education specialists, are not qualified to carry out physical assessments and so, for a variety of reasons relating to restrictions imposed on professional domains, it can be difficult to establish practice and uptake tends to be lower.

In Hungary, where there has been a long history of movement training programmes,[33] the ground is more fertile for the acceptance of other methods that complement existing knowledge. Magdalena Zweegman, INPP Principal for Hungary, has worked in cooperation with an oncologist and the Department for Rehabilitation at Semmelweiss Hospital to implement a modified version of the standard INPP programme for post-oncology brain cancer patients for whom there was no cure. Although the results are empirical, individual case studies indicate that remarkable improvements can be made in the control of balance and coordination, leading to greater independence and improved quality of life. This is an area for ongoing research in the future.

In Italy, Manolo Dominguez, the INPP Principal for Italy, is Director of Instituti Fay – an organisation, which started in Spain, based on the principles and methods established at the Institutes for Human Potential in Philadelphia by Temple Fay, Glen Doman and Carl Delacato. Insitituti Fay specialises in providing intensive rehabilitation programmes for individuals suffering from brain injury. Where appropriate, the INPP programme is integrated into a more intensive and multi-factorial programme as well as being used with children who present with specific learning difficulties.

These are just a few examples of how cultural differences and individual professional experience are enabling the INPP method to be applied in new ways.

The INPP today

In 2022, the INPP's core focus remains the assessment and remediation of NMI in practice, the training of teachers to implement the modified version of the INPP programme in schools and the training of other professionals in the influence of NMI on learning, achievement and emotional well-being.

Social pressures have increased on parents, many needing to return to work within a year of a child's birth. Despite the benefits of nursery care, evidence suggests that problems associated with NMI seem to be on the rise.

Besides the studies cited above which investigated the incidence of NMI in children in mainstream primary schools, evidence released by organisations involved in assessing and remediating language delay suggests that there is also an increase in the number of children from socially deprived backgrounds who enter the school system with immature language skills (Department of Education 2010). Immature language skills are linked to poorer educational outcomes and are recognised as providing an indication of well-being in relation to difficulty in forming friendships, making social connections and behaving appropriately (Waldfogel and Washbrook 2010).

> Early language acquisition impacts on all aspects of young children's non-physical development. It contributes to their ability to manage emotions and communicate feelings, to establish and maintain relationships, to think symbolically, and to learn to read and write. While the majority of young

> children acquire language effortlessly, a significant minority do not.
>
> The UK prevalence rate for early language difficulties is between 5% and 8% of all children, and over 20% for those growing up in low-income households. The high prevalence among disadvantaged children is thought to contribute to the achievement gap that exists by the time children enter school and continues until they leave. It is well known that language difficulties predict problems in literacy and reading comprehension, but less well known that they may be indicative of problems in children's behaviour and mental health as well. For example, oral language difficulties are typically present in the educational profiles of young offenders. We believe the fundamental link between language and other social, emotional and learning outcomes makes early language development a primary indicator of child wellbeing. (Law and Asmusson 2017)

Speech is not only a feature of language but also a motor skill. Both language and motor skills develop in a context of social and physical interaction and experience. Motor aspects of speech depend on coordination of the fine muscles of the lips, tongue and swallow mechanism with breathing for clear articulation. Neuromotor immaturity, other neurological factors, hearing deficit and auditory-processing difficulties can each contribute in different ways to a history of delayed speech. Social and environmental factors such as prolonged use of dummies, insufficient one-to-one conversation and interaction in the early years, access to reading materials, being read to as a child, and overexposure to e-media and background noise can all interfere with a child's natural propensity to develop speech. Parents may be unaware of the importance of all of the above in early development, and there is a growing need to educate new generations of parents (who have grown up in the technological age) in how the environment and parental time and interaction can either enhance or interfere with the development of motor skills and/or speech. Increasingly, the INPP's work has come to encompass education and training for parents as well as various professions in the reasons why all aspects of child development are important.

Levels of professional training offered by the INPP

- One-day course for teachers in the use of 'Assessing Neuromotor Readiness for Learning. The INPP Developmental Screening Test and School Intervention Program'.
- One-day course for clinicians and health practitioners (medical background) in the use of 'Neuromotor Immaturity in Children and Adults. The INPP Screening Test for Clinicians and Health Practitioners'.
- One-year postgraduate practitioner training course comprising three teaching and one examination module; the basic entry criterion is a first (bachelor's) degree in a subject allied to education, medicine or psychology.

Appendices

Studies and Selected Papers

An Oral Presentation to INPP Practitioners on a CPD Day in the 1990s

Lawrence Beuret
(Reproduced by permission of Lawrence Beuret)

Case 1: Adolescent 1

Adolescent 1 was referred for evaluation for possible NDD because of unusual scatter in scores on the WISC-III (Weschler Intelligence Scale for Children).

He was 16 years of age. He had no history of any difficulty in learning to read but he had never shown any interest in reading outside school. There was no sign of visual disturbances such as skipping of lines when reading, but he complained of headaches and concentration drifting after 15–30 minutes of reading.

He was not aware of specific writing difficulties, but he had not made the complete transition from printing to cursive writing. At the time of first assessment he ranked 17th from the bottom of a class of 675.

Neurodevelopment assessment revealed a lack of head-righting reflexes. Amphibian and segmental rolling reflexes were slightly underdeveloped and traces of an ATNR, TLR and Moro reflex were still present, but the primitive reflex scores were not sufficiently high to account for his presenting problems.

After six weeks on a reflex stimulation/inhibition programme, it was reported that reading was easier, there was no sign of headache or eye strain and he was able to remember details of what he had read. His writing had changed entirely to cursive script and he was attaining a B grade average in three classes. He had also bought a book to read for pleasure.

Case 2: Adolescent 2

Adolescent 2 was 13 years of age at the time of assessment. His presenting symptom was difficulty with fine motor coordination.

At five years of age, testing had indicated that he might belong in the range of 'gifted' children, but it was noted that his movements were very tense and he had difficulty getting written work done.

At ten years of age, he was not doing written assignments or keeping on task.

By 11 years, he was actively resisting writing anything down. At the time of assessment (13 years) he avoided writing and, if pressed, would run sentences together without punctuation or capital letters. When writing, he had to prop his head up with one hand. When assessed, he did not have the usual history consistent with writing problems, such as early fine motor difficulties, complaints of hand or arm pain with prolonged writing, or poor penmanship.

His reflex profile showed only a minimal level of ATNR, certainly not consistent with the level of writing difficulty that he was experiencing. He did have underdeveloped head-righting reflexes, amphibian reflex and segmental rolling reflexes from the shoulders.

Two areas of his history raised the suspicion of inadequate postural reflex involvement:

- the need to support his head when writing
- running of sentences together without punctuation or capitalisation

Two months after he started a reflex stimulation/inhibition programme, his mother reported that he was less resistant about writing and had begun to use capital letters and punctuation correctly. He was also sitting in a normal position to write.

Case 3: Adult 1

Adult 1 was 30 years of age and had been referred for assessment by a psychiatrist for problems with attention. He had been prescribed Ritalin™ in the past but had not responded to it.

He had experienced reading problems since the first grade but was not considered learning disabled. He had received tutoring between the first and twelfth grades and had struggled through high school and college. Reading more than two pages resulted in fatigue, loss of focus, headache and eye irritation. Vision therapy had helped at nine years of age but had not solved all of these problems. At the age of 30 his reading level was equivalent to sixth grade.

He did not suffer from motion sickness (a common indicator of underlying neurodevelopmental problems in adolescents and adults if it persists beyond puberty), but he complained of difficulty focusing and keeping his place if he tried to read in a car.

When writing, he often mixed printing and cursive script, and prolonged writing resulted in word omissions and spelling errors. By 14 years of age he was experimenting with drugs and at the time of assessment was enrolled in Alcoholics Anonymous.

His reflex profile showed minimal traces of primitive reflex activity. Oculo- and labyrinthine head-righting reflexes were underdeveloped, as were the amphibian and segmental rolling reflexes. Testing for the labyrinthine head-righting reflexes had resulted in feelings of vertigo. In addition to a reflex assessment, he undertook the Minnesota Multiphasic Personality Inventory.

The initial MMPI profile (solid line) showed significant elevations on the scales shown in Figure A1. Retesting at five and eleven months after the commencement of a reflex stimulation/inhibition programme showed the profile to be within normal limits (dotted line in Figure A1).

Other changes of significance as treatment progressed were:

- ability to read and focus for one hour or more.
- improved ability to recognise unfamiliar words that would previously have been skipped over
- cessation of lower-back tension
- improved organisational skills at work
- parents and Alcoholics Anonymous sponsor both commented on increased energy and productivity
- golf improved

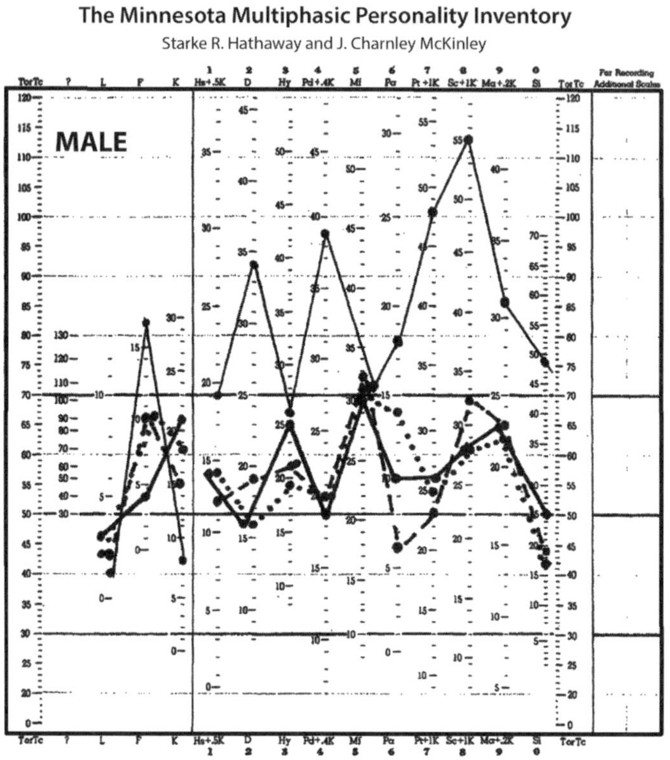

Figure A1: MMPI showing change in profile with significant criteria before and after an INPP programme.

- able to enjoy documentaries and not just the CNN and sports TV he used only to watch
- auditory processing improved

After 30 weeks on the programme, the subject was able to absorb more information the first time he read something. He was studying for the stockbroker's exam and doing well on practice tests.

Additional research

Several schools have carried out small independent studies into the efficiency of 'The INPP Developmental Exercise Program for Use in Schools' (Goddard Blythe 1996).

At Mellor Primary School the reading age of eight- to ten-year-olds in the experimental group improved from 6.3 years in October 1999 to 8.6 years in July 2000 compared with a gain only from 6.8 to 7.8 years in the control group (Pettman 2001).

At Knowle Church of England School in Solihull, children in the experimental group made a gain of 14 months in reading compared with eight months in the control group (Preedy et al. 2003).

At St Margaret Mary Roman Catholic School in Carlisle all children were assessed using the DAP test at the beginning and the end of the programme. The DAP test has been in use since 1923, when Burt (1921) first suggested that children's drawings relate to intelligence. It has been shown to correlate with other intelligence tests such as the Binet and the Wechsler. The drawings also reveal information about a child's general awareness of space and of their own body. Without such awareness the child has no frame of reference for performing such skills as writing, reading and athletic ability, all of which require movements in space.

The children's drawings showed a marked improvement in the use of space, and proportion – such as head size. They showed more awareness of the neck, hands, fingers, eyelashes and details of clothing. Some of the children made a gain of 50 points on the percentile rating scale. The most immature drawings were the ones that showed the greatest improvements. Results from schools where the programme has been used suggest that there does exist a specific group of children who are underachieving as a direct result of immature physical skills (Inspiring Partners 2006).

The North Eastern Library Board, Northern Ireland, using the INPP school programme, completed a highly detailed study involving 672 children. The results were made available in 2005 and will be found on the INPP's website.[34] ■

Table A1: Historical indicators of NMI

Historical indicators of neuro-developmental delays

Pregnancy

- Hyperemesis (severe sickness)
- Severe viral infection during the first 12 weeks or between 26 and 30 weeks
- Excessive alcohol consumption and/or drug abuse
- Radiation
- Accident or infection
- Threatened miscarriage
- Hypertension
- Placental insufficiency (small for dates)
- Smoking
- Toxoplasmosis
- Severe stress
- Uncontrolled diabetes

Birth

- Prolonged labour or precipitive labour
- Placenta previa
- High forceps or ventouse extraction
- Breech
- Cesarian
- Cord around the neck
- Feta! distress
- Premature (more than 2 weeks early) or post mature (more than 2 weeks late)

Newborn disorders

- Low birth weight (under 5 lbs)
- Incubation
- Distorted skull
- Prolonged jaundice
- Requiring rescusitation
- Blue baby
- Heavy bruising
- Problems with feeding the first 6 months

Infancy

- Illnesses involving a high fever, delirium or convulsions in the first 18 months
- Adverse reaction to any of the innoculations
- Late at learning to walk (later than 18 months)
- Late at learning to talk (later than 18 months)

Childhood and school history

- Travel sickness-headache or nausea, especially while reading in car, boat or plane.
- Difficulty learning to ride a two-wheel bicycle
- Difficulty learning to read
- Difficulty learning to write, or in making the transition from printing to cursive script
- Difficulty in learning to tell the time (clock face v. digital clock)
- Poor hand–eye coordination

Rarely will a single factor by itself indicate Neuro-Developmental Delay. As with primitive reflexes, it is only where a cluster of factors exist that NDD may be present. Indicators of NDD are not limited to the above list.

Table A2: Development and transformation of the reflex system

Reflex	Emerges	Inhibition	Transformation
1. Uterine withdrawal reflexes	5–7 weeks in utero	9–32 weeks in utero	Moro reflex
2. Moro reflex	9–12 weeks in utero	2–4 months neonate	Adult 'startle' response (Strauss reflex)
3. Palmar reflex	11 weeks in utero	2–3 months neonate	Voluntary release progressing to a 'pincer' grip
4. Plantar reflex	11 weeks in utero	7–9 months neonate	Adult Plantar
5. Asymmetrical tonic neck reflex	c. 18 weeks in utero	3–9 months neonate	Amphibian reflex
6. Asymmetrical tonic neck reflex	20 weeks in utero	3–9 months neonate	Adult Plantar
7. Rooting reflex and 8. Suck reflex	24–28 weeks in utero	3–4 months neonate	Adult suck reflex and subsequent development of mature sucking and swallowing movements essential for speech and clear articulation
9. Tonic labyrinthine reflex forwards	12 weeks in utero	3–4 months neonate	Head-righting reflex Landau reflex
10. TLR-backwards	Emerges at birth	2–4 months neonate	Head-righting reflexes
11. Babinski reflex	1 week neonate	12–24 months	Adult Plantar
12. Stepping reflex	1 week neonate	6 months	Inhibited by 6 months at the latest
13. Abdominal reflex	4 weeks neonate	Remains	Is indicative of increasing maturity in the upper pyramidal tract and thus is associated with balance and muscle tone
14. Landau reflex	4–6 weeks neonate	3 years	Control of balance between flexor and extensor muscles
15. Head-righting reflexes	2–4 months	Remains	The basis of balance, oculomotor functioning orientation and spatial awareness

Elective Mutism: The Unchosen Silence

Sally Goddard

(First published as an INPP Monograph in 1991)

The term 'selective mutism' – formerly described as 'elective mutism' – implies a voluntary refusal to speak in certain situations. *The Diagnostic and Statistical Manual of Mental Disorders (DSM IV)* (American Psychiatric Association 1994) describes its characteristics as follows:

> The essential feature of selective mutism is the persistent failure to speak in specific social situations, (e.g. school, with playmates) where speaking is expected, despite speaking in other situations. (This diagnosis should not be given if it lasts for less than a-month, the child has no knowledge of the subject being discussed, or suffers from other forms of language or developmental disorders, or schizophrenia.) Instead of communicating by standard verbalisation, children with this disorder may communicate by gestures, nodding or shaking the head, or pulling or pushing, or in some cases by monosyllabic, short or monotone utterances, or in an altered voice.
>
> Associated features include: Excessive shyness, fear of social embarrassment, social isolation and withdrawal, clinging, compulsive traits, temper tantrums or other controlling or oppositional behaviour, particularly in the home.
>
> *[Please note that information contained in this paper was based on knowledge at the time and was a working hypothesis.]*

Selective/elective mutism is a separate condition from autism, but in certain circumstances it may be viewed as a minor form of autism or a manifestation of a particular autistic type of behaviour. One autistic 17-year-old, who had been unable to talk since the age of six, was later able to write down her experiences of being locked in a silent world (Hocking 1990).

The following original text was written without punctuation of any kind. Minimal punctuation has been inserted by the writer to facilitate easier reading.

> Caroline wanted to talk so much, but it seemed to be an impossible task. 'Do you think she will ever talk?' was the question that everyone always asked her mother

and her teacher, to which they replied. 'There is no reason why she shouldn't. All the apparatus is there. She used to talk when she was a little girl.' Some people found this hard to believe. They thought her parents must be deluding themselves and that she had always been silent. But she had spoken. She could remembers quite clearly the times she had said things to her Mommy. 'Look at the moon!' she said one day, caught by the sudden beauty of it in the daytime sky. She must have been about six years old at the time, lost in her misery, but still responsive to beauty coming unawares from the heavens. She could remember other times when she had tried to say things, but had been caught in the black web of her unhappiness and unable to utter a sound. It is very difficult to explain the way in which her fear gripped her vocal chords. It felt as though unseen hands were pressing on her throat struggling to extinguish life itself. Such a little place for the air to come and go, and so little room for the mysterious life force to exist. That area of her body seemed so especially vulnerable, so very exposed, that it must be protected at all costs, even the cost of silence. It seemed to save valuable air for the process of life itself. There was none to spare for eventual speech, so speech had to go. No one realised that this was one of the fears behind the silence: this sense of tight breathlessness that seemed to suffocate and threaten what little life there was with extinction. This was a real feeling when she was a tiny girl, but it was not until she was nearly grown up that she had the detachment to describe it. It was the same with so many feelings now that she was older. She could give a description to the things that had hurled great doubts and fears at her small mind. She had the words to describe what it had all been like. That's why she felt it was so important to write a book to explain. As her teacher had said, she was in a position to help others. Real experience, ably described, was worth a ton of suppositions by well-meaning experts. What hurt so much was the widely held belief that students of psychiatry seemed to hold: If you were silent you could not understand. If you didn't use language you couldn't express any thoughts. But how did they know that a lot of speechless people hadn't got heads full of beautiful expressive language that they couldn't use, because no one had found the key to their confidence.

It would be very easy to analyse this girl's feelings in terms of psychological aetiology, but it is the purpose of this paper to argue that elective mutism has an underlying physical basis and to examine the underlying mechanisms that in certain situations may inhibit the organs of speech production.

Two of the most powerful images that this girl's description evokes are those of fear and of breathlessness. Many phrases in the English language imply a connection between fear and the inability to talk: 'petrified', 'speechless with fear', 'frozen to the spot', 'tongue-tied' and 'struck dumb' – each one a recognition of a normal, momentary response to extreme fear. The question that poses itself here is: Why should certain individuals experience such extreme fear in the course of their day-to-day living, even to the extent that they cannot operate or interact effectively with the outside world?

An explanation may be found in the concept of NDD. Neurodevelopmental delay encompasses a variety of symptoms, of which elective mutism may be one. These symptoms emanate from an arrested or omitted stage of development during either the foetal or the infantile period. Subsequent development proceeds normally thereafter, but an underlying weakness or immaturity remains within the central nervous system which may cause other systems in the body to misfire under certain conditions. The existence and extent of NDD is measured by the presence and the strength of primitive reflexes beyond the normal age of inhibition and by the absence of postural reflexes. The latter should have developed to allow the individual to manipulate and interact effectively in the environment. Active primitive reflexes beyond the first year of life and/or underdeveloped postural reflexes after the age of three-and-a-half years are signposts of central nervous system maturity.

During normal development, the primitive reflexes should emerge, strengthen, fulfil a function and then undergo inhibition during the first year of life. There should be a strict chronology, sequence and rhythm to this reflex structure, so that by a certain age specific milestones should have been achieved. Any interruption of the sequence will result in the early reflexes remaining locked in the system, causing the emergence of subsequent reflexes to be disturbed and further central nervous system development to be built upon eccentric foundations.

The earliest known reflexes to emerge are those that appear five to seven weeks after conception and that form a group of 'withdrawal reflexes'. These constitute the earliest observed realisation of tactile awareness in the embryo, who, when barely visible to the naked eye, will respond to tactile stimulation in the mouth region with a rapid amoebic-like withdrawal movement of the whole organism. It has been suggested (Goddard 1989b) that the early withdrawal reflex may be a manifestation of the FPR, described in detail by Kaada (1986), which can have important implications in later life if it is not inhibited during the gestational period.

Capute (1986) divides the primitive reflexes into five categories:

- intrauterine reflexes that appear and are suppressed during intrauterine development (not present at birth)
- intrauterine/birth reflexes
- reflexes that appear during later intrauterine development, are present at birth and are inhibited by six months of age
- postural reflexes
- reflexes that appear during late infancy following inhibition of the primitive reflexes

The withdrawal reflexes belong to the first category and should be inhibited at the time of the emergence of the Moro reflex 9–32 weeks after conception. This suggests that the Moro reflex itself plays an inhibitory role for the preceding reflex and that only the development of a full and strong Moro reflex will complete this task. If the Moro reflex fails to develop fully during this period, then both the withdrawal reflexes and the Moro reflex could remain locked and active in the system beyond the normal age of inhibition.

How can the presence of these two reflexes impair later functioning – and particularly the mechanisms of speech – if they remain active at the subcortical level beyond the age of inhibition?

Kaada (1986) described the characteristics of the FPR using the analogy of the 'terrified rabbit' who becomes frozen to the spot at which he has experienced sudden fear. In the animal kingdom this may serve the useful purpose so that the motionless animal will not attract the attention of its predator. For humankind, such behaviour is a maladaptive response to situations with which the individual is unable to cope.

Its accompanying characteristics are also significant. Activation of the FPR results in immediate motor paralysis accompanied by an inability to breathe out. Muscle tone is reduced and there is lack of response to external stimuli. A pain-suppressing mechanism is released, together with bradycardia and peripheral vasoconstriction. Kaada (1986) states that the FPR is 'a reflex present in the entire animal kingdom which is temporarily released from cortical control as a result of extreme fear'. If it fails to undergo full inhibition at the correct time in humans, then it remains active at the subcortical level, lowering the threshold of fear in the individual such that it can be activated by minor stimuli that present no actual threat to the individual at all.

The Moro reflex should emerge between nine and 32 weeks after conception, be fully present at birth and undergo inhibition after three to four months of neonate life. At nine to twelve weeks, other vital systems in the body are also developing: the vestibular system, the cerebellum and the hypothalamus. If the Moro reflex, which is the foetus's primitive alerting response to stress or threat, does not develop fully at this time, it is possible that the foetus's stress responses may be inadequate. For example, Odent (1986) describes how the entire hormonal profile for later life is regulated during this dynamic period of development:

> At an early stage of foetal life the pituitary gland, which controls all other endocrine glands, can secrete all the known pituitary hormones. When the foetus is 11–12 weeks old, the vessels that will become the hypothalamus and the pituitary glands come together. By that time, the hypothalamus is already controlling the pituitary, and by the time the foetus is three months old, the day-to-day variations in the stress hormone ACTH [adrenocorticotropic hormone] are already well established.

Specific hormonal states at an age when the basic adaptive system has not reached maturity may set the hormonal levels for life. For instance, constant unalleviated stress in the foetus or baby will result in the release of stress hormones and regulate the hypothalamus in such a way that the seeds for future conditions such as poor stress tolerance and hypertension are sown.

The hypothalamus acts as a bridge between the brain and the hormonal system: it belongs to both and plays a leading role in responses to psychological stress. Together with the limbic lobe, it stimulates the pituitary axis, the reticular activating system and the sympathetic arm of the autonomic nervous system – three separate circuits that respond to unfamiliarities and to challenge. Activation of these three circuits leads to the release of the stress hormone ACTH together with other hormones from the brainstem and sympathetic nerves, which result in a rise in heart rate, dilation of the pupils and increased discharge of the reticular activating system, which in turn leads to an increase in muscle tension, a rise in blood pressure and heart rate and the inhibition of reflex bradycardia. These are all the physical symptoms of the activated Moro reflex, which has sometimes been referred to as the initiator of the fight or flight mechanism. The Moro may also be regarded as a release mechanism from an activated FPR.

What might be the result of both the FPR and the Moro reflex remaining active at the subcortical level in an individual?

We would have a person with a low fear threshold and a low stress threshold. A person who may be hypersensitive to touch, sound, specific frequencies of sound, and changes in their visual field, smell and possibly taste. They may be able to compensate and overcome their hypersensitivity in many situations, but this will involve conscious overriding of instinctive reflexive responses by the cortex. They will become quickly fatigued, and with the fatigue their ability to compensate will be reduced and so a reflexive response will be more easily elicited. Which particular reflex is elicited will depend upon the circumstances. In certain situations both reflexes will be overcome by conscious control and the individual will react rationally and effectively. At other times, the situation may provoke the Moro or overreaction response. On another occasion the withdrawal reflexes will claim priority and the individual will find it impossible to respond at all. Elective mutism may be the result of the latter scenario.

What remains to be answered, however, is this: Why should specific social situations provoke such extreme fear?

Where the FPR and the Moro reflex remain, later reflexes in the hierarchical structure may also be aberrant to some degree. The TLR may remain in its residual or retained form, so that any movement of the head forwards or backwards beyond the midplane point will result in automatic flexion or extension of the arms and the legs – a response that can only be controlled by conscious muscular effort. In that case, balance in the upright position will tend to be unstable or inconstant. Furthermore, the labyrinthine and oculo-head-righting reflexes that should be present at six months of age will not develop fully. This in turn will affect oculo-motor functioning.

The TLR also exerts a direct influence upon the labyrinth. The labyrinth is a complex organ for attaining balance, which through the movement of fluid in three orthogonal tubes operates rather like a spirit level (carpenter's level), activating special nerves that send signals to the brain concerning movement of the head. The vestibular apparatus then detects changes of the direction and position of the head in space, particularly when the movement starts and stops. Information from the vestibular apparatus is combined with information from other sensory channels.

Both prenatally and after birth, the vestibular system controls body image impression and also kinaesthesia (the sensation of bodily movement in space).

The vestibular apparatus is also a filtering point for sound. The ear acts as a collecting organ not only for sound stimuli but also for those stimuli that are responsible for coordinating the vestibular portion of the labyrinth (Tomatis 1980). If, as a result of aberrant reflexes, the vestibular system is dealing with conflicting messages from other sensory channels, this sensory conflict may interfere with the transmission of auditory stimuli from the ear to the language-processing centres in the cortex. The addition of a TLR to an FPR and a Moro reflex imposes a new set of problems on the individual. Balance is not under automatic control, oculo-motor functioning may be erratic and there may be issues with accurate sound discrimination, so that the individual suffers from the 'cocktail party deafness' phenomenon. A string of words may sound like a meaningless unit. Individual conversation within a group may be perceived as a conglomerate of jumbled sounds that do not immediately make sense. This condition is sometimes referred to as 'auditory delay' or 'auditory confusion'. Such an individual may have a heightened sensitivity to certain frequencies of sound and a lesser sensitivity to other frequencies, with the result that parts of words are not easily registered and miscellaneous sounds may intrude more readily on the listener's consciousness. Under these circumstances the environment becomes disorientating and bewildering. Each of us has known at some time how unpleasant and frightening it is to be lost in a strange place. The child with a strong TLR, Moro reflex and FPR knows what it is like to feel lost many times in each waking day. In such situations the FPR can be easily elicited.

The vestibular apparatus is also linked to the vagus or tenth cranial nerve at the level of the medulla (Blythe 1990). The vagus nerve contains both sensory and motor fibres. The sensory fibres convey sensitivity to part of the external ear and carry afferent impulses from the pharynx and the larynx and the internal organs of the thorax and abdomen. The motor fibres and accessory nerves serve the striated muscles of the palate, the larynx and the pharynx. If a child is already overloaded by outside stimuli, their compensatory mechanisms are stretched to capacity and so little energy is available for verbal expression. Far too much attention is concentrated upon making sense of conflicting perceptions. The confused vestibular system innervates the vagus nerve and its impulses to the organs of speech production.

Overaction of the vestibular system alerts earlier aberrant reflexes. The withdrawal reflexes come into play, and the child cannot talk. The FPR impedes breathing and affects the muscles for speech, which fall into momentary paralysis. The child has the ability to talk – but not in this particular environment. Their filtering system for outside stimuli is inadequate. Their ability to categorise and discriminate and thus to make sense of their environment is impaired. With this information in mind, the 17-year-old girl's descriptions of fear and of breathlessness quoted at the beginning of this paper start to make sense.

The situation may be further complicated by the presence of one other reflex – the ATNR. The ATNR can still be elicited after six months when a child is asleep Where it persists when the child is awake beyond six months of neonate life, several areas of functioning may be impaired. In its primitive form the reflex is elicited as the baby turns their head to one side. The limbs on the side to which the head has turned will extend as the occipital limbs flex.

When a child starts to learn fine motor activities such as writing, control of the writing hand will be affected each time the child turns their head to focus on the writing hand. Hand–eye coordination generally may be immature. Balance may be thrown when the child is in an upright position, since any movement of the head in a lateral direction will result in stiffening of the limbs on one side. Smooth eye movements may be affected to the extent that eyes, head and body cannot move independently of one another and can only operate as a unit, such that saccades can only be accomplished with head and/or body tracking. The continued presence of the ATNR will also interfere with the establishment of unilaterality of brain functioning (Gesell and Ames 1947). Tasks that involve crossing the midline may present difficulties (Bobath 1975). A dominant ear and a dominant language centre may never have been fully established and so the child will switch erratically from left to right hemisphere for receptive and expressive language tasks.

Both the left and the right hemispheres in the brain have language centres, but the left side is the most efficient for most people. The left side of the brain is also responsible for the execution of methodical, sequential tasks, whereas the right side is responsible for scanning and targeting. If a child has an inadequate filtering mechanism, then the cortex is easily overloaded by information that should have been screened earlier in the receiving line. It should have reached the cortex partly categorised, with miscellaneous information filtered out. If this has not occurred, then the left side of the brain will be greatly overworked performing tasks that should have been completed earlier in the receptive process. The processing may then need to switch to the right-brain language centre, which the child cannot utilise as immediately or as fluently. The brain may continue switching from right to left functions. Receiving, processing and expression of language are not automatic tasks for this child in any situation that involves too many stimuli. The child reaches overload far too quickly. With overload comes confusion: confusion generates fear, and so the FPR may be activated and once again the child is unable to speak.

If we return to the earlier DSM III definition of elective mutism, the interpretation may be rather different in the light of these reflexes. 'Refusal to speak' may be seen as 'inability to speak' and 'including at school' may be replaced by 'especially at school' where the child does not perceive the environment to be a safe one because they cannot make sense of it. On the other hand, their willingness to communicate via gestures and nodding starts to seem perfectly reasonable. The associated features also warrant further examination. Fear paralysis reflex will induce excessive shyness, social isolation and withdrawal, together with a fear of school. Compulsive traits and negativism tend to be an attempt to establish order and security in an insecure and frightening world. Albeit these are self-defeating strategies for the individual in that situation, they provide some temporary reassurance of self-control in a world that has no safe framework for them in which they can operate effectively. Both DSM III's and DSM IV's listing of 'temper tantrums' as another symptom presents the second half of the puzzle: a child with these issues experiences sensory overload more quickly than others do; unable to integrate sensory impressions with appropriate verbal responses fast enough to meet the immediate demands of the environment, they revert to non-verbal forms of communication. In this context, behaviour is language.

Fear paralysis reflex invokes a state of withdrawal and temporary paralysis. The Moro reflex, on the other hand, elicits an overreactive response to certain stimuli. Where the FPR remains active in the system at the subcortical level, the Moro reflex will also remain active. (If it does not, then there is no safety mechanism to arouse the individual from the FPR, and in extreme cases death will result. Sudden infant death syndrome may be one example of this.) Children who have disappeared into the withdrawal state may only emerge from that state either with a violent outburst of anger or with tears of frustration or with hyperactivity. If, finally, the Moro reflex is activated, it releases them from their paralysed state. Such children are the product of an unresolved conflict between two opposing reflexes that should not even be present beyond the age of four months of neonate life.

Other forms of elective mutism may also be part of this conflict. The individual is unable to verbalise feelings or to recount events that have a traumatic content. The associated feelings or sensations are so strong that the individual becomes imprisoned in a silence that both locks in the feeling and forms part of the pathway to shock. One eleven-year-old girl later asked, 'Why couldn't you see that the way I was, was telling you what I was saying?' as if the silence spoke more loudly and more eloquently than any words could have. In such situations it is as if the fright, fight or flight reaction is activated but the 'fright' or 'freeze' element acts like a brake on the fight or flight response. The fear paralysis reaction traps feelings inside the body preventing the fight or flight mechanism from acting and releasing internal excitation. The effect is rather like the brake and accelerator of a car being applied at the same time. Repetition of an emergency situation without the ability to fight or flee, may result in states of extreme withdrawal (helplessness) and depression, since the activated feelings are turned inwards but will not go away. Individuals of this type will find most forms of therapy extremely threatening, since the only release mechanism they know is an explosive and cataclysmic one that they constantly fight to control.

Blythe (1971; 1976) found that the true emotional regressive phase of the hypnotic state would be interrupted if speech was introduced and the subject was expected to talk during regression. It was as if in the process of speech the patient lost contact with the feelings. Elective mutism would appear to be the other side of the same coin: where bodily and perceptual sensation is too great, the pathway to speech becomes strangled.

The INPP has achieved improvement with a small number of elective mutes on a reflex inhibition programme. Initially, the aim was to stimulate an existing Moro reflex until it is present in its fully retained form. This gives the child a second chance to utilise the Moro reflex – both as an inhibitor to its predecessor, the FPR, and to give the child the full release mechanisms they may never have had in any previous stage in their life. Paradoxically, as the Moro reflex reaches its fully retained form many of the symptoms of overreactivity and oversensitivity actually abate, as if, at last, the body can utilise to the full its instinctive channels of response to danger.

Brunnström (1962; 1970) may provide one explanation for this. She worked as a physical therapist promoting mobility in children and adults with severe cerebral palsy. She provoked primitive movement patterns that she had observed to be present following either pyramidal tract damage or that are normally present in the foetus. She stated that:

> A patient may be able to perform voluntary flexor and extensor movements, only by utilising the facilitating effect of one or the other of these reflexes. When a conflict between will and inhibitory reflex impulse exists, the will does not always gain supremacy. (Brunnström 1970)

Finally, the majority of the children in question have marked vestibular problems.

Vestibular stimulation would seem to be an obvious starting point for a rehabilitation or remediation programme. However, practitioners of the INPP method and occupational therapists using the A Jean Ayres sensory motor-training programme have observed that a number of the children who require vestibular stimulation either cannot tolerate it or only benefit from it to a limited degree. Where the FPR and Moro reflexes are still present, vestibular stimulation may activate one or both of them, such that the patient either finds it too distressing or that it reinforces faulty existing compensatory strategies. There may be improvement in gross muscle coordination and balance, but there is rarely a spillover into educational performance. If, however, vestibular stimulation is added after the FPR and Moro reflex have been inhibited, the individual is less sensitive and the programme is far more effective and there will be concomitant improvement in educational performance.

All of the above suggests that there is a physical basis for elective mutism. Accepting that there are cases of both elective mutism and traumatic mutism which are the result of psychological factors, I nevertheless believe that for the majority the psychological factors are secondary. Where both an FPR and a Moro reflex remain active in the individual, certain social situations will present extreme threat. Extreme threat will engender vulnerability in the susceptible individual. Such vulnerability will be accompanied by fear – fear may activate early primitive reflexes at any time in the case of 'elective mutism' – paralysing the organs of speech in specific situations. ■

Why Do Children Roll and Tumble?

Sally Goddard

(First published in First Steps *magazine, Australia)*

The first of all the senses to develop is the sense of balance. It is vital for posture, movement and a sense of 'centre' in space, time, motion, depth and self. All other sensation passes through the balance mechanism (vestibular system) at brainstem level before it is passed on to a specialised region higher in the brain. Hence, all the other senses a child will depend upon for learning are linked to balance.

To the newborn baby, perception and motion are the same thing. They are not aware that sound and movement, vision and touch are separate sensations, since for them these sensations all fuse together as a single experience or feeling. Thus motion is the child's first language, and the more eloquent they become in this primary language, the quicker they will develop other powers of expression, exploration and development.

Stimulation of the balance mechanism is an integral part of the embryo's growth from the moment of conception. Every movement that the mother makes is felt in the cushioned environment of the womb. After birth the feelings continue to be sensed through a vast repertoire of movement patterns, from lying, kicking, rolling and sitting, to crawling and creeping on the hands and knees, walking, running hopping, skipping, swinging, rolling and tumbling. It is through movement that further connections are made between the vestibular apparatus and higher centres of the brain. It takes until the age of seven or eight years for the balance mechanism, the cerebellum and the corpus callosum to be myelinated; during these early years vestibular stimulation is a natural ingredient in every normal child's play.

The infant begins with constant repetition of arm and leg movements, practising extension and flexion of the muscles and training hand–eye coordination. The eight-month-old who rolls back and forth across the floor with no particular goal in sight is preparing their balance for sitting, standing and eventually walking. As far as they are concerned, when they move, the world moves with them, and when they stop, the world stands still once more. Creeping on hands and knees then acts as an important bridge, enabling them to combine the use of vestibular, proprioceptive and visual systems for the first time. Walking then increases not only mobility, but allows the child to roam with independent use of the hands. These are the early building blocks for learning which must then be practised and integrated with other systems. Thus, in the early years, movement is the child's main vocabulary, and language is body based. Voluntary control of movement can only develop though the broadening of movement horizons.

The three-to-six-year-old child who constantly hops, skips and twirls while walking down the street is still learning to control their balance, for the most advanced level of balance is the ability to stay still. The action of not moving requires whole body functions and muscle groups to operate together without continuous adjustment and signifies the advent of mature postural control. The child who cannot stay still knows instinctively that their balance still needs practice. The child who cannot stay on the pavement if there is a low wall running alongside it, but who must climb from one level to another and back again, is still teaching themself muscle control, depth perception and visual motor integration skills. Somersaults and cartwheels further facilitate the separation of motion from other sensations, for it is only when a child has control of movement that they can pay full attention to other experiences.

Hyperactivity and attention deficit may be two signs of immaturity in vestibular functioning. As parents, teachers and caretakers, we tend to implore our hyperactive children to 'sit still' and to 'be quiet'. It has been shown that hyperactive children who are allowed to spin for 30 seconds in either direction show an increased capacity for attention for up to 30 minutes afterwards, which suggests that they need vestibular stimulation to get their brain into gear.

Our eyes operate from the vestibular circuit in the brain. Our ears share the same cranial nerve, and the sense of touch is integrally linked to the vestibular system through the movement across hair cells whose receptors are located in the dermis of the skin. If motion is a child's first language, then sensation is the second. Only when both motion and sensation are integrated can the higher language skills of speech, reading and writing develop fluently. Children who roll and tumble are engaged in their first lesson towards becoming the Einsteins of the future. ■

Glossary

Accommodation: Ability to focus quickly from near to far distance and vice versa.

Acoustic stapedius reflex: The contraction of the stapedius pulls the ossicles – the tiny bones in the ear – away from the eardrum and so lessens the impact of sound vibrations. The nerve that controls this muscle mingles with fibres of the facial nerve. In this way, it interacts with the nerves that control facial expression and those that bring information from the skin of the external ear (Kandel et al. 1991).

Afferent: Information leading to the brain.

Ambilaterality: Relating to or affecting both sides.

Anxiety as a secondary consequence of vestibular–visual mismatch: The functional relationship between the visual and vestibular systems is experienced in many ways. For example, if the vestibular system is stimulated as a result of rotation or rocking, the sensation of dizziness gives the temporary illusion that the visual world is moving. If you are seated in a waiting train at a railway station and the train alongside you starts to move away, the brain is fooled by the visual stimulus into thinking that the body is moving. Discrepancy between what is sensed and what is real results in disorientation which can subsequently be experienced as anxiety.

Apraxia: See *praxis.*

Archicerebellum: Ancient cerebellum.

Axon: The extension of a nerve cell along which impulses travel away from the cell body.

Babkin response: The stimulus for this reflex consists of deep pressure applied simultaneously to the palms of both hands while the infant is in an appropriate position, ideally supine. The stimulus produces a reflex of flexion or forward bowing of the head, opening of the mouth and closing of the eyes. The reflex can be demonstrated in the newborn but should be inhibited after four months of age. It shows a neurological link between the mouth and the hands, which also becomes obvious in the palming movements of the hands a child makes while nursing. (Kittens do this when being fed.) Like many reflexes, it can be elicited in either direction.

Basal ganglia: Three small masses of nerve tissue – the caudate nucleus, the putamen and the globus pallidus. Located at the base of the brain, they are involved in the subconscious regulation of movements.

Bradycardia: Slow heartbeat rate.

Brainstem: The range of bulges that form the central core of the brain running from the top of the spinal cord into the middle of the brain. It comprises the medulla, pons and midbrain.

Cephalo-caudal: From head to toe sequence of development in the infant.

Cerebellar damage: Can cause paralysis in affected regions of the body. Cerebellar dysfunction can result in clumsiness affecting visual motor performance and manual dexterity. Hence the cerebellum used to be known as 'the patron saint of the clumsy child' (Restak 1991). As the cerebellum is the regulator of the postural reflexes, cerebellar-dependent functions will be affected if the postural reflexes fail to develop. Equally, cerebellar dysfunction may interfere with the development of postural reflexes. The cerebellum also plays an important role in sequential and rote learning and in short-term memory. This may be one reason why medication aimed at the cerebellum and the vestibular apparatus, according to Levinson (1984), can dramatically improve sequential memory.

Cognition: The interpretation and understanding of information derived from perception.

Corpus callosum: A wide, thick nerve tract, consisting of a bundle of commissural fibres, beneath the cerebral cortex. It functions as the connective pathway that connects the left and right hemispheres of the brain, allowing information to pass between them. One of the major differences between men and women can be seen here, since the corpus callosum develops to be 40 per cent larger in women than in men. This may go some way to explaining men's tendency to be more single-minded in their approach to tackling problems, whereas woman tend to be more able to be aware of a number of factors simultaneously.

Crawling: Moving forward using arms and legs with belly and chest on the ground.

Creeping: Crawling on hands and knees. The terms 'creeping' and 'crawling' are sometimes used interchangeably.

Cross-laterality: The condition of people whose hand, foot, eye or ear dominance is not uniformly right or left sided.

Cutaneous: Pertaining to the skin.

dB (decibels): Measure of volume of sound.

Dendrites: Short fibres that branch out from the cell body and pick up incoming messages.

Dermis: Top layer of the skin.

Disinhibition: Occurs after trauma or in degenerative diseases such as Alzheimer's disease when reflexes re-emerge in the reverse chronological order of their inhibition in the first year of life.

Dominance: Supremacy of one side over another within the brain. This refers to the two cerebral hemispheres, but it can be applied to other parts of the body, where there are twos, such as the hands, ears, eyes and feet. Cerebral dominance occurs in the brain but lateral preference (preferred hand, foot, eye, etc.) can emerge from cerebral dominance modified by experience.

Dysdiadochokinesia: difficulty performing rapid, alternate movements, e.g. fine muscle movement in the hands or feet. This will affect handicraft activities and may also be linked to speech defects.

Dyslexia: Difficulty in reading. Generally used only in cases where there is normal intelligence but the usual methods of teaching have failed.

Dyspraxia (or apraxia): The inability to select responses in an appropriate order and orient them for proper execution, even though no paralysis exists.

Extension: Movement away from the body.

Exteroceptive: Relating to stimuli that are external to the body.

Efferent: Information or commands from the central nervous system to the body.

Figure-ground effect: Inability to separate and categorise conflicting visual information, e.g. walking up an open staircase or crossing a slatted bridge where the water can be seen through the boards.

Flexion: Bending towards the front centre of the body.

Fixation: Focusing of the eyes on a stationary point and holding that focus.

Frequency: Hearing depends on air waves that move with a regular rhythm through the air. An example of this is when the skin of a drum is struck and it starts to vibrate, forcing the skin to move in one direction and then springing back in several diminishing repetitions until its movement finally dies away. Each outward movement of the skin compresses the air and, as the skin retracts, the air can expand again. This repeated cycle of compression and expansion through the air moves to a regular rhythm at so many cycles per second. If the cycle occurs 200 times per second, the sound frequency will be described as 200 hertz (Hz).

Homeostasis: The state of steady internal, physical and chemical conditions maintained by living systems.

Homolateral: One side of the body at a time – for example, walking swinging the arm and leg on the same side. In the adult, homolaterality may cause a soldier to be unable to march or a dancing partner to seem to have two left feet.

Humours: Hippocrates introduced the concept of the four humours as part of a process of combining naturalistic knowledge, philosophy and ancient science to arrive at a holistic understanding of the human body and its relationship with the world around it. The four humours related to the four elements and to the seasons and were thought to be mirrored in temperament: blood (sanguine); yellow bile (choleric); black bile (melancholic); phlegm (phlegmatic). It was believed that health depended on the four humours being balanced in quantity and strength.

Hyper: Oversensitive, inadequate filtering of extraneous sensations.

Hyperacuity: A sensory capability that transcends sampling limits set by discrete receiving elements. This may include hypersensitivity to specific sounds.

Hypertonus: Extensor muscles exert greater influence than the flexor muscles.

Hypo: Undersensitive, inadequate sensations received.

Hypotonus: Weak muscle tone.

Hz (hertz): Vibrations per second, a measure of the pitch of a sound heard, e.g. 125Hz is perceived as a low sound, 8,000Hz as a high sound.

Infant: From the Latin *infans*, meaning unable to speak.

Infrasound: Sounds below 20Hz.

Inhibition: Suppression of one function through the development of another. The first function becomes integrated by or within the second.

Interoceptive: Perception of sensation from inside the body.

In utero: In the mother's womb.

Kinaesthesis: See *Proprioception*.

Lateral line receptor: A sensory system found in many kinds of fish and some amphibians which informs the animal of water motion in relation to body surface.

Limbic system: Part of the old cortex and its primary related nuclei. It is shared by all mammals and is associated with smell, autonomic functions and certain aspects of emotion and behaviour.

Medulla: Plays a critical role in transmitting signals between the spinal cord and the higher parts of the brain and in controlling autonomic activities such as heartbeat and respiration.

Midbrain: The uppermost part of the brainstem. The term is sometimes used to include all the structures just below the cortex, sometimes even including the cerebellum.

Muscle tone: Balance between flexor and extensor muscles.

Myelin: A soft fatty substance surrounding a nerve fibre.

Myelination: The process by which axons acquire myelin.

Neocerebellum: New cerebellum.

Neonate: Newborn and the first two weeks after birth.

Neural development: In infancy neural development determines when each reflex emerges and when it becomes inhibited. Thus, the presence or absence of reflexes at key stages in development may be used as diagnostic signposts of central nervous system maturity.

Neural pruning: A natural process that occurs at different developmental stages and involves removing neurons that are no longer used or useful to the brain.

Neurodevelopmental delay: The presence of primitive reflexes beyond the normal age at which they are inhibited and/or the absence of postural reflexes.

Neuron: An individual nerve cell. Neurons are the smallest units of the nervous system.

Neurotransmitter: A chemical substance made, stored and released by neurons. Neurotransmitters are chemical messengers between neurons at synapses.

Occipital: Relating to the back of the head.

Oculo-motor function: The ability to adjust and coordinate eye position during movement. Several movements assist with this process: saccades, smooth pursuit, fixation, accommodation vestibulo-ocular reflex and optokinetic reflex. Control of eye movements is important for accurate visual perception.

Ontogenetic: Refers to the developmental history of an individual organism.

Opisthotonus: A form of spasm in which the head and heels are bent backward and the body bowed forward.

Otoliths: Minute crystalline particles suspended in a gelatinous mass into which the hair cells of the utricle and saccule of the inner ear project. They are under the influence of gravity and exert traction on the cilia of the hair cells during movements of the head and body.

Palaeocerebellum: Old cerebellum.

Parasympathetic nervous system: Increases salivary gland secretions, decreases the heart rate, promotes digestion and dilates the blood vessels. It is the opposite partner of the sympathetic nervous system.

Perception: The registering of sensory information in the brain. Cognition is the interpretation and understanding of that information.

Phylogenetic: Relating to the evolutionary development and diversification of a species, organism or group of organisms.

Pons: A group of nerves, located above the medulla and below the midbrain, that function as a connection between the cerebrum and cerebellum.

Poor pupillary adaptation to light: In poor lighting conditions pupils automatically dilate to allow more light to enter the eye; conversely, in bright light pupils should automatically contract to reduce the amount of light entering the eye. Failure to contract adequately when light intensity increases may result in photosensitivity.

Praxis: The brain's ability to select responses, arrange them in an appropriate order and orient them for proper execution.

Proprioception: Information derived from relative tension in the muscle spindles and joints pertaining to the position of body parts. This supports awareness of where different parts of the body are and enables one to carry out complex manoeuvres without conscious awareness. Though often used interchangeably with 'kinaesthesis', the term 'proprioception' encompasses all sensations involving body position, either at rest or in motion, whereas 'kinaesthesia' refers only to sensations arising when active muscle contraction becomes involved.

Reflex: Involuntary movement in response to a stimulus and the entire physiological process activating it.

Reflex inhibition programme: A series of exercises based upon foetal and infant movement patterns. Its purpose is to inhibit aberrant primitive reflexes. It is tailored specifically to the individual's needs.

Reticular activating system: A complex network of nerve fibres, occupying the central core of the brainstem, that function in states of wakefulness and alertness.

Saccades: Rapid eye movements that accurately take the eye from fixation point to fixation point when a person reads a line of text. Saccadic eye movement also serves the function of erasing the prior visual image.

Sacrum: Five vertebrae fused together at the lower end of the spinal column to form a triangular bone which lies between the haunch bones and forms the back wall of the pelvis.

Scoliosis: Abnormal curvature of the spine.

Simian: Apelike.

Soft signs of neurological dysfunction: Provide indications of immaturity in the functioning of the central nervous system but do not provide information about the aetiology/location/source of the areas involved.

Sympathetic nervous system: Network of nerve fibres that, especially under stress, ready the body for either flight or standing to fight. It does so by increasing the heartbeat, quickening the breath and enhancing the supply of oxygen to the muscles by syphoning the blood supply from the skin to deep muscle. It works in a balancing act with the parasympathetic nervous system to keep the body in a state of metabolic equilibrium.

Synapse: Functional junction between neurons. Can be either electrical or chemical in nature. Neurotransmitters act as chemical messengers across these junctions.

Tactile defensive: A pattern of observable behavioural and emotional responses that are sensitive, negative, avoidant and disproportionate in response to certain types of tactile stimuli that most people would not find to be painful.

Threshold: The point at which a stimulus is strong enough to cross over a synapse.

Transverse midplane: Divides the body into cranial and caudal regions (head and tail). Movement through the midplane involves flexion and extension of the head.

Unilaterality: Dominance of one side of the brain over the other.

Ventral: Relating to the underside of the body.

White noise: Continuous background sensation that is always present and intrudes upon other sensations. It can be an auditory, visual or tactile sensation.

References

Allen, MS, Walter, EE and Swann, C (2019). Sedentary behaviour and risk of anxiety: A systematic review and meta-analysis. *Journal of Affective Disorders* 242: 5–13.

Amen, D (2013). *Healing ADD: The Breakthrough Program That Allows You to See and Heal the 7 Types of ADD.* New York: GP Putman.

American Psychiatric Association (1994). *Diagnostic and Statistical Manual of Mental Disorders* (DSM IV). Washington.

Ames, LB (1967). *Is Your Child in the Wrong Grade?* New York: Harper & Row.

Anderson, DI, Campos, JJ, et al. (2001). The flip side of perception–action coupling: Locomotor experience and the ontogeny of visual postural coupling. *Human Movement Science* 20 (4–5): 461–87.

Andrich, P, Shihada, MB, Vinci, MK, Wrenhaven, SL and Goodman, GD (2018). Statistical relationships between visual skill deficits and retained primitive reflexes in children. *Optometry & Visual Performance* 6 (3): 106–11.

Arnheim, R (1969). *Visual Thinking.* Berkeley: University of California Press.

Ayres, AJ (1989) *Sensory Integration and the Child.* Los Angeles: Western Psychological Services.

Aziz Rahman M, Hoque N, Sheikh M, Salehin M, Beyene G, Tadele Z, et al. (2020). Factors associated with psychological distress, fear and coping strategies during the COVID-19 pandemic in Australia. *Global Health* 16: 1–15.

Bachman, ML (1991). *Dalcroze Today – An Education Through and Into Music.* Oxford: Clarendon Press.

Bai, DL and Bertenthal, BI (1992). Locomotor status and the development of spatial search skills. *Child Dev.* 63: 215–26.

Bakker, DJ (1990). *Neurophysiological Treatment of Dyslexia.* Oxford: Oxford University Press.

Barsch, RH (1968). *Achieving motor perceptual efficiency: A space orientated approach to learning.* Seattle: Special Child Publications.

Begley, S. (1992). Mapping the brain. *Newsweek*, 20 April, 40–4.

Bein-Wierzibinski, W (2001). Persistent primitive reflexes in elementary school children: Effect on oculomotor and visual perception. Paper presented at 13th European Conference of Neuro-developmental Delay in Children with Specific Learning Difficulties, Chester, UK.

Bein-Wierzibinski, W. (2004). *Räumlich konstruktive Störungen bei Grundschulkindern von 2004*. Peter Lang.

Bell, C and Magendie, F (1820). On the nerves of the orbit. *Philosophical Transactions of the Royal Society* 113: 289–307.

Bender, L (1946). Instructions for the use of the visual–motor gestalt test. New York: American Orthopsychiatric Association.

Bender, ML (1976). Bender–Purdue reflex test. San Rafael, CA: Academic Therapy.

Benett, R (1988). *The Hidden Moro*. Unpublished document.

Berg, A and Fitzgerald, LS (2013). Neurophysiological training in children with motor difficulties. *Fysioterapeuten* 5: 20–4.

Berkow, R and Fletcher, AJ (eds) (1987). *The Manual of Diagnosis and Therapy,* 15th edn. Rahway, NJ: Merck, Sharp & Dohme Research Laboratories.

Berkowitz, PH and Rothman, EP (1960). *The Disturbed Child*. New York: New York University Press.

Bernhardsson, K and Davidson, K (1982). *Ett Annorlundo siit att hjiilpa med inliirningssviirigheter*. Gothenburg: Educational Psychology Department, Gothenburg Education Authority.

Bernhardsson, K and Davidson, K (1983). *Different Way of Helping Children with Learning Difficulties: A Final Report from the Dala Clinic*. Gothenburg: Gothenburg Educational.

Bertenthal, BI, Campos, JJ and Barrett, KC (1984). Self-produced locomotion: An organiser of emotional, cognitive and social development in infancy. In *Continuities and Discontinuities in Development*, ed. R Emde and R Harmony, 175–210. New York: Plnum.

Berthoz, A (2000). *The Brain's Sense of Movement*. Cambridge, MA. Harvard University Press.

Beuret, LJ (1992). The role of neuro-developmental delays in advanced academic failure. Paper presented at 4th European Conference of Neuro-developmental Delay in Children with Specific Learning Difficulties, Chester, UK, 6–8 March.

Beuret, LJ (2000). The role of postural reflexes in learning, pt.2. Paper presented at 12th Conference of Neuro-developmental Delay in Children with Specific Learning Difficulties, Chester, UK, 10–12 March.

Beuret, LJ (2009). The effects of neurodevelopmental delay in adults and in adolescents. In *Attention, Balance and Coordination: The A B C of Learning Success*, ed. SA Goddard Blythe. Chichester, UK: Wiley-Blackwell.

Birnbaum, MH (1994). Behavioral optometry: A historical perspective. *Optometric Extension Programme* 65 (4): 255–64.

Bloedel, JR and Brachfa, V (1997). Duality of cerebellar motor and cognitive function. *International Review of Neurobiology* 41: 613–34.

Blythe, P (1971). *Hypnotism, Its Power and Practice.* London: Arthur Barker.

Blythe, P (1973). *Stress disease: The growing plague.* London: Arthur Barker.

Blythe, P (1974). *Drugless Medicine.* London: Arthur Barker.

Blythe, P (1976). *Self Hypnotism.* London: Arthur Barker.

Blythe, P (1980). An organic basis for neurosis and the existence, detection and treatment of secondary neurosis. Gothenburg: Swedish Institute for Neurophysiological Psychology.

Blythe, P (1990a). The evolution of a theory of neuro-developmental delay in children with specific learning difficulties and neurological dysfunction in adults suffering from emotional disorders, together with the emergence of neuro-developmental re-education. Chester, UK: INPP.

Blythe, P (1990b). A physical basis for panic disorder. Lecture at 4th International Conference of Neurological Dysfunction in Children and Adults, Guernsey, September.

Blythe, P and Goddard Blythe, SA (2012). Correcting clinical facts: Abnormal reflexes in behavioral optometry and vision therapy. *Journal of Behavioral Optometry* 23 (5–6): 138–42.

Blythe, P and McGlown, DJ (1979). *An Organic Basis for Neuroses and Educational Difficulties.* Chester, UK: Insight.

Blythe, P and McGlown, DJ (1980). *The Clinician's Handbook for the Remediation of Organic Brain Dysfunction.* Chester, UK: Insight.

Bobath, B (1975). *Abnormal Postural Reflex Activity Caused by Brain Lesions.* London: William Heineman,

Bobath, K and Bobath, B (1955). Tonic reflexes and righting reflexes in the diagnosis and assessment of cerebral palsy. *Cerebral Palsy Bulletin,* 16 May, 3–10.

Brunnström, S (1962). Training the adult hemiplegic patient: Orientation of techniques to patients' motor behaviour. In Approaches to treatment of patients with neuromotor dysfunction. 3rd International Congress, World Federation of Occupational Therapists.

Brunnström, S (1970). *Movement Therapy in Hemiplegia: A Neuro-Physiological Approach.* New York: Harper & Row.

Burt, C (1921). *Mental and Scholastic Tests.* London: PS King.

Butler Hall, B (1998) Discovering the hidden treasures in the ear. Paper presented at 10th European Conference of Neuro-developmental Delay in Children with Specific Learning Difficulties, Chester, UK, 6–8 March.

Campos, JJ, Anderson, DI, Barbu-Roth, MA, Hubbard, EM, Hertenstein, MJ and Witherington, D (2000). Travel broadens the mind. *Infancy* 1: 149–219.

Capute, AJ (1986). Early neuromotor reflexes in infancy. *Pediatric Annals*, 15 March, 217–26.

Capute, AJ, Shapiro BK, Palmer, FB, Accardo, PJ and Wachtel, RC (1981). Primitive reflexes, a factor in non-verbal language in early infancy. In *Language Behaviour in Infancy and Early Childhood*, ed. RE Stark. Amsterdam: Elsevier.

Chevalier, N, Kurth S, Doucette, MR, Wiseheart, M, Deoni, SCL, Dean, DC, O'Muircheartaigh, J, Blackwell, KA, Munakata, Y and LeBourgeios, MK (2015). Myelination is associated with processing speed in early childhood: Preliminary insights. *PloS One* 10 (10).

Cottrell, S (1987). The Moro Revisited. Unpublished document.

Cottrell, S (1988). Aetiology, diagnosis and treatment of asthma through primitive reflex inhibition. Paper presented at 2nd International Conference of Neurological dysfunction, Stockholm, October.

Courchesne, E, Townsend, J and Saitoh, O (1994). The brain in infantile autism. Posterior fossa structures are abnormal. *Neurology* 44: 214–23.

Cratty, BJ (1973). *Movement, Behavior and Motor Learning*. London: Henry Kimpton.

Cripe, C (2009). The fab four in neurodevelopment. Presentation to INPP European Conference, Chester, UK, 4–5 April.

Crutchfield, CA and Barnes, MR (1993). *Motor Control and Motor Learning in Rehabilitation.* Atlanta: Stokesville.

Daniels, JC, and Diack, H (1962). *The Standard Reading Tests.* London. Chatto & Windus.

De Klein, A and Magnus, R (1924). Experimentell Physiologie des Vestibulapparatus. *Handbuch der Neurologie*, des, Ohresheilkunde.1.[Q317]

Delacato, CH (1959). *The Treatment and Prevention of Reading Problems.* Springfield, IL: Charles C Thomas.

Delacato, CH (1974). *The Ultimate Stranger, The Autistic Child.* Novato, CA. Academic Therapy.

DeMyer, W (1980). *Techniques of the Neurological Examination.* New York: McGraw-Hill.

Department of Education (2010). Investigating the role of children's early educational outcomes. Research Report 134.

Diamond, S, Balvin, R and Diamond, R (1963) *Inhibition and Choice.* New York: Harper & Row.

Doman, G, Le Winn, EB and Wilkinson, R (1977). Temple Fay M.D., revisited: 'The other side of a fit.' A bill of particulars on seizures and on discontinuing anti-convulsant drugs. *In-Report 6.*

Draper, LT (1993). *Lecture Notes on Neurology.* Oxford: Blackwell Scientific.

Emery, M (1987). The social and neurophysiological effects of television and their implications for marketing practice: An investigation of adaptation to the cathode ray tube. PhD thesis, University of South Wales.

Faulkner, P (1988a). The detection of neuro-physiological factors in children with reading problems. Paper presented at 2nd International Conference of Neurological Dysfunction, Stockholm, October.

Faulkner, P (1988b). Handwriting Difficulties and CNS Dysfunction in Children of High Intelligence. Unpublished document.

Field, J (1992). *Accommodating the Neuro-Developmentally Delayed Child within the Classroom.* Worcester: Field.

Field, J and Blythe, P (1988). *Towards Developmental Re-education.* Worcester: Field.

Finger, S (2000). *Minds Behind the Brain: A History of the Pioneers and Their Discoveries.* New York: Oxford University Press.

Fiorentino, MR (1981). *Reflex Testing Methods for Evaluating C.N.S. Development.* Springfield, IL. Bannerstone House.

Flourens, MJP (1824). *Recherches Éxperimentales sur les Proriétés et Les Functions du Système Nerveux des Animaux Vertebras.* Paris: Crevot.

Frostig, M (1970). *Movement Education: Theory and Practice.* Chicago: Follett.

Fukuda, T (1961). Studies on human dynamic postures from the viewpoint of postural reflexes. *Acta Otolaryngol. Suppl.* 161: 1–52.

Gaddes, WH (1980). *Learning Disabilities and Brain Function: A Neurophysical Approach.* New York: Springer Verlag.

Galaburda, AM (2001). Dyslexia and the brain. Paper presented at 5th British Dyslexia Association International Conference, York, April.

Galaburda, AM, LeMay, M, Kemper, TL and Geschwind, N (1978). *Right/Left Asymmetries in the Brain.* Cambridge, MA: Harvard University Press.

Galant, S (1917). Der Rückgratreflex: Ein neuer Reflex im Säuglingsalter mit besonderer Berücksichtigung der anderen Reflexvorgänge bei den Säuglingen. Inaugural dissertation, Basler Druck- & Verlagsanstalt.

Galley, PM. and Forster, AL (1987). *Human Movement.* Edinburgh: Churchill Livingstone.

Ganong, F (1997). *Review of Medical Physiology.* Stamford, CT: Appleton & Lange.

Gazzaniga, S (1973). Brain theory and minimal brain dysfunction. *Annals of the New York Academy of Sciences* 205.

Gershon, M. *The Second Brain.* New York: Harper Collins

Gesell, A (1947). *The First Five Years of Life: A Guide to the Study of Pre-School Children.* Part 1. London: Methuen.

Gesell, A and Ames, L (1947). The development of handedness. *Journal of Genetic Psychology* 70: 155–75.

Gibson, EJ (1988). Exploratory behavior in the development of perceiving, acting, and the acquiring of knowledge. *Annu. Rev. Psychol.* 39: 1–41.

Gieysztor, EZ, Choińska, AM and Paprocka-Borowitz, M (2018). Persistence of primitive reflexes and associated motor problems in healthy pre-school children. *Archives of Medical Science* 14 (1): 167–73.

Gieysztor, EZ, Sadowska, L and Choińska, AM (2017). The degree of primitive reflex integration as a diagnostic tool to assess the neurological maturity of healthy preschool and early school age children. *Nursing and Public Health* 7 (1): 5–11.

Gieysztor, EZ, Choińska, A, Kowal, M, Pecuch, A, Borowicz, W and Paprocka-Borowicz, M (2019). The level of primitive reflex integration in children who play a musical instrument. *Polish Journal of Pediatrics* 5 (94): 293–98.

Goddard, SA (1989a). *The Continued Presence of the Fear Paralysis Reflex and Its Effect Upon Subsequent Central Nervous System Development.* Chester, UK: INPP.

Goddard, SA (1989b). *The Fear Paralysis Response and its Interaction with the Primitive Reflexes.* Chester, UK: INPP.

Goddard, SA (1990). A developmental basis for learning difficulties and language disorders. Paper presented at 2nd European Conference of Neuro-Developmental Delay in Children with Specific Learning Difficulties, Chester, UK, 2–4 March.

Goddard, SA (1991). Elective mutism – the unchosen silence. Paper presented at 3rd European Conference of Neuro-developmental Delay in Children with Specific Learning Difficulties, Chester, UK, 1–3 March.

Goddard, SA (1995). The role of primitive survival reflexes in the development of the visual system. *Journal of Behavioral Optometry* 6 (2): 31–35.

Goddard, SA (1996). *A Teacher's Window into the Child's Mind.* Eugene, OR. Fern Ridge Press.

Goddard, SA (2002). *Reflexes learning and behavior.* Eugene, OR: Fern Ridge Press.

Goddard Blythe, SA (1996). *The INPP screening test and developmental exercise programme for use in schools with children with special needs.* Chester, UK: INPP.

Goddard Blythe, SA (2001). Neurological dysfunction as a significant factor in children diagnosed with dyslexia. Paper presented at 5th International British Dyslexia Association Conference, University of York, 18–21 April.

Goddard Blythe, SA (2004). *The Well Balanced Child.* Stroud, UK: Hawthorn Press.

Goddard Blythe, SA (2005). Releasing educational potential through movement: A summary of individual studies carried out using the INPP test battery and developmental exercise programme for use in schools with children with special needs. *Child Care in Practice* 11 (4): 415–32.

Goddard Blythe, SA (2008). *What Babies and Children Really Need.* Stroud, UK: Hawthorn Press.

Goddard Blythe, SA (2009) *Attention Balance and Coordination: The ABC of Learning Success.* Chichester, UK: Wiley-Blackwell.

Goddard Blythe, SA (2011a). *The Genius of Natural Childhood.* Stroud, UK: Hawthorn Press.

Goddard Blythe, SA (2011b). Neuromotor immaturity as an indicator of developmental readiness for education. In *Movement, vision, hearing: The basis of learning,* ed. EM Kuleesza, 131–5. Warsaw: Wydawnictwo Akademii Pedagogiki Specjalnej im. Marii Grzegorzewskiej.

Goddard Blythe, SA (2012). *Assessing Neuromotor Readiness for Learning: The INPP Developmental Screening Test and School Intervention Programme.* Chichester, UK: Wiley-Blackwell.

Goddard Blythe, SA (2014). *Neuromotor Immaturity in Children and Adults: The INPP Screening Test for Clinicians and Health Practitioners.* Chichester, UK: Wiley-Blackwell.

Goddard Blythe, SA (2018). *Movement – Your Child's First Language.* Stroud, UK: Hawthorn Press.

Goddard Blythe, SA and Hyland, D (1998). Screening for neurological dysfunction in the specific learning difficulty child. *British Journal of Occupational Therapy* 61 (10): 459–63.

Goddard Blythe, SA, Duncombe, R, Preedy, P and Gorely, T (2021). Neuromotor readiness for school: The primitive reflex status of young children at the start and end of their first year at school in the United Kingdom. *Education* 50 (5): 3–13.

Gold, SJ (1986). *When Children Invite Child Abuse.* Eugene, OR. Fern Ridge Press.

Gold, SJ (1998). *If Kids Just Came With Instruction Sheets.* Eugene, OR. Fern Ridge Press.

González, SR, Kenneth, MS, Ciuffreda, LC, Hernández, LC and Esaclante, JB (2008). The correlation between primitive reflexes and saccadic eye movements in 5th grade children with teacher-reported problems. *Optometry and Vision Development* 39 (3): 140–5.

Griffin, P (2013). Is there a link between neuromotor immaturity and educational attainment? *Open Doors Therapy.*

Guyton, AC (1991). *Basic Neuroscience – Anatomy and Physiology.* Philadelphia: WB Saunders.

Hallett, M and Grafman, J (1997). Executive function and motor skill learning. *International Review of Neurobiology* 41: 297–323.

Harte, S (2015). Physical development and national curriculum levels – the incidence of neuromotor immaturity (NMI) in London primary schools and the relationship between NMI and national curriculum measures of achievement. Paper presented at Child Development in Education Conference, London, October.

Hebb, DO (1949). *The Organisation of Behavior.* New York: Wiley.

Hepper, PG and Shahidullah, SB (1994). Development of fetal hearing. *Archives of Disease in Childhood* 71: F81–7.

Herbert, J, Gross, J and Hayne, H (2007). Crawling is associated with more flexible memory retrieval by 9-month-old infants. *Dev. Sci.* 10: 183–189.

Higgins, CI, Campos, JJ and Kermoian, R (1996). Effect of self-produced locomotion on infant postural compensation to optic flow. *Dev. Psychol.* 32: 836–41.

Hobson, Allan P (1988) *The Dreaming Brain.* New York: Basic Books.

Hocking, B (1990). *Little Boy Lost.* London: Bloomsbury.

Holt, KS (1991). *Child Development.* London. Butterworth-Heinemann.

Horobin, K and Acredolo, LP (1986). The role of attentiveness, mobility history, and separation of hiding sites on Stage IV search behavior. *J. Exp. Child Psychol.* 41: 114–27.

Hubbard, DG (1971). *The Skyjacker: His Flights of Fantasy.* New York/London. Collier Macmillan.

Hurst Vose, R (1981). *Agoraphobia.* London: Faber & Faber.

Hutton, JS; Dudley, J; Horowitz-Klaus ,T; de Witt ,T and Holland, SK (2020). Associations between screen-based media use and brain white matter integrity in preschool-aged children. *JAMA Pediatr.* 174 (1).

Inspiring Partners (2006). St Aidans School Sport Partnership: Learn to move, move to learn. *Youth Sport Trust.*

Ivanović, L, Ilic-Stosovic, S, Nikolic, S and Medenica, V (2018). Does neuromotor immaturity represent a risk for acquiring academic skills in school-age children? *Military-Medical and Pharmaceutical Review* 76 (10): 1062–70.

Ivry, RB and Keele, SW (1989). Timing functions of the cerebellum. *Journal of Cognitive Neuroscience* 1: 136–52.

Johanneson-Alvegård, C (1990). Application of neuro-psychological principles within the Swedish state school system. Presentation to 4th European Conference of Neuro-developmental Delay in Children with Specific Learning Difficulties, Chester, UK, 6–8 March.

Johansen, KV (1993). *Lyd, Horelseog Sprogudvikling.* Gudhjem, Denmark: Dyslexia Research Lab.

Johansson, B, Wendenberg, E and Westin, B (1964). Measurement of the tone response by the human fetus. *Acta Otolaryngol* 57: 188–92.

Kaada, B (1986). *Sudden Infant Death Syndrome: The Possible Role of the Fear Paralysis Reflex.* Oxford: Oxford University Press.

Kandel, E, Schwartz, JH and Jessell, TM (1991). *Principles of Neural Science,* 3rd edn. Norwalk, CT: Appleton & Lange.

Kavale, K and Mattson, DP (1983). One jumped off the balance beam. *Journal of Learning Disabilities* 16 (3): 165–73.

Kephart, NC. (1960). *The Slow Learner in the Classroom*. Columbus, OH: Merrill.

Kermoian, R and Campos, JJ (1988). A facilitator of spatial cognitive development. *Child Dev.* 59: 908–17.

King, LJ and Schrager, OL (1999). A sensory and cognitive approach to the assessment and remediation of developmental learning and behavioral disorders. Paper presented at Symposium on a Sensory/Cognitive Approach to the Assessment and Remediation of Developmental Learning and Behavioral Disorders, Atlanta, 19–20 March.

Kiphard, EJ (2000). Intervention program using the German psycho-motor approach with exceptional children. Paper presented at 13th European Conference of Neuro-developmental Delay in Children with Specific Learning Difficulties, Chester, UK, 10–12 March.

Klein, DP (1980). Anxiety reconceptualised. *Compr. Psychiatry* 21: 411–27.

Kohen-Raz, R (1986). *Learning Disabilities and Postural Control*. London: Freund.

Kretch, KS, Franchak, JM and Adolph, KE (2014). Crawling and walking infants see the world differently. *Child Dev.* 85 (4): 1503–18.

Krugman, HE (1971). Brain wave measures of media involvement. *Journal of Advertising Research* 11 (1): 3–9.

Krugman, HE (2000). Memory without recall, exposure without perception. *Journal of Advertising Research* 40 (6): 49–54.

Kushima, M, Kojima, R, Shinohara, R, Horiuchi, S, Otawa, S, Ooka, T, Akiyama, Y, Miyake, K, Yokomichi, H and Yamagata, Z (2022). Japan environment and children's study group. Association between screen time exposure in children at 1 year of age and autism spectrum disorder at 3 years of age: The Japan environment and children study. *JAMA Pediatr.* 176 (4): 384–91.

Kuss, DJ and Lopez-Fernandez, O (2016). Internet addiction and problematic internet use: A systematic review of clinical research. *World Journal of Psychiatry* 6 (1): 143–76.

Landsberg, PG (1975). Bradycardia during human diving. *South African Medical Journal* 49(15): 626–30.

Lane, C (2012). *Self-Voice: A Major Rethink*. London: ARROW Tuition.

Large, M (2006). Switch on the kid's telly, switch off their brains. *Parliamentary Brief* (London) 10/11. December.

Larsell, O (1947). The cerebellum of myxinoids and petromyzonts including developmental stages in the lampreys. *Journal of Comp. Neurology* 86: 395–445.

Law, J and Asmusson, K (2017). Language as a child well-being indicator. *Early Intervention Foundation*, 27 September.

Lecanuet, JP, Granier-Deferre, C and Busnel, M (1988). Fetal cardiac and motor responses to octave-band noises as a function of central frequency, intensity and heart rate variability. *Early Hum Dev.* 18: 81–93.

Lefroy, R (1990). *Improving Literacy Through Motor Development.* Palmyra, Australia: Dunsborough Enterprises.

Leiner, HC, Leiner, AL and Dow, RS (1986). Does the cerebellum contribute to mental skills? *Behav. Neuroscience* 100: 443–54.

Leiner, HC, Leiner, AL and Dow, RS (1993). Cognitive and language functions of the human cerebellum. *Trends in Neuroscience* 16: 444–7.

Le Mée, K (1994). *Chant.* London: Random House.

Levinson, HL (1981). *A Solution to the Riddle Dyslexia.* New York: Springer-Verlag.

Levinson, HL (1984). *Smart But Feeling Dumb.* New York: Warner Books.

Levinson, HL (1986). *Phobia Free.* New York: M Evans.

Levinson, HL (1989). A cerebellar–vestibular explanation for fears/phobias: Hypothesis and study. *Perceptual and Motor Skills* 68: 67–84.

Levinson, HL (1991). *The Upside-Down Kids.* New York: M Evans.

Lloyd B (1994–95). Adapting and applying INPP exercises and sound therapy into school. Presentation at INPP Associate Supervision Days, Chester, UK.

Lorente de No, R (1933). Vestibular–ocular reflex. *Archives of Neurology and Psychiatry* 30: 245–91.

Ludwig, AM (1975). Sensory overload and psychopathology. *Diseases of the Nervous System*, July, 357–60.

Machover, K (1942). *Personality Projection Through the Drawing of a Human Figure.* Springfield, IL: Charles C Thomas.

MacLean, P (1978). *A Mind of Three Minds: Educating the Triune Brain.* Chicago: National Society for the Study of Education.

Madaule, P (1993). *When Listening Comes Alive.* Norval, ON: Moulin.

Madejewska, M, Choińska, AM, Gieysztor, EZ and Trafalska, A (2016). Neuromotorical assessment of children aged 4–7 from the Kamienna Góra district based on Sally Goddard tests. *Piel. Zdr. Publ.* 6 (3): 179–86.

Marlee, R. (2008). Neurological developmental delay research programme. Report prepared for Behaviour Support Service Schools and Family Support Division, Children's Services Directorate, Northumberland County Council, Morpeth, UK.

Matuszkiewicz, M and Gałkowski, T (2021). Developmental language disorder and uninhibited primitive reflexes in young children. *Journal of speech, language, and hearing research* 64 (3): 935–48.

McGlown, DJ (1971). The diagnosis of 'organic brain dysfunction' in children of educational age. Unpublished thesis.

McGlown, DJ and Blythe, P (1980). *Developmental Check List and Evolution of Primitive and Postural Reflexes*. Chester, UK: INPP.

McPhillips, M and Sheehy, N (2004). Prevalence of persistent primary reflex and motor problems in children with reading difficulties. *Dyslexia* 10: 316–38.

McPhillips, M, Hepper, PG and Mulhern, G (2000). Effects of replicating primary reflex movements on specific reading difficulties in children: A randomised, double-blind, controlled trial. *The Lancet* 355 (2).

Merzenich, MM, Jenkins, WM, Johnston, P and Tallal, P (1996). Temporal processing deficits of language-learning impaired children ameliorated by training. *Science*, 5 January, 77–81.

Micklethwaite, J (2004) Study investigating the efficacy of the INPP developmental exercise programme for use in schools at Swanwick Primary School, Derbyshire. Report prepared for the Department for Education and Skills (DfES) Best Practice Research Scholarship.

Ministry of Human Resource Development (2020). The New Education Policy 2020. https://www.mhrd.gov.in/sites/upload_files/mhrd/files/NEP_Final_English_0.pdf.

Moro, E (1918). Das erste Trimenon. *Münchener Medizinische Wochenschrift* 65: 1147–50.

NEELB 2004. An evaluation of the pilot INPP movement programme in primary schools in the North-Eastern Education and Library Board (NEELB), Northern Ireland. Final Report. Compiled by Brainbox Research Ltd, Leeds.

Nicolson, RI and Fawcett, AJ (1994). Comparison of deficits in cognitive and motor skills among children with dyslexia. *Annals of Dyslexia* 44 (1): 147–64.

Nicolson, R, Fawcett, A and Dean, P (1994). Impaired performance of children with dyslexia on a range of cerebellar tests. *Annals of Dyslexia* 46: 259–83.

Noica, D (1912). Sur les réflexes cutanés du dos. *Revue Neurologique* 23: 134–7.

O'Dell, N and Cook, P (1996). *Stopping Hyperactivity – A New Solution*. New York: Avery,

Odent, M (1986). *Primal Health*. London: Century Hutchinson.

Odent, M (1991). Early expression of the rooting reflex. Paper presented at 3rd European Conference of Neuro-developmental Delay, Chester, UK, 1–3 March.

Oosterveldt, WJ (1991). The development of the vestibular system. Presentation to 3rd European Conference of Neuro-developmental Delay in Children with Specific Learning Difficulties, Chester, UK, 1–3 March.

Pandya, A and Lodha, P (2021). Social connectedness, excessive screen time during COVID-19 and mental health: A review of current evidence. Front. *Hum. Dyn.*, 22 July. https://doi.org/10.3389/fhumd.2021.684137

Panksepp, J (1998). *Affective Neuroscience: The Foundations of Human and Animal Emotions.* Oxford: Oxford University Press.

Pavlides, O and Miles, T (1987). *Dyslexia Research and Its Applications to Education.* Chichester, UK: Wiley.

Pecuch, A, Gieysztor, E, Wolańska, E and Paprocka-Borowicz, M (2021). Primitive reflex activity in relation to motor skills in healthy preschool children. *Brain Sciences* 11 (8): 967.

Peiper, A (1963). *Cerebral Function in Infancy and Early Childhood.* New York: Consultants Bureau.

Petr, B, Konicarova, J and Raboch, J (2021). Disinhibition of primitive reflexes in attention deficit and hyperactivity disorder: Insight into specific mechanisms in girls and boys. *Front. Psychiatry*, 8 November.

Pettman, H (2001). The effects of developmental exercise movements on children's persistent primary reflexes and reading difficulties: A controlled trial. Mellor Primary School, Leicester. Final Report, Best Practice Research Scholarship Study. Department of Education and Skills.

Piaget, J (1954). *The Construction of Reality in The Child.* New York: Basic Books.

Posner, MI and Raichle, ME (1994). *Images of Mind.* New York: Freeman.

Preedy, P, O'Donovon, C, Scott, J and Chapman, E (2003). Exercises for learning. A beacon project between Knowle CE Primary School and Kingsley Preparatory School.

Preedy, P, Duncombe, R and Gorely, T (2020). Physical development in the early years: The impact of a daily movement programme on young children's physical development. *Education* 3–13 50: 289–303.

Preedy, P, Sanderson, K and Ball, C (eds) (2017). *Early Childhood Education Redefined: Reflections and Recommendations on The Impact of Start Right.* Abingdon, UK: Routledge.

Pulgar Marx, I (1955). *Revista Espanola de Pediatra* 11: 317.

Pyfer, J and Johnson, R (1981). Factors affecting motor delays. In *Adapted physical activity*, ed. RL Eason, TL Smith and F Caron. Champaign, IL: Human Kinetics.

Restak, R (1991). *The Brain Has A Mind of Its Own.* New York: Harmony Books.

Rider, B (1972). Relationship of postural reflexes to learning disabilities. *American Journal of Occupational Therapy* 26 (5): 239–43.

Righarde, L and Frantz, K (2005). *Delivery Self-Attachment.* Los Angeles: Geddes.

Rorschach, H (1964). *Psychodiagnostics.* Berne: Hans Huber.

Savan, A (1999). The effect of background music on learning. *Psychology of Music* 27 (2): 138–46.

Schilder, P (1933). The vestibular apparatus in neuroses and psychoses. *Journal of Nervous and Mental Disease* 78: 1–23, 137–64.

Schore, AN (1994). *Affect Regulation and the Origin of the Self.* Hove, UK: Laurence Erlbaum.

Schrager, OL (2001). Posture and balance; important markers for children's learning development. Paper presented at 13th Conference of Neuro-developmental Delay in Children with Specific Learning Difficulties, Chester, UK, 10–11 March.

Shaskan, DA and Roller, WL (1985). *Paul Schilder: Mind Explorer.* New York: Human Sciences Press.

Shaywitz, SE (1996). Dyslexia. *Scientific American*, November, 77–83.

Shepherd, GM. (1994). *Neurobiology.* Oxford: Oxford University Press.

Shepherd, R (1990). *Physiotherapy in Pediatrics.* Oxford: Butterworth-Heinemann.

Sherrington, C (1906). *The Integrative Action of the Nervous System.* New Haven: Yale University Press.

Silvester, E (2006). Commentary in DVD, *Learn to Move, Move to Learn.* St Aidan's School Sport Partnership, Youth Sport Trust.

Skeffington, AM (1943). Visual rehabilitation. In *Analytical Optometry.* Santa Ana, CA: Optometric Extension Programme Foundation.

Skeffington, AM, Lesser, SK and Barstow, R. (1947–50). Nearpoint optometry. *Optom. Extension Prog.* 3–5.

Snider, RS and Stowell, A (1944). Receiving areas of the tactile, auditory, and visual systems in the cerebellum. *Journal of Neurophysiol.* 7: 331–57.

Snowdon, D (2001). *Aging with Grace.* London: Fourth Estate.

Steffert, B (1997). Sign minds and design minds. Paper presented at 9th European Conference of Neuro-developmental Delay in Children with Specific Learning Difficulties, Chester, UK, 15–16 March.

Stehli, A (1992). *The Sound of a Miracle: A Child's Triumph over Autism.* London: Fourth Estate.

Steinbach, I (1994). How does sound therapy work? Paper presented at 6th European Conference of Neuro-developmental Delay in Children with Specific Learning Difficulties, Chester, UK, 11–13 March.

Storr, A (1993). *Music and the Mind.* London: HarperCollins.

Strauss, H (1929). *Journal of Psychology* 38: 111.

Sugden, DA and Henderson, E (2007). Movement Assessment Battery for Children, 2nd edn.

Suggate, S and Bruce, T (2019). *Reclaim Early Childhood: The Philosophy, Psychology and Practice of Steiner Waldorf Early Years Education.* Stroud UK: Hawthorn Press

Tansley, AE (1967). *Reading and Remedial Reading.* London: Routledge & Kegan Paul.

Telléus, C (1980). En komarativ studie av neurologisk skillnader hos born medoch utan lsoch skrivovarigheter. Master's thesis, Gothenburg University.

Thelan, F (1979), Rhythmical stereotypes in normal human infants. *Animal Behavior* 27: 699–715.

Thomas, A and Saint Anne Dargassies, S (1952). *Etudes Neurologigues sur le Nouveau-né et le Jeune Nourisson*. Paris: Masson et Cie.

Tomatis, AA (1980). Audio-psycho-phonology: A new challenge. Lecture given at Potchefstrom University, South Africa, April.

Torgerson, S (1983). Genetic factors in anxiety disorders. *Arch. Gen. Psychiatry* 40: 1085–9.

Trevor-Roper, P (1987). *The World Through Blunted Vision*. London: Penguin.

Uchiyama, I, Anderson, DI, Campos, JJ, Witherington, D, Frankel, CB, Lejeune, L, et al. (2008). Locomotor experience affects self and emotion. *Dev. Psychol.* 44: 1225–31.

Valenstein, E (2002). The discovery of chemical neurotransmitters. *Brain and Cognition* 49 (1): 73–95.

Veras, R (1975). *Children of Dreams, Children of Hope*. Chicago: Henry Regnery,

Virchow, R (1949). Zur pathologischen Physiologie des Bluts. 4. Farblose, pigmentirte und geschwänzte, nicht specifische Zellen im Blut. Virchows. *Arch. Pathol. Anat. Physiol. Klin. Med.* 2: 587–98.

Waldfogel, J and Washbrook, E (2010). *Low Income and Early Cognitive Development in the U.K.* London: Sutton Trust.

Whitmore, K, Hart, H and Willems, G (eds). *A Neurodevelopmental Approach to Specific Learning Disorders*. London: Mac Keith Press.

Whytt, R (1751). *An Essay on the Vital and Other Involuntary Motions of the Animal*. Edinburgh: Hamilton, Balfour & Neil.

Wilkinson, G (1994). The relationship of primitive postural reflexes to learning difficulty and underachievement. MEd thesis, University of Newcastle upon Tyne.

Wisbey, A (1977). Sounding out dyslexia. *World Medicine*, October.

Zivan, M, Bar, S, Jing, X, Hutton, J, Farah, R and Horowitz-Kraus, T (2019). Screen-exposure and altered brain activation related to attention in preschool children: An EEG study. *Trends Neurosci. Educ.* 17: 100117.

Notes

1 Neural development – not chronological age – determines at what time each reflex emerges and at what time it becomes inhibited. Thus the presence or absence of reflexes at key stages in development may be used as diagnostic signposts of central nervous system maturity.

2 This is because in bright light the pupils should automatically contract to reduce the amount of light entering the eye. In dim light, they should rapidly dilate to allow maximum light to reach the retina. Failure to do this may result in photosensitivity.

3 P Blythe, personal communication, 1985.

4 A study published in 2021 examined the incidence of primitive reflexes in children with early speech disorders, later school difficulties and signs of neuromotor immaturity (NMI). Whereas signs of general NMI in this group were significant, the palmar, rooting and spinal Galant reflexes were not significantly present (Matuszkiewicz and Gałkowski 2021). However, clinical observation of a large number of children over a period of many years has shown a correlation between difficulties with dysdiadochokinesia in the fingers with mirroring movements in the mouth to be present in children with a history of early speech delay. This is not necessarily the result of the palmar and oral reflexes being present, but may reveal a continued hand–mouth connection, which should have become uncoupled.

5 V Dickson, personal communication, 1991.

6 K Phillips, contribution to INPP seminar, Chester, UK, 1994.

7 LJ Beuret, personal communication, 1989.

8 'Creeping' and 'crawling' are sometimes used interchangeably. In this book, 'crawling' refers to crawling with the tummy in contact with the floor, and 'creeping' refers to creeping on hands and knees.

9 The word 'attitude' comes from French, in which it originally referred to the manner in which the body is held. It has become more widely used to refer to emotional and psychological stance, which may or may not be linked to postural abilities.

10 P Blythe, personal communication, 1992.

11 The ability to adjust focus between different visual distances is sometimes described as 'accommodation'.

12 Reflex movements provide a child with their earliest movement vocabulary.

13 M Portwood, personal communication to P Blythe, 2001.

14 One of the major differences between men and women can be seen here, since the corpus callosum develops to be 40 per cent larger in women than in men. This may go some way to explaining men's tendency to be more 'single-minded' in their approach to tackling problems, where women can be more aware of a number of factors at the same time.

15 The functional relationship between the visual and vestibular systems is experienced in many ways. For example, if the vestibular system is stimulated as a result of rotation or rocking, the sensation of dizziness gives the temporary illusion that the visual world is moving. If you are seated in a waiting train at a railway station and the train alongside you starts to move away, the brain is fooled by the visual stimulus into thinking that the body is moving. Discrepancy between what is sensed and what is real results in disorientation which can then be experienced as anxiety.

16 On mass cutaneous withdrawal reflexes, see Chapter 1.

17 Insufficient tactile experience can also occur in old age and situations of loneliness and isolation. When one is deprived of the warm touch of another loving human being, immune functioning and mood regulation can also become depressed.

18 Fathers can also play a part in this. This will be explored further in Chapter 6.

19 Some children who initially either have left-ear preference or show no clear ear preference when first tested become more left-eared for a short period of time when they begin auditory discrimination training, which suggests that it may be developmentally normal to be left-eared at certain stages of language acquisition and that right-ear preference is an indication of maturity in language development. This would fit with Allan Schore's theory of continuous interchange between the left and right hemispheres of the cortex during the learning stages of new skills.

20 A Duighan, personal communication, 1994.

21 Report provided by Meersbrook Primary School, 2018–19.

22 https://www.movementforlearningproject.co.uk/

23 The word 'discipline' derives from the Latin *disciplina*, which originally meant 'instruction' or 'knowledge'.

24 N Rowe, personal communication, 1996.

25 J Middlemiss, personal communication, 1987.

26 J Ten Hoopen, personal communication, 1995.

27 K Lorenz cited in https://www.premierhealth.com/your-health/articles/health-topics/screen-addiction-affects-physical-and-mental-health#:~:text=Screen%20use%20releases%20dopamine%20in,negative%20impact%20of%20your%20life

28 Source cannot be traced.

29 https://www.apa.org/monitor/2020/04/cover-kids-screens#:~:text=AAP%20calls%20for%20no%20screen,of%20screen%20time%20per%20day

30 E Keeling, personal communication, 2001.

31 S Dubin, personal communication, 2012.

32 T Hansen-Lauff, personal communication, 1996.

33 The Peto Institute in Budapest provides one example. Started by Dr Andras Peto in 1945, it teaches children who have cerebral palsy and cannot control their bodies properly to lead more independent lives by means of conductive education.

34 https://www.inpp.org.uk/research-publications/research/

Index

A

B

E

F

G

R

S

W

X

Z

Other books by Sally Goddard Blythe

Published by Wiley-Blackwell:

Attention, Balance and Coordination: The ABC of Learning Success

Assessing Neuromotor Readiness for Learning: The INPP Developmental Screening Test and School Intervention Programme

Neuromotor Immaturity in Children and Adults: The INPP Screening Test for Clinicians and Health Practitioners

Other books by Sally Goddard Blythe

Published by Hawthorn Press:

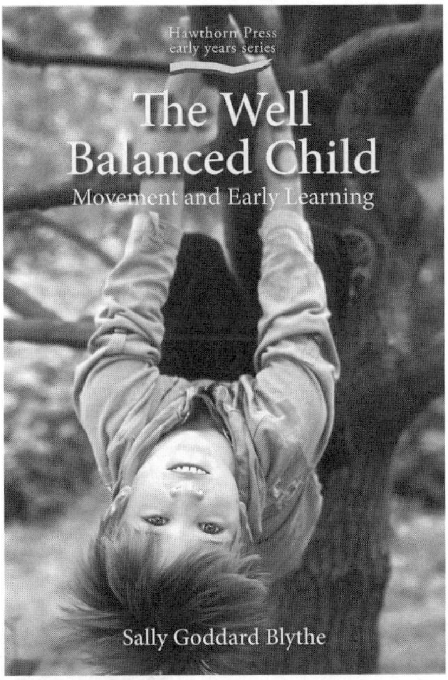

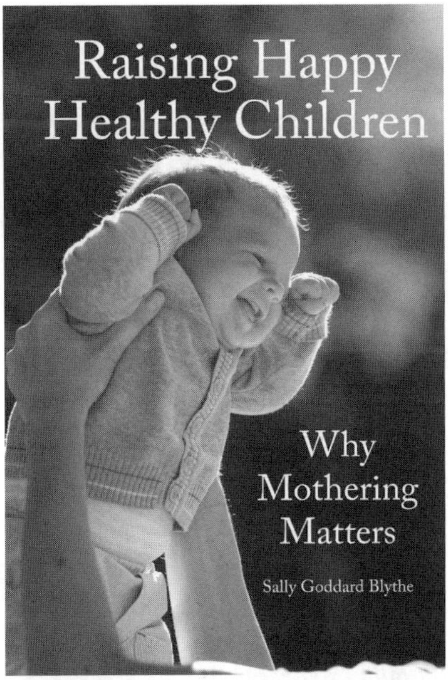

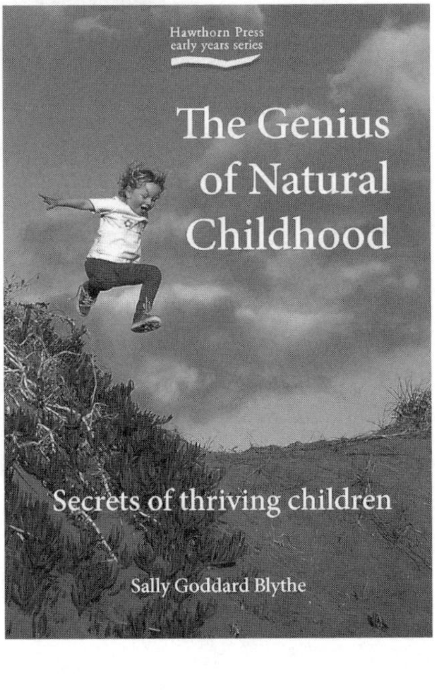

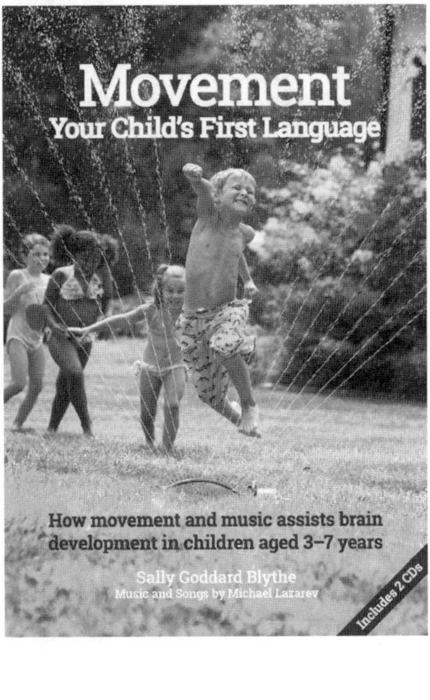

Other books published by Hawthorn Press

Reclaim Early Childhood

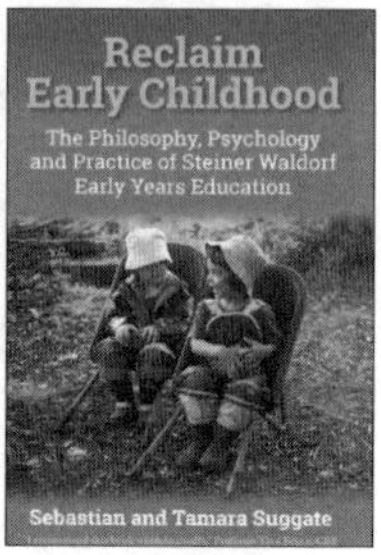

The Philosophy, Psychology and Practice of Steiner Waldorf Early Years Education

Sebastian and Tamara Suggate

224 pages;
234 × 156mm; Paperback;
ISBN: 978-1-912480-10-4

Games Children Play II

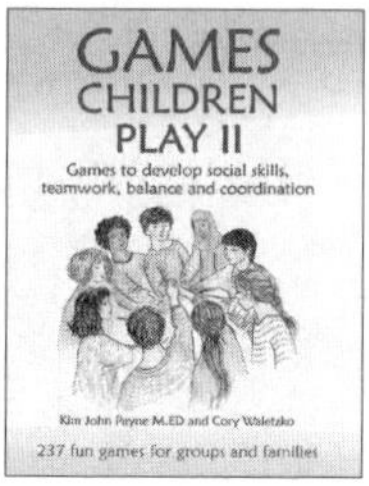

Games to develop social skills, teamwork, balance and coordination

Kim John Payne M.ED and Cory Waletzko

264 pages;
246 x 189mm; Paperback;
ISBN: 978-1-912480-52-4

Simplicity Parenting

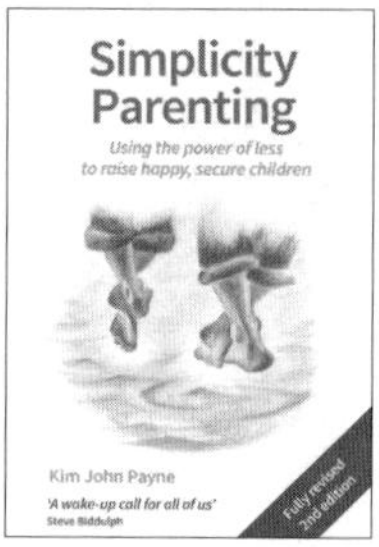

Using the power of less to raise happy, secure children

Kim John Payne

352 pages;
234 x 156mm;
Paperback.
ISBN: 978-1-912480-03-6

Stories to Light the Night

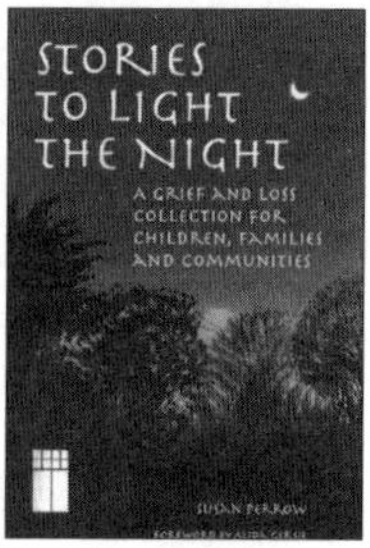

A Grief and Loss Collection for Children, Families and Communities

Susan Perrow

192 pages;
234 x 156mm;
Paperback;
ISBN: 978-1-912480-27-2

Ordering Books

If you have difficulties ordering Hawthorn Press books from a bookshop, you can order direct from our website www.hawthornpress.com, or from our UK distributor BookSource: 50 Cambuslang Road, Glasgow, G32 8NB, Tel: (0845) 370 0063, E-mail: orders@booksource.net.

Details of our overseas distributors can be found on our website.

Hawthorn Press
www.hawthornpress.com